The World Health Report 1997

Conquering suffering Enriching humanity

Report of the Director-General

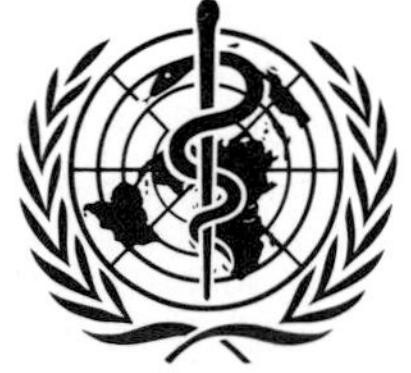

World Health Organization

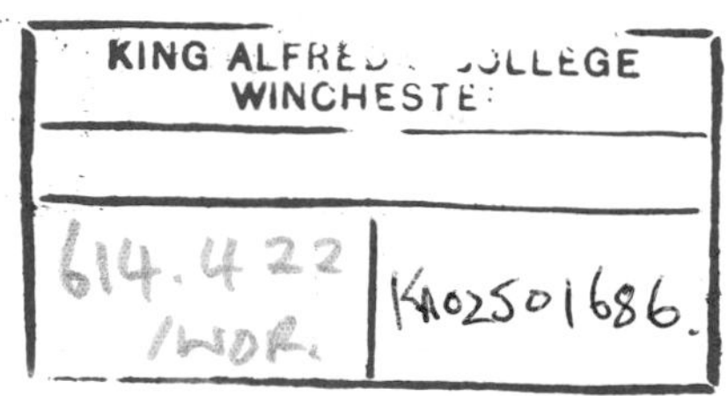

WHO Library Cataloguing in Publication Data

The world health report 1997: conquering suffering, enriching humanity
1. World health 2. Chronic disease
3. Cost of illness 4. Health priorities
5. Risk factors 6. Age factors
7. World Health Organization

ISBN 92 4 156185 8 (NLM Classification: WA 540.1)
ISSN 1020-3311

Information concerning this publication can be obtained from:
Office of World Health Reporting
World Health Organization
1211 Geneva 27, Switzerland.
Fax: (41-22) 791 4870

Design and layout by WHO Graphics
Printed in France
97/11275 – Sadag – 15000

Contents

Message from the Director-General

Increased longevity without quality of life is an empty prize. Health expectancy is more important than life expectancy.

In today's rapidly changing world, some traditional attitudes towards human health, suffering and disability need to be urgently reviewed.

For example, infectious diseases can no longer be regarded as restricted to developing countries. This is clear from the evidence of their international resurgence and the intercontinental spread of AIDS. Nor can chronic noncommunicable diseases continue to be judged only as problems of the richer nations. They are emerging at an alarming rate in poorer regions, unwelcome additions to the infections which still flourish there.

Until now, the term for this phenomenon – the "double burden" of disease – has usually been applied only to developing countries. But it can no longer be confined to these countries alone; it has expanded into a double threat to global health. In the battle for health in the 21st century, infectious diseases and chronic diseases are twin enemies that have to be fought simultaneously on a global scale.

We dare not turn our back on infectious diseases, for they will return with a vengeance if we do. The lessons of AIDS, tuberculosis, malaria, cholera and *Escherichia coli* food-poisoning outbreaks must not be forgotten. In addition to the many millions of people a year who are killed by infectious diseases, hundreds of millions of others are afflicted by them. This was the theme of *The World Health Report 1996*.

But neither can we ignore the growing burden in suffering and disability represented by noncommunicable diseases and conditions – cancer, circulatory disease, metabolic and hormonal imbalances, mental disorders, musculoskeletal conditions – most of which are chronic; they invariably afflict the sufferer with pain and disability, for years and even decades. This, too, is the plight of hundreds of millions. Confronting these chronic conditions, and the crisis of suffering that goes with them, is the theme of *The World Health Report 1997*.

Health is being increasingly affected by a number of factors over which the individual has little control, and over which the conventional health sector also has little sway: social and economic circumstances, labour-saving technologies, and the information and communication revolutions. People in poorer countries are now acquiring many of the unhealthy lifestyles and behaviours of the industrialized world: sedentary occupations, inadequate physical activity, unsatisfactory diets, tobacco, alcohol and drugs. Populations in richer countries continue to live with all these risks. Problems are aggravated by the international spread of misleading information about consumer products. All these factors together will lead to a global increase in premature ill-health from chronic diseases.

Worldwide, life expectancy has increased dramatically during the last decades of the 20th century. But in celebrating our extra years, we must recognize that increased longevity without quality of life is an empty prize, i.e. *health* expectancy is more important than *life* expectancy.

Unlike many infectious diseases, the majority of chronic diseases are preventable but cannot as yet be cured. The emphasis must therefore be on preventing their onset, delaying their development in later life, reducing the suffering that they cause, and providing the supportive social environment to care for those disabled by them.

The World Health Report 1995 showed that many countries are experiencing not merely an epidemiological transition, but an epidemiological polarization – a widening gap in health between rich and poor. The poorer an individual is, the more probable it is that he or she will become ill and die young of an infectious disease; the richer the person, the greater are the odds of suffering and dying from a chronic disease at an advanced age.

These facts raise a fundamental issue. Global health priorities which emphasize infectious diseases, will benefit the poor much more than the rich. However, as these diseases are controlled, and as the population ages, chronic diseases which cause suffering and disability increasingly take over.

Any further improvements in health thus demand integrated, comprehensive action addressing all the determinants of ill-health. Countries, particularly in the developing world, can no longer afford to deal with the two challenges of infectious and chronic diseases sequentially, as in the past. They must address them simultaneously, and the international community must help them to do so. Developed countries, for their part, cannot focus exclusively on chronic diseases and ignore the dangers of infectious diseases.

The expression "double burden" has a second connotation, referring to the obligation on the workforce to provide for two sets of dependants: children and the elderly. Although the number of child dependants may decrease, the total burden of responsibility on the working population will grow due to the increasing number of the elderly. It is therefore vitally important to protect this key sector of society from premature ill-health and disability, in order that their productivity – essential for the support of their dependants and for economic development – can be safeguarded. Preventive measures in adulthood also improve the prospects of a healthier old age, thereby allowing people to remain socially productive for longer and reducing the burden of elderly dependence.

In identifying priorities for action, this report looks towards key forms of chronic diseases that are major causes of death or avoidable ill-health and disability. These are areas in which actions or interventions that have a direct and tangible effect on individual health – that make a difference, and make it sooner rather than later – are possible.

At almost every stage of chronic disease, exciting opportunities are available to do just that. The time has come to seize those opportunities – in preventing chronic diseases, treating them, curing them; in renewing attacks on the many risk factors that contribute to them; in improving standards of care, and access to that care.

Together, these opportunities form a realistic basis for conquering suffering, reducing its social and economic costs to families and society, and thereby enriching humanity.

Hiroshi Nakajima, M.D., Ph.D.
Director-General
World Health Organization

Chapter 1

The state of world health

Chronic diseases kill more than 24 million people a year – equal to almost half of all deaths worldwide.

Dramatic increases in life expectancy, combined with profound changes in lifestyles, are leading to global epidemics of cancer and other chronic diseases. For instance, the number of cases of cancer is expected to at least double in developing countries during the next 25 years, and there is likely to be a similar rise in cases of diabetes. The result will be a huge increase in human suffering and disability. In addition to the many millions dying prematurely from these diseases each year, hundreds of millions of people will face many years of chronic disability and suffering, with profound socioeconomic consequences. Already, chronic diseases kill more than 24 million people a year – equal to almost half of all deaths worldwide.

Life expectancy, health expectancy

The dramatic increases in life expectancy achieved during the 20th century are certain to have profound consequences for humanity far into the new millennium. Half a century ago, the great majority of the global population died before the age of 50. Today, the great majority survive well beyond that age. Average life expectancy in developing countries is now 64 years, and is projected to reach 71 years by the year 2020. It is already higher in many industrialized countries. A child born in Japan today, for example, can expect to live to be 80 years old.

These are outstanding landmarks on the pathway of human evolution, and could not have occurred without the tremendous advances in medicine and public health, in science and technology, that have occurred since the beginning of this century. Such advances are continuing at a remarkable pace, and offer real hope for a better and healthier future for mankind.

But while extending our life span is desirable in itself, it is much more so if it can be accompanied by freedom from additional years of suffering poverty, pain or disability. Unfortunately, for many millions of people, there is as yet no such freedom. The quality of human life is at least as important as its quantity. Individuals are entitled to be concerned not so much about their *life* expectancy as about their *health* expectancy – and are rightly demanding to be better informed about it.

Health expectancy can be defined as life expectancy in good health, and amounts to the average number of years that an individual can expect to live in such a favourable state. For all of us who look forward to a longer life than that of our predecessors, it is vital to realize that increased longevity does not come free. While the ideal vision for everyone may be to lead a physically and mentally healthy life well into old age, every year many millions die prematurely or are disabled by diseases and conditions that are to a large extent preventable. Longer life can be a penalty as well as a prize. A large part of the price to be paid is in the currency of chronic disease, the main subject of this report.

The World Health Report 1996 – Fighting disease, fostering development showed the enormous burden that infectious diseases impose on humanity, particularly in the developing world, killing about 17 million people a year and afflicting hundreds of millions of others. This toll continues despite vaccines, medicines and other preventive and curative treatments which save millions of lives every year.

The health transition

In the industrialized world, infectious diseases are well under control, thanks to progress in areas such as clean water and sanitation, immunization, and firmly-established health services. It is noninfectious diseases – particularly cancer, circulatory diseases, mental disorders including dementia, chronic respiratory conditions and musculoskeletal diseases – that now pose the greatest threat to health in terms of life lost and disability in developed countries. These are essentially the chronic diseases that strike later in life, and which, as life expectancy increases, will become more prevalent.

Globally, chronic diseases are responsible for almost half of the 52 million or so deaths that occur every year. Among adults, the leading causes are circulatory diseases, including heart disease and stroke, which kill more than 15 million people. Cancer kills more than 6 million; chronic obstructive pulmonary disease almost 3 million. All impose heavy burdens of disability, social cost and economic loss.

But the same threat is also growing in developing countries, for as life expectancy there also increases, so too does the certainty that people will become more and more prone to diseases that are more common among older age groups. Already, the outlook for most individuals in the developing world is that if they do manage to survive the infections of infancy, childhood and maturity, they will become exposed in later life to noninfectious diseases that threaten to shorten or disable their remaining years.

Health researchers often refer to this situation as the "epidemiological transition" – the changing pattern of health in which poor countries inherit the problems of the rich, including not merely illness but also the harmful effects of tobacco, alcohol and drug use, and of injuries, suicide and violence.

The phenomenon is also sometimes known as the "double burden". The description is all too accurate: hundreds of millions of people now live under two shadows – the long-familiar one of infectious diseases, such as malaria or tuberculosis, and in addition the new and growing shadow of noninfectious, chronic diseases, for which they lack adequate treatment, and of the social ills that all too frequently accompany socioeconomic development.

Increasingly, health is influenced by social and economic circumstances over which the individual has little control, and over which the conventional health sector also has little sway. As a result, many countries are now experiencing not merely an epidemiological transition, but an "epidemiological polarization" – a widening gap in health terms between rich and poor. This was the theme of *The World Health Report 1995 – Bridging the gaps*.

For richer, for poorer?

That report showed that infectious diseases are more prevalent among poorer and rural people, while middle- and upper-income urban dwellers – whose life expectancy is higher – are more exposed to noninfectious diseases and conditions. In other words, the poorer an individual is, the more probable it is that he or she will become ill and die of an infectious disease; the richer the person, the greater are the odds of suffering and dying from a noninfectious disease. Furthermore, as the gaps in life expectancy clearly demonstrate, the poor die young, while the rich die old.

These facts raise a fundamental issue: global health priorities which emphasize infectious diseases will benefit the poor much more than the rich. Shifting priorities significantly away from infectious diseases towards chronic diseases would benefit the rich at the expense of the poor, and further widen the gaps that currently exist between them. This would be in direct conflict with the goals of equity in health. The aim is to achieve adequate health for all, rather than simply to achieve still better health for those whose health is already adequate.

The aim is to achieve adequate health for all, rather than simply to achieve still better health for those whose health is already adequate.

Any further improvements in health thus demand integrated, comprehensive action addressing all the determinants of ill-health. Countries, particularly in the developing world, can no longer afford to deal with the two challenges of infectious diseases and chronic diseases sequentially, as in the past: they must address them simultaneously, and the international community must help them to do so. While these will certainly be challenges reaching far into the future, they already exist today, and must be confronted today.

Indeed, separating infectious and noninfectious diseases creates something of a false division. It is becoming more and more difficult to establish a firm borderline between them. For example, several forms of cancer are known to be linked to infectious agents, and infections also play a role in some cardiovascular diseases – rheumatic heart disease, for instance.

Perhaps more important is the recognition that physical and mental health are interrelated. Physical illness frequently has serious psychological consequences. It is little wonder, given how much long-term pain and distress chronic diseases impose on individuals, that depression and other affective disorders are themselves emerging as major disease burdens. At the same time, there is mounting evidence that some mental disorders, such as dementia, have a biological basis.

Curing and caring

One crucial and controversial difference between infectious and chronic diseases needs to be recognized. The history of medicine and public health shows that infectious diseases can be cured – eliminate or destroy the infectious agent, and the disease is defeated. The eradication of smallpox is the supreme example, but many other infectious diseases are steadily being defeated, among them poliomyelitis and leprosy. This could not be achieved without strong community participation – immunization campaigns, for example, cannot succeed without active community support.

Chronic diseases, however, are another matter. With a few exceptions, they have not so far lent themselves so easily to cure. They are less open to direct community action. They do not spread from person to person. Every case of chronic disease represents a burden borne by one individual who, depending on circumstances, may or may not have access to treatment or support (*Box 1*).

Box 1. Essential drugs for chronic diseases

Many chronic diseases can be treated effectively with drugs, and every year more of these drugs enter the market, especially in industrialized countries. Some of the new drugs, but not all, represent real therapeutic advances; most are very expensive. They are often taken for long periods, if not for life, which leads to high treatment costs and increased chances of unwanted side-effects. Chronic diseases are increasingly prevalent in developing countries and the need for drugs to treat them is therefore also rising, although they often remain untreated, because people either have no access to regular medical care or cannot afford it.

The best way to ensure the availability of and equitable access to essential drugs, including those for chronic diseases, is to develop standard treatment protocols and lists of essential drugs for different levels of health care, and to use these as the basis for the supply of drugs, for the training and supervision of health workers, and for reimbursement schemes. Essential drugs should be selected on the basis of evidence and in accordance with the criteria used for compiling the WHO *Model list of essential drugs*, which is updated every two years.

The need for drug selection is not restricted to developing countries. Health care costs in general, and drug costs in particular, are rising everywhere. Most of the increased drug cost is due to the use of new medicines, and many of these are for chronic diseases. In order to ensure an optimal use of limited resources, a careful evaluation is needed of their cost-effectiveness in relation to existing treatment alternatives. Some industrialized countries have developed very detailed procedures for this difficult process. One example is the pharmaceutical benefit scheme in Australia, which requires proof that a drug is more cost-effective than existing treatments, before it is being approved for reimbursement. It is interesting to note that the list used in the Australian scheme contains approximately the same number of active ingredients as the national list of essential drugs in Zimbabwe.

Another example is the Scottish intercollegiate guidelines network, which is developing national treatment protocols entirely on the basis of evidence. For every treatment recommendation, the strength of the supporting scientific evidence is indicated according to four levels – the strength of the evidence defines the strength of the recommendation. The main objective of the Scottish guidelines is to attain the highest standards in health care, rather than cost-containment. Some of the recommendations lead to increased health care cost, for example in the treatment of diseases which are generally known to be underdiagnosed and undertreated (e.g. diabetic retinopathy).

These two examples show that essential drugs are not for poor countries only or for rural areas only. The concept of essential drugs is just as valid in developed countries, in teaching hospitals, and in health insurance schemes. It is as valid for the treatment of cancer, cardiovascular diseases and metabolic disorders as it is for malaria, acute diarrhoea and pneumonia.

Premature mortality and disability from chronic diseases are more common than in previous times. The trend is a reflection of the way our lives are changing.

Despite enormous investments in cancer research, and great progress in that field in recent years, the most common cancers stubbornly resist medical control. Intertwined as they are with heredity and natural ageing, occurring gradually and stealthily as they often do over decades, they and other chronic diseases pose far greater problems for medical science than do many infectious diseases.

This stark fact demands a realistic response: if the majority of chronic diseases cannot as yet be cured, the emphasis must be on preventing their premature onset, delaying their development in later life, reducing the suffering that they cause, and providing the supportive social environment to care for those disabled by them.

This must be particularly true of dementia sufferers. Today there are an estimated 29 million people worldwide with dementia, and the number will rise dramatically in the coming years with an ageing population. Already robbed of their memories and rendered helpless by the disease, the last thing they have to lose is their dignity. They will need from health professionals, families and society an extra degree of care with compassion.

Today there are an estimated 380 million people aged 65 years or more, including around 220 million in developing countries. By 2020, the figures are projected to reach more than 690 million and 460 million respectively. It is also forecast that by the same year chronic diseases may be responsible for a large proportion of deaths in the developing world. Cancer and circulatory disease, which have long been dominant in the industrialized world, are already the major causes of death in South-East Asia.

Hazards of living

The development of these diseases is seldom, if ever, due to one single cause. Vulnerability to them may be inherited – an area which geneticists have only begun to explore, but undoubtedly of great importance. In addition, many lifestyle and environmental factors are known to increase the risks – factors such as smoking, heavy alcohol consumption, inappropriate diet, and inadequate physical activity. These are at least to some extent within the control of the well-informed individual. But there are others, such as the effects of poverty; poor reproductive and maternal health; undernutrition in infancy and childhood; genetic predisposition; environmental pollution; and unhealthy living and dangerous or stressful working conditions, over which the individual alone has little control.

The ascendancy of chronic diseases is not simply a question of age, although natural ageing plays a fundamental role, or of genetic predisposition. Today, premature mortality and disability from chronic diseases are more common than in previous times. The trend is also a reflection of the way our lives are changing in response to a changing world. For instance, the rapid emergence of middle classes in many developing countries has brought with it unhealthy dietary and behavioural changes.

In many parts of the world, lifestyles are undergoing radical changes – from physical, outdoor labour to sitting at a desk or working in a factory, from rural life to urban existence, from traditional diet to convenience foods, from strict codes of sexual behaviour to more permissive standards, from negligible consumption of alcohol and/or tobacco to daily or heavy consumption of one or both.

Tobacco-related deaths – primarily from lung cancer and heart disease – already amount to 3 million a year, or 6% of total deaths. Other cancers are also linked to smoking. Researchers estimate that during the 1990s, 30 million people will have been killed by smoking, more than half of them while in middle age. While in the past most of these deaths have been in industrialized countries, there are ominous trends in the developing world, where there are estimated to be about 800 million people who smoke, and that number is increasing.

Major work-related illnesses include cardiovascular diseases, respiratory diseases, cancer, musculoskeletal disorders, and reproductive and psychological disorders. Occupational injuries alone affect more than 120 million persons and cause at least 200 000 deaths a year. Up to 350 different substances have been identified as occupational carcinogens. In western Europe alone, some 16 million people are exposed to carcinogenic agents at work.

The interplay of these and other factors is complex and is only gradually being investigated and understood. So too are the interaction between one chronic disease and another, and the genetic components that either predispose some individuals to certain diseases or offer protection against them.

For example, inherited predisposition is important in some common diseases of later life, including coronary heart disease and diabetes mellitus. The number of people suffering from diabetes worldwide is projected to more than double from 135 million now to almost 300 million by 2025.

Millions of people are born every year with hereditary diseases, such as haemophilia or cystic fibrosis, which may require lifelong treatment. Of some 140 million infants born each year, about 4 million enter the world already disabled by major congenital anomalies. Reproductive health, including the health of the mother before, during and after pregnancy is fundamental to the well-being of her infant, and influences that child's development into adulthood.

Largely at the other end of the age spectrum, hundreds of millions of adults suffer from mental illnesses ranging from chronic depression and schizophrenia to Alzheimer disease, and huge numbers are disabled for many years by musculoskeletal disorders such as rheumatoid arthritis, back pain and osteoporosis.

Making a difference

Although many chronic diseases most commonly appear only after middle age, some strike much earlier. This report examines them, or the factors influencing them, across the entire human life span. Many of the seeds of adult disease are sown in infancy, childhood and adolescence. Children are vulnerable to a wide range of chronic diseases, including rheumatic heart disease, asthma, and some forms of cancer.

At every stage, opportunities exist for prevention or treatment, for promoting healthy behaviour, for cure or for care. Major efforts have also been made, and continue to be made, in these fields, in attacking risk factors, in promoting health as a component of social policies, and in protecting the environment through pollution control.

As this report shows, there is much that remains to be done, and must be done now – in preventing chronic diseases, treating them, curing them; in renewing attacks on the many risk factors, including those outlined above, that contribute to them; in alleviating suffering and reducing disability; in improving standards of care, and access to that care.

Throughout, the report attempts to keep the health of the individual as the centre of interest. Indeed, a key approach to the preparation of the report has been the recognition that the impact of disease on the individual is fundamental to improving health for the community at large.

One person's suffering can often be overshadowed by the social ramifications of disease in general. In such circumstances, the individual may feel neglected, or forgotten. Involving that person to a greater degree in the protection of his or her health is increasingly necessary.

In terms of setting priorities, the report considers chronic diseases that are major causes of death or avoidable ill-health and disability. These are areas where actions or interventions that have a direct and tangible effect on individual health – that make a difference, and make it sooner, rather than later – are possible.

In recent years action may often have been less direct, requiring legislation or regulation, with slower repercussions for individual health. At the same time, the report outlines what individuals can do to take care of their own

At every stage, opportunities exist for prevention or treatment, for promoting healthy behaviour, for cure or for care.

health, and how the family and society can support them.

Future [illegible] be mere repeti[illegible] cation mes[illegible]ugh to say simply: don't smoke, don't drink excessively, take exercise and consume a better diet. These messages are indispensable. If followed, they will help substantially in reducing the risks of some chronic diseases; but in terms of prevention they will not in themselves be enough. Enabling people to adopt healthy lifestyles, and creating supportive environments for health are two core elements of health promotion action. But such action requires time to produce results.

Research into the biological origins of disease is essential to prevention, and the importance of treatment and rehabilitation for those who have already contracted disease cannot be overlooked.

Latterly, the emphasis has been on protecting and promoting health rather than on prevention, treatment, cure and rehabilitation. The global trends in chronic disease indicate that shorter-term approaches, such as the development of new drugs, treatments and vaccines, are urgently needed. Research into the biological origins of disease is essential to prevention, and the importance of treatment and rehabilitation for those who have already contracted disease cannot be overlooked.

Following a general section giving an overall assessment of the global health situation in 1996, this report deals with the chronic diseases that are leading causes of death and disability. It gives a brief description of each disease, and estimates the global numbers affected by it; identifies risk factors that contribute to it; and explains the methods of prevention, detection, diagnosis and treatment. Together, these methods form a basis for reducing and conquering suffering, reducing its social and economic costs to families and society, and thereby enriching humanity.

The global situation – 1996 update

The global political situation

The global trends towards democratization continued unabated during 1996. Many countries carried out popular elections, considered to be reasonably free and fair, to choose their governments. These elections laid the foundations for increased participation of people in building their nations, deciding on development priorities, shaping the style of governance and determining its degrees of transparency and accountability.

Although the transition towards democracy has in some instances frustrated popular hopes and aspirations, people have in general not given up pursuing this goal. But the pace of progress was being cautiously set. In an ageing world, the proportion of the elderly among electorates is increasing. Their empowerment through education and information should ensure, in a democratic environment, that their interests and priorities are reflected in health and welfare policies and programmes.

Liberal democracy has given billions of people the right to express their opinions freely and openly. Thanks to modern communication media, there has been rapid and wide diffusion of information on many of the issues that are fundamental to human development.

Unfortunately many nations and states where sharp differences among ethnic and religious groups were set aside in the pursuit of economic development, now experience bitter feuds that lead to new social divisions. Political maps are being redrawn as numerous ethnic and political groups emerge, make claims and parcel out new territories. The increase in the number of Member States of WHO from 170 in 1991 to 190 in 1996 partly reflects this phenomenon.

A number of local conflicts and threats to peace became internationally known owing to almost immediate global media communication. The flow of arms to many of these areas afflicted by civil violence has been increasing, and major victims have been civilians, primarily women and children (*Box 2*).

In many cases, massive new population movements within and across international borders have also taken place. It is estimated that in December 1995, more than 26 million people belonged to "populations of concern to UNHCR", which include in addition to more than 13 million refugees, persons granted temporary protection and those allowed to stay in another country on humanitarian grounds. More than 40% of refugees (5.7 million) were in Africa and about 35% (4.5 million) in Asia.

As emergency relief and humanitarian assistance are provided to these people, another battle must be fought to overcome the difficulties they face in having access to preventive and curative care, to food and water and to rehabilitation in a context of general anarchy when basic infrastructure is disrupted or destroyed and human and material resources are diverted elsewhere. A major concern is the outbreak of epidemics of diseases such as cholera, dysentery, meningitis, malaria, typhus and measles, as well as the spread of antibiotic resistance among the displaced populations.

WHO, in collaboration with UNHCR and UNICEF and other national and international nongovernmental organizations, undertakes activities to contain and control epidemics during complex emergencies and mass population movements, through early detection and timely response using surveillance systems adapted to the population groups concerned and local situations, bearing in mind the need to strengthen local capability (*Box 3*). The International Committee of the Red Cross has been focusing on developing capability in "war surgery" through training seminars and transmitting its experience to wider medical and health circles through publications and videos. Many of the refugees suffer mental distress as a result of problems and difficulties encountered before, during or after the flight from their home regions. At each stage of these journeys, specific steps – such as organizing programmes dealing with the trauma of political violence – have been taken to lessen their risk of ill-health.

Box 2. Victims of armed conflict

In the 50 years since the end of the Second World War, over 20 million people have died in more than 150 local wars in Africa, Asia, Europe and Latin America. In countries such as Bangladesh, Cambodia, China, Iran, Iraq, Nigeria, Rwanda and Viet Nam, at least one million people have been killed in each conflict.

In the past decade, around 2 million children have died as a result of war, and many times that number have been displaced from their homes. In situations of armed conflict, deaths of children are 24 times higher than in times of peace. An estimated 4 million children have been disabled because of armed conflict, many of them from injuries caused by landmines. It is projected that from 117 million to 138 million children could be vulnerable to the indirect effects of such conflicts by the year 2000.

Since 1945 so-called "conventional" weapons have directly caused the deaths of more than 230 million people. During this period the percentage of direct war deaths among civilians has increased steadily, and in recent years approximately nine times as many civilians as military personnel have been killed by weapons during war. Landmines and the blinding laser (which can burn out a human retina) are among those which cause the most concern. Wounds caused by landmines are extremely difficult to treat. The majority of the victims are civilians.

In addition to the health consequences of the direct use of arms, there are those attributable to militarization and arms even if the weapons are never used. Even wealthy countries suffer the consequences of diversion of resources to military purposes, but developing countries are the most affected, suffering delay or reversal of economic development and deprivation of essential nutrition, housing, education and health services. Most modern weapons are manufactured in industrialized countries and many of them (amounting to more than $35 billion) are sold or given to developing countries.

The world economy

The growth of the world economy accelerated slowly during 1996. Global economic and financial conditions were considered to be encouraging on the whole, despite a disappointing performance in Europe generally. The strength of economic activity was particularly impressive in the emerging market economies of the developing world with an increasing number of them reaping the benefits of structural reforms and a favourable macroeconomic situation. In most of the economies in transition, the

Box 3. WHO in Rwanda

In November and December 1996, the massive and sudden return of nearly 1.2 million Rwandan refugees from eastern Zaire and the United Republic of Tanzania to Rwanda surpassed the capacity of the government of Rwanda and the international community to take care of them, resulting in significant threats to health. WHO responded immediately at the field level by coordinating health activities and monitoring their health status.

Potential for epidemics. Cases of cholera and dysentery, and deaths due to severe diarrhoea were frequently reported. One of the main concerns was the spread of drug resistance which could significantly affect the treatment of these diseases. Sporadic outbreaks of meningitis had occurred in the past in Rwanda, but were contained thanks to an efficient early detection system.

Threat of other infectious diseases. Malaria and acute respiratory diseases were the two most common causes of morbidity in the country. HIV prevalence was high among the general population, with sexually transmitted diseases one of the 10 most common causes of morbidity. Cases were poorly managed, and condoms rarely provided at the peripheral level. The treatment and control of tuberculosis cases was hampered by a shortage of drugs.

Weakness of health care services. Only 43% of the health facilities had the minimum necessary equipment. Some hospitals reported an increase of 60% in the occupation of beds after the repatriation movement. Facilities at health centres for delivery and postdelivery care were rudimentary and often unsatisfactory. The significant number of women among the returnee population increased the need for antenatal, natal and postnatal care services. The massive return of the refugees exacerbated the shortage of drugs in most of the health centres as well as of beds, mattresses, gloves, needles and other pieces of equipment.

Lack of health care personnel. Most health facilities were reported to be understaffed. The Ministry of Health estimated that 80 additional medical doctors and 80 nurses needed to be recruited. The health management structures were not functional in some areas, mainly those bordering eastern Zaire, due to the insecurity which prevailed before the massive repatriation.

WHO provided prompt assistance to Rwanda and the subregion by:

- sending experts in the areas of epidemiology, public health, water and sanitation to provide technical support in response to the urgent situation;
- recruiting United Nations volunteer medical officers to provide medical care in the district health facilities in the communes that received the greatest number of refugees;
- conducting, at the request of the Ministry of Health, a rapid assessment of the health situation in Rwanda after the massive influx of returnees;
- coordinating the activities of nationals and nongovernmental organizations in districts and communes;
- assisting the Ministry of Health in elaborating the health component of the Government Emergency Programme for Repatriation and Resettlement of Returnees;
- providing essential drugs and other medical supplies for the control of cholera and malaria;
- supporting laboratory diagnosis of cholera in Rwanda, including drug sensitivity testing.

move towards capitalism was becoming increasingly successful, with the private sector responding to macroeconomic stability, market forces, and to countries' integration into the world economy. Overall the global economic expansion is expected to continue at a satisfactory pace during the rest of this decade, stimulated by the growing interaction of countries in world trade, foreign direct investment and capital markets – the globalization process.

The global economic decline of the early 1990s seemed to have ended, with the world's gross output of goods and services growing at about 2.5% in 1996, that is, for the third consecutive year. At least 109 countries with a combined population of 5.3 billion (all but about 300-400 million of the world's people) saw their per capita output rise in real terms during 1996.

Developing countries continued to experience a rise in per capita GDP in 1996. There were 75 countries with a combined population of at least 4.3 billion in this group in 1996 compared to 50 countries in 1993. The least developed countries in particular have made significant progress in this regard. At least 21 out of the 48 least developed countries (with about 80% of the total population of these countries) registered growth in per capita GDP in both 1995 and 1996. This compares impressively with the experience of the early 1990s, when only about a dozen least developed countries, with about half the population, were in this category. The gain in countries with rising per capita GDP has been most pronounced in Africa, where the percentage of the population living in countries with growing per capita GDP increased from 67% in 1995 to over 87% in 1996. The total output of the economies in transition was one-third less in 1995 than in 1990. Whereas these economies in central and eastern Europe and the Baltic States began to grow from 1994, the output of the newly independent States continued to decline, and the prospects for positive growth in the near future are uncertain. Developed countries experienced a growth rate of about 2% in 1996 with an uneven growth and labour market performance. Inflation was successfully contained, but unemployment remained stubbornly high, notwithstanding respectable economic growth, and became a major concern in many of these countries. Overall, the short-term outlook for the global economy is a continued but modest increase, with growth rates in real terms for 1997 projected at more than 6% for the developing countries, 3% for the economies in transition and 2.5% for the developed countries.

The global economic environment for developing countries has also been relatively favourable over the past five years. Growth in world trade averaged more than 6% annually during 1991-1995, which is more than the growth of world output during this period. Private capital inflows to developing countries quadrupled, yet marked disparities in growth in capital inflows persisted among and within developing regions. The extent to which countries benefited from the increased integration of the world's goods and capital markets was also highly uneven (*Table 1*). Available data reveal, however, that the fastest growing regions over the past five years also showed the greatest advances in integration with the world economy. A boost to international trade was given both by the establishment of the World Trade Organization (WTO) at the beginning of 1995 and by the creation of several new regional economic groups. As a result of trade liberalization, a growing number of developing countries are expected to experience gains in real income as a result of their increasing integration in the global economy.

Among the many individual trade agreements that WTO administers, several have implications for the health sector, particularly those regarding standards. Aimed at ensuring that national health and safety regulations are not used as a disguised form of protectionism, the agreements on technical barriers to trade and on sanitary and phytosanitary measures encourage countries to use internationally agreed quality and safety standards. They cover such health-related items as pharmaceuticals and biologicals, together with food products – a major export of developing countries – and their application should lead to the production of safer, higher-quality goods. Pharmaceuticals are further affected by the agreement on intellectual property rights, by virtue of which their patenting has become compulsory. The eventual impact of that measure on the continuing availability of low-cost drugs in developing countries remains to be seen.

To guard against the risk of financial interests taking precedence over public health and to enable national authorities to handle the impact of an expansion of international trade in services, UNCTAD and WHO in 1996 jointly launched a project on international trade in health services. Following a global analysis and case studies, the plan is to examine the problems and opportunities that developing countries face in the sector of trade in health services, as well as associated social advantages and disadvantages, as a basis for strengthening the capacity of developing countries to maximize net benefits.

Many developing countries have succeeded in establishing markets for their goods in both developed economies and developing countries. Current international economic conditions are providing an opportunity for growth from which many countries have been

Table 1. Growth and integration, 1991–1995[a]

Region	Real GDP growth per capita 1991–1994 (%)	Real GDP growth 1991–1994 (%)	Speed of integration index	Export growth per capita 1991–1995 (%)	Foreign direct investment flows as a share of GDP 1993–1995 (%)
East Asia	8	9.4	0.77	14.1	3.1
South Asia	1.8	3.9	0.87	8.4	0.3
Latin America and the Caribbean	1.6	3.6	-0.23	7.2	1.1
Middle East and North Africa	-0.3	2.4	-0.19	0.4	0.4
Sub-Saharan Africa	-2.2	0.7	-0.46	-1.6	0.9
Europe and Central Asia	-9.3	-9	0.46	1	1.4

[a] Ranked by real GDP growth per capita.
Source: World Bank, *Global economic prospects and the developing countries 1996.*

able to benefit. The challenge now is to translate this growth into reductions in unemployment and poverty.

Though some progress has been made in reducing poverty in the developing world since 1987, overall gains have been small and uneven. Recent studies by the World Bank indicate that while overall poverty (its threshold level being an income of less than $1 per capita per day), fell slightly from 30% of the world population in 1987 to 29% in 1993, the number of people living on less than $1 a day rose by about 85 million to 1.3 billion in 1993. Significant progress has been made in reducing the number and share of households with low incomes in South and East Asia and in the Eastern Mediterranean and northern Africa in the last decade; they are more or less static in Latin America and in sub-Saharan Africa, but are rising in eastern Europe and central Asia.

There is hope that poverty in the world can be considerably reduced during the next decade.

There is hope that poverty in the world can be considerably reduced during the next decade. This will depend on political commitment and sustained action, at national and international levels, for implementing the World Bank's *The heavily indebted poor countries (HIPC) debt initiative – a program of action* and country-focused activities for achieving at least the global target of the Organization of Economic Cooperation and Development for shaping the 21st century.

Success in these efforts would ironically pose great challenges for the control of "diseases of affluence" such as chronic and debilitating diseases. For, with even small improvements in living standards, people become exposed to a lifestyle and behaviour such as consumption of high-fat foods, alcohol and tobacco, a more sedentary life and inadequate physical activity. Several studies have shown that not only poverty but also affluence can lead to a wide variety of causes of death, disease and disability.

Population and its growth

One encouraging statistic from the United Nations Population Division's 1996 assessment of world population prospects was that the average annual increase of the global population fell from 87 million persons during the period 1985-1990 to 81 million during 1990-1995.

The population increased globally by more than 80 million during the year, reaching a total of 5.8 billion in mid-1996. It increased by 17 million children and adolescents aged 0–19, 55 million adults aged 20-64, and 9 million elderly aged 65 and above (of which 3 million aged 75 and above). The age group 0–19 years grew by about 0.7% during the year, while the elderly population grew by about 2.4%; the adult population increased by 1.8%. The increase in the elderly population aged 65 and above consisted of more women (4.7 million) than men (4.2 million) during the year.

Fertility

The world population in 1995 was about 29.5 million fewer (34 million less in developing countries and about 4.5 million more in developed countries) than assessed in 1994. This was because in 1990-1995 fertility declined to 3 children per woman instead of 3.1 as predicted. If this trend continues, the population of 9.4 billion in 2050 may well be nearly half-a-billion less than the 1994 projection. The population of developing countries is now estimated to have grown by about 1.8% per annum between 1990 and 1995 instead of 2.1% in 1980-1985 – due to a decline in fertility in a number of countries of south-central Asia and sub-Saharan Africa. For example fertility declined in Bangladesh, Côte d'Ivoire, India, Kenya, Syria and Turkey. Added to this fertility decline was the higher mortality in countries affected by wars, such as Burundi, Iraq, Liberia and Rwanda, and by the spread of AIDS.

Population ageing

The number of people aged 65 years and above increased to 380 million, accounting for 7% of the total global population of 5.8 billion in 1996; those aged above 80 years formed more than 16% of the over-65s. While the proportion of females among those aged 65 and above was about 55%, among those aged 80 and above it was 65%.

Between 1990 and 1995, the population aged 65 and above increased by 14% globally; by 17% in developing countries and 11% in the least developed countries; but by only about 10% in developed countries. Compared with 1996, by the year 2020 the over-65 population is projected to increase by 82% globally; by about 110% in the least developed and developing countries; and by about 40% in the developed countries. In 1996, less than 5% of the population were aged 65 and above in 102 countries. By 2020, this will be the case in only 68 countries. Among those over 80 years, there will be a more rapid increase in the number of women than men. A major challenge will be to develop innovative ways of tackling the special health and welfare problems of elderly women.

Education

The context for educational development in the 1990s has been profoundly affected by recent changes in the world political and economic order. These changes include the emergence of new democratic governments, the continuing globalization of the world economy, expansion of the service sector and the rapidity of new information and communication technologies – all of which call for new knowledge, skills and attitudes. About 103 million children aged 6-11 need a place in primary school in the developing regions during the 1990s. The World Declaration on Education for All adopted in March 1990 broadened the scope of basic education to include early childhood development, primary education, nonformal learning (including literacy and life skills) for youth and adults, and learning conveyed through the media and social action. A global assessment for the period 1990-1995 indicated that there has been definite progress in basic education. Programmes for early childhood development which integrate education, health and nutrition components are a fast-growing area of basic education reaching more than 56 million children in the developing regions, i.e. about one out of five in the 3-6-year age group.

The single most positive and significant feature of the mid-decade balance sheet was, however, in primary education in most developing countries. Enrolments increased from 496 million pupils in 1990 to 545 million pupils in 1995 – with the pace of enrolment growth being twice as fast during 1990-1995 as in the 1980s; sub-Saharan Africa and South Asia enrolled the most additional pupils – some 33 million since 1990. In spite of economic hardship, many countries affected by serious declines in enrolment during the 1980s appeared to have reversed the downward trend. Compared with an estimated 128 million school-age children with no access to schooling in 1990, the number of out-of-school children in the 6-11 age group in all developing countries in 1995 was some 110 million. Sub-Saharan Africa was the only region where the number of out-of-school children continued to grow.

Most developing countries still lack the capacity to monitor learning achievement in primary schools. Grade repetition and drop-out continue to be serious obstacles to universal primary education. Against this background, developing countries in 1995 had an estimated 870 million illiterate youth and adults aged 15 years and over – some 4 million more than in 1990. The overall adult literacy rate increased from 75% in 1990 to 77% in 1995; however, nearly two-thirds of all illiterate adults were women, a proportion that has not changed since 1990. In developing countries, there was an increase in female enrolment from about 225 million in 1990 to about 250 million in 1995. Literacy rates among women have in-

A major challenge will be to develop innovative ways of tackling the special health and welfare problems of elderly women.

creased slightly to 71% in 1995 but lag behind men's literacy rates in nearly all developing countries. The nine high-population countries – Bangladesh, Brazil, China, Egypt, India, Indonesia, Mexico, Nigeria and Pakistan – which account for more than 70% of the world's illiterate adults, have identified the provision of basic education through mass media as one of the main areas whose potential has yet to be fully exploited. Education plays a key role in tackling ill-health, particularly when it includes "life skills" related to central issues of daily life, such as health, hygiene, nutrition, the environment and civil rights. Positive developments such as those outlined above and progress towards "education for all", though not spectacular, augur well for the control of diseases and reduction of suffering in the future.

The estimated number of homeless people worldwide varies between 100 million and 1 billion.

Environment, housing and homelessness

Housing-poverty contributes significantly to ill-health. The term describes households that lack safe shelter, piped water and adequate sanitation and drainage. An estimated 1 billion rural households lack water supplies. Several hundred million people rely on simple latrines. At least 600 million urban dwellers in Africa, Asia and Latin America live in life- and health-threatening homes and neighbourhoods. The estimated number of homeless people worldwide varies between 100 million and 1 billion, depending on how homelessness is defined. The estimate of 100 million includes those who sleep outside or in public buildings or in overnight shelters. The 1 billion estimate includes those in refugee camps or in insecure or temporary accommodation.

Homelessness rose in the developed world during the 1980s. In the United States, the number of shelter beds available for the homeless in cities of over 100 000 inhabitants nearly tripled during that period – from 41 000 to 117 000. In the United Kingdom, the number of households recognized as homeless by public authorities rose from around 20 000 in 1970 to 117 900 in 1986 and to 167 300 in 1992. In the early 1990s, 1.8 million people in the 12 countries of the European Union depended in the course of a year on public or voluntary services for temporary shelter, or slept outside. At least another 15 million people lived with more than two persons per room, in substandard housing.

The dwelling-place is a critical component of the interaction between people and their environment. Studies in developed countries show that people spend more than 90% of their time indoors; there are few similar studies in developing countries.

The construction of water and sanitation facilities represents only a fraction, often relatively small, of the total effort necessary to achieve the desired health benefits, particularly reducing risks of infection. Many water resource development projects have failed to establish any health objectives or even to consider the likely indirect health outcomes of the projects. Concern about the possible carcinogenic risks arising from exposure to chemical contaminants in drinking-water focuses mainly on certain pesticides, halogenated organic compounds and inorganic compounds. The causal association between high arsenic concentrations in drinking-water and skin cancer is now well established. Furthermore, elevated mortality from several cancers, including bladder cancer, has been observed in populations exposed to high concentrations of arsenic in drinking-water. Procedures for the collection, disposal and treatment of wastes can be sources of carcinogenic hazard. For example, chemical agents may be present in the gases and particulates emitted during waste incineration, or in leachates from landfill sites that find their way into surface water and groundwater.

There are tens of thousands of man-made chemicals in common use throughout the world, and each year up to 2000 new chemicals are introduced onto the market. An estimated 50 million people work on plantations in developing countries and are in direct contact with pesticides. Over 500 million more are exposed through traditional agriculture and as seasonal workers. Even the theoretically nonexposed population may suffer toxic effects through food or water contamination with pesticides. Examples of the most dramatic pesticide-related incidents include methyl contamination of seeds in Iraq (over 6000 people affected and over 400 deaths) or the contamination of flour with parathion in Colombia (600 affected and 88 deaths). The consequences of chronic poisoning with heavy metals include heart failure, kidney disorders and hypertension arising from exposure to cadmium, and cardiovascular disease associated with exposure to arsenic. Exposure to high levels of lead has a direct toxic effect on the heart. The risk could grow in urban areas in developing countries with the rising number of vehicles using leaded petrol, despite restrictions.

Four years after the accident at Chernobyl nuclear power station, increased incidence of thyroid cancer was observed in children in Belarus and Ukraine. This was much sooner than would have been predicted from the radiation studies of Japanese survivors of the atomic bomb. Thyroid cancer is normally rare in children, but more than 420 cases were observed in children aged under 15 in Belarus between 1986 and 1995, compared to only 3 cases during 1981-1985. The main sources of nonionizing radiation are ultraviolet radiation from the sun and artificial light sources, and natural and human-made electromagnetic fields. Over 100 000 malignant melanomas of the skin are estimated to occur globally each year. The main risk at present, however, arises from excessive exposure to ultraviolet light, particularly as a result of sunbathing.

About 3 million deaths are estimated to be accountable to air pollution globally each year. Evidence, mostly from industrialized countries, links outdoor air pollution with cardiovascular diseases and asthma. Heart failure has been linked to airborne particles, carbon monoxide, and sulphur dioxide levels. Some lung diseases, such as pneumoconiosis, are caused by inhalation of industrial dusts.

Food security and nutrition

Hunger persists at a time when global food production could meet the needs of every person on the planet. Freedom from hunger and malnutrition, essential to the enjoyment of the highest attainable standard of health, is among the fundamental rights of human beings. Current food availability for the world as a whole was estimated by the Food and Agricultural Organization (FAO) at 2720 calories per person per day in 1990-1992, up from 2300 calories in 1961-1963. Food availability has increased in all regions, except sub-Saharan Africa. It is projected that by 2010, even developing countries as a group will have achieved the per capita food availability of 2730 calories.

Progress towards increasing food security has been uneven within and among countries, leaving an unacceptably large number of undernourished or food-insecure individuals. Increased production and distribution supplemented by food aid can help promote food security. Nutritional status, however, reflects not only the quantity of food available and consumed but also its quality, including safety, and the extent to which the body transforms food into nutrients that will protect and promote health and enable people to function to their potential capacity. Malnutrition must therefore be considered from two points of view: undernutrition and obesity.

Progress towards increasing food security has been uneven, leaving an unacceptably large number of undernourished or food-insecure individuals.

While over 800 million people are estimated to lack access to food to meet their daily basic needs for energy and protein, more than 3 billion people are deficient in essential micronutrients such as iodine, vitamin A and iron. These deficiencies lead to poor physical and cognitive development as well as to lowered resistance to illness, brain damage, blindness and even death. More than half of the deaths occurring annu-

Life expectancy at birth for both sexes continued to improve globally, reaching a global value of 65 years by 1996.

ally among children aged under 5 in developing countries are associated with malnutrition.

Simultaneously, these countries are also currently experiencing a different type of nutrition crisis: diet-related chronic diseases and disorders. Too often, one type of malnutrition is being exchanged for, or – worse still – being superimposed upon another in many of these countries. It is increasingly recognized that cultural aspects of food production, distribution and preparation play a crucial role in the promotion of good nutrition, apart from the types of food themselves.

Obesity, or overweight, is a lifestyle risk factor associated with increased morbidity and mortality from chronic diseases such as circulatory diseases, cancer, diabetes and chronic musculoskeletal and respiratory diseases. In many cases these diseases are preventable. An increase in glucose intolerance among school-age children is linked to consumption of sugary soft drinks and is an example of unhealthy dietary habits. More often than not, obesity is the result of unhealthy eating habits coupled with a sedentary way of life. When intake of energy with food exceeds energy expenditure, the excess is stored in the form of body fat. Energy storage is part of the body's natural protection against famine and is fundamental for survival when food is scarce. However, when energy storage becomes the rule rather than the exception, it leads to obesity, which can be described as the point beyond which increasing body fat storage is associated with elevated health risks.

Interventions focus on weight-loss therapy. Weight loss is difficult to sustain, but is likely to benefit health in the long term if it is sustained. Many overweight individuals who lose an appreciable amount of body weight regain it later. Repeated attempts to lose weight may thus lead to "weight cycling", which itself may be associated with adverse health consequences.

A recent FAO study predicts that the trends towards increasing per capita food supplies will continue in most developing countries, and that the incidence of undernutrition may fall by the year 2010 to a fairly low level of 12% of the total population. It is therefore likely that increasing incidence of obesity may evolve as a major concern with far-reaching implications for health, in view of the massive burden of disability and death that would result from diet-related heart disease, cancer and other chronic diseases. The Rome Declaration on World Food Security and the World Food Summit Plan of Action adopted in November 1996 have also set the objective of ensuring that food supplies are safe, appropriate and adequate to meet the energy and nutrient needs of the population. Adequate nutrition, achieved through regular consumption of an adequate and balanced diet, is indispensable for good health and essential to avoid many of the diet-related chronic diseases.

Life expectancy and mortality

Life expectancy at birth for both sexes continued to improve globally, reaching a global value of 65 years by 1996 (63 for men and 67 for women). In 50 countries, it was under 60 years for both sexes. In 53 countries, the value was less than 60 for men and in 48, it was less than 60 for women.

Estimates of life expectancy at birth between 1980 and 1995 are available for 171 WHO Member States. Between 1980 and 1995, life expectancy at birth increased by about 4.6 years globally for both sexes, with an increase of about 4.4 for men and 4.9 for women. There were increases of at least 5 years for men in 74 countries, and for women in 80. In three Member States, the increase represented 10 years or more; in 74, the increase was between 5 and 10 years; in 94 it was less than 5. In 10 countries, however, there was a decrease, 7 of which are economies in transition and 3 developing countries.

A significant trend in global mortality can be observed if the patterns of death in 1960 and 1996 are compared. Of 50 million deaths in 1960, 19 million were in children under 5, whereas the number had declined to 11 million for the same age group in 1996. On the

Table 2. Global health situation: mortality, morbidity and disability, selected causes for which data are available, all ages, 1996 estimates

Diseases/conditions (based on ICD-10)	Number (000) Deaths	Cases New (incidence)	Cases All (prevalence)	Disabled persons (permanent and long-term)
ALL CAUSES	**52 037**			
Certain infectious and parasitic diseases (selected), of which:	**17 312**			
Acute lower respiratory infection (ALRI)	3 905	394 000[a]	...	...
Tuberculosis	3 000[b]	7 400[b]	...	...
Diarrhoea (including dysentery)	2 473	4 002 000[a]	...	...
Malaria	1 500-2 700	300 000-500 000	...	...
HIV/AIDS	1 500	3 100	22 600	...
Hepatitis B	1 156	...	...	...
Measles	1 010	42 000	...	...
Whooping cough (pertussis)	355	40 000	...	...
Neonatal tetanus	310	385	...	...
Trypanosomiasis, African (sleeping sickness)	150	200	300	100
Dengue fever/dengue haemorrhagic fever	138	3 100	...	...
Leishmaniasis (total), of which:	80	2 000	3 820	...
Leishmaniasis, visceral (kala-azar)	80	500	1 270	...
Leishmaniasis, cutaneous and mucocutaneous	...	1 500	2 550	...
Amoebiasis (*Entamoeba histolytica*)	70	48 000	...	...
Hookworm diseases (ancylostomiasis and necatoriasis)	65	...	151 000	...
Rabies (dog-mediated)	60	60[c]	...	...
Ascariasis (roundworm)	60	...	250 000	...
Onchocerciasis (river blindness)	47	...	17 655	770
Trypanosomiasis, American (Chagas disease)	45	300	18 000	...
Meningococcal meningitis (see also bacterial meningitis)	40	...	400	50
Schistosomiasis	20	...	200 000	...
Japanese encephalitis	10	40	...	8
Trematode infections (foodborne)	10	...	40 000	...
Trichuriasis (whipworm)	10	...	45 530	...
Poliomyelitis, acute	7	20	...	10 600
Cholera (1996 notifications)[d]	6	120	...	...
Leprosy	2	530	1 260	3 000
Yellow fever (1995 notifications)	0.2	1.0	...	...
Plague (1995 notifications)	0.1	1.9	...	...
Giardiasis	...	500	...	...
Endemic treponematoses	...	460	2 600	260
Dracunculiasis (guinea-worm infection)	...	130	140	...
Hepatitis C	...	...	170 000[e]	...
Trachoma	...	...	152 420	5 600
Lymphatic filariasis	...	...	119 100	119 100
Sexually transmitted diseases (selected), of which:				
Syphilis	...	12 000	28 000	...
Gonococcal infection (gonorrhoea)	...	62 000	23 000	...
Chlamydial infections, including lymphogranuloma (venereum)	...	89 000	85 000	...
Chancroid	...	2 000	2 000	...
Trichomoniasis	...	170 000	113 000	...
Anogenital herpes	...	20 000	...	...
Anogenital warts	...	30 000	...	...
Others (including emerging diseases e.g. influenza, Ebola, Lassa)	683	...	...	...

[a] Figure refers to episodes.
[b] Subject to revisions following completion of country-specific estimates.
[c] In addition, 10 million people receive treatment every year.
[d] As at 31 January 1997.
[e] Based on studies reviewed, the prevalence is 3% of the world population.

Diseases/conditions (based on ICD-10)	Number (000)			
		Cases		
	Deaths	New (incidence)	All (prevalence)	Disabled persons (permanent and long-term)
Malignant neoplasms (cancers) – all sites	**6 346**	**10 320**	**17 930[f]**	
Trachea, bronchus and lung	989	1 320	1 205	...
Stomach	776	1 015	970	...
Colon and rectum	495	875	1 850	...
Liver	386	540	265	...
Breast (female)	376	910	2 810	...
Oesophagus	358	480	270	...
Mouth and pharynx	324	575	1 075	...
Cervix	247	525	1 560	...
Lymphomas	232	395	735	...
Pancreas	227	200	125	...
Leukaemia	217	280	370	...
Prostate	194	400	1 015	...
Bladder	143	310	780	...
Ovary	129	190	455	...
Kidney	92	165	360	...
Larynx	91	190	505	...
Body of the uterus	67	170	600	...
Melanoma of skin	39	115	315	...
Other malignant neoplasms	965	1 665	2 665	...
Diseases of the blood and bloodforming organs and certain disorders involving the immune mechanism (selected), of which:				
Thalassaemias and sickle cell disorder	240	290	2 320	...
Haemophilia	...	10	420	...
Anaemia, of which:	...	...	1 987 300	...
Iron deficiency anaemia	...	...	1 788 600	...
Endocrine, nutritional and metabolic diseases (selected), of which:	**943**			
Diabetes mellitus	571	10 540	135 000	...
Malnutrition including protein-energy malnutrition (PEM)	372[g]	...	200 000[h]	...
Iodine deficiencies (disorders of thyroid gland), of which:	...	...	...	120 800
Goitre	...	...	760 000	76 000
Cretinoids	...	...	...	33 600
Cretinism	...	...	...	11 200
Mental and behavioural disorders (selected), of which:	**323**			
Dementia	200	2 610	29 000	15 950
Alcohol dependence syndrome	103	75 000	120 000	...
Substance abuse (drug dependence syndrome)	20	...	28 000	...
Schizophrenic disorders	...	4 500	45 000	27 000
Mood (affective) disorders	...	122 865	340 000	146 000
Anxiety disorders	...	...	400 000	...
Mental retardation (all types)	...	...	60 000	36 000
Diseases of the nervous system (selected), of which:	**203**			
Bacterial meningitis (excluding neonatal meningitis)	120	...	1 100	145
Parkinson disease	58	305	3 765	2 635
Multiple sclerosis	25	105	2 505	750
Epilepsy	...	2 000	40 000	10 000
Diseases of the circulatory system (selected), of which:	**15 300**			
Ischaemic (coronary) heart disease	7 200	...	...	...
Cerebrovascular disease	4 600	...	9 000	...
Other heart diseases (e.g. peri-, endo-, and myocarditis and cardiomyopathy)	3 000	...	...	...
Rheumatic fever and rheumatic heart disease	500	...	12 000	...
Hypertensive disease	...	...	690 600	...

Diseases/conditions (based on ICD-10)	Number (000)			
		Cases		
	Deaths	New (incidence)	All (prevalence)	Disabled persons (permanent and long-term)
Diseases of the respiratory system (selected), of which:	**2 888**			
Chronic obstructive pulmonary disease (COPD)	2 888	...	600 000	...
Asthma	...	...	155 000	...
Diseases of the musculoskeletal system and connective tissue (selected), of which:				
Neck and back disorders	...	...	1 039 200[i]	...
Arthritis and arthrosis, of which:	...	...	354 500	...
Osteoarthritis	...	...	189 500[j]	...
Rheumatoid arthritis	...	...	165 000	...
Pregnancy, childbirth and the puerperium (selected), of which:	**585**	**76 500**		
Haemorrhage	145	14 000	...	...
Indirect obstetric causes	115	13 200	...	...
Sepsis	89	11 800	...	...
Abortion	76	19 900	...	...
Hypertensive disorders in pregnancy	73	6 900	...	...
Obstructed labour	45	7 200	...	...
Other direct obstetric causes	42	3 500	...	...
Certain conditions originating in the perinatal period (selected), of which:	**3 745[k]**			
Prematurity	1 150	...	...	...
Birth asphyxia	940	...	...	...
Congenital anomalies	520	3 600	...	...
Neonatal sepsis and meningitis	460	...	...	...
Birth trauma	440	...	...	...
Other causes	235	...	...	...
External causes (selected), of which:	**1 058**			
Suicide	833	...	...	...
Occupational injuries due to accidents at work	225	125 000	...	12 500
Occupational diseases	...	160 000	...	...
Other and unknown causes	**3 094**			
Visual disability, of which:				**179 200**
Blindness (total):	...	...	44 800	44 800
Onchocerciasis-related	...	45	290	290
Cataract-related	...	...	19 340	19 340
Glaucoma-related	...	...	6 400	6 400
Trachoma-related	...	...	5 600	5 600
Vitamin A deficiency-xerophthalmia	...	...	2 850	2 850
Other	...	...	10 320	10 320
Hearing loss (41 or more decibels)				**121 000**

[f] Figures refer to 5-year prevalent cases (patients who are still alive between 0 and 5 years after diagnosis).
[g] To this figure should be added:
(i) 732 000 deaths in the neonatal period diagnosed as due to low birth weight and attributable to intrauterine growth retardation;
(ii) 500 000 under-5 deaths listed as terminal infections (usually diarrhoea, respiratory infections or measles), but basically due to severe malnutrition.
[h] Figure refers to children under 5.
[i] 30% of global population aged 20 and above.
[j] 50% of elderly show radiographic changes. The percentage of those with symptomatic and potentially symptomatic osteoarthritis is even greater.
[k] Total number of deaths is about 5 million, which includes 755 000 deaths from neonatal pneumonia (under ALRI), 310 000 deaths from neonatal tetanus and 60 000 deaths from diarrhoea.

Fig. 1. Deaths and population in the world by age, 1965–2025

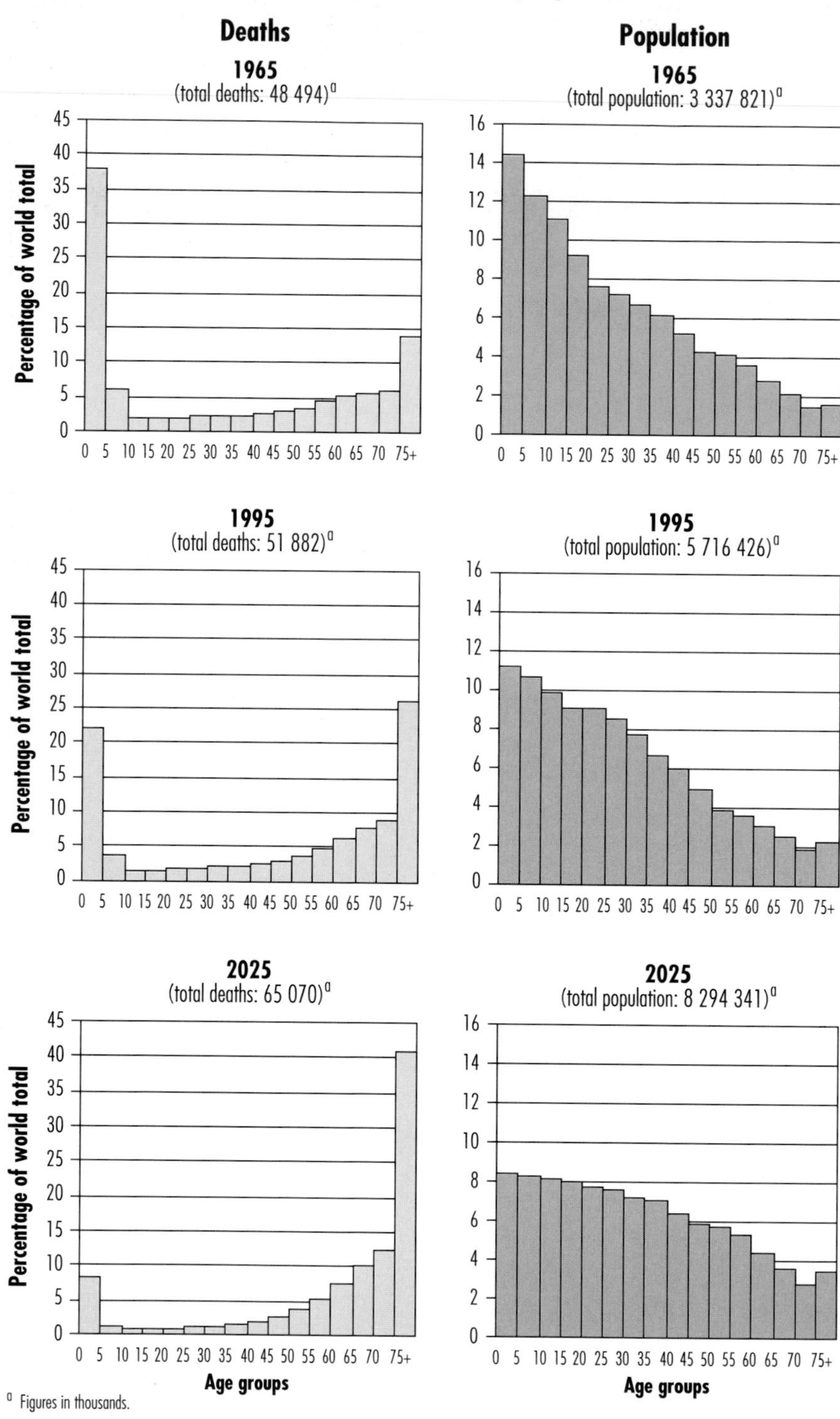

[a] Figures in thousands.

other hand, from 12 million deaths in those aged 65 and above in 1960, the figure had increased to 22 million in 1996. While in 1960 most deaths occurred in those aged under 50, they now occur in those aged 50 and above.

The ratio of deaths among those aged 65 and above to deaths among those aged 15 or less has increased from 0.9 in 1980 to 1.6 in 1996. Whereas 16 years ago, there were equal numbers of deaths in both age groups, now there are three deaths among the elderly for two among children and adolescents. If the trend continues, it is expected that by the year 2025, more than 60% of all deaths will be among those aged 65 and above, more than 40% being among those aged 75 and above, while 10% of the population will be aged 65 and above, and more than 3% aged 75 and above. The population distributions by age for 1965, 1995 and 2025 given in *Fig. 1* show the ageing of the population.

An approximate distribution by cause of the estimated 52 million deaths worldwide in 1996 is given in *Table 2*. Of these deaths, over 17 million were ascribable to infectious and parasitic diseases; more than 15 million to circulatory diseases; over 6 million to malignant neoplasms; and about 3 million to respiratory diseases. *Fig. 2* gives an approximate distribution of deaths worldwide in 1996.

Deaths due to three major killers – circulatory diseases, malignant neoplasms (cancers) and noninfectious respiratory diseases – globally account for more than 24 million or about 40% more than those due to infectious and parasitic diseases. Heart disease and stroke are the leading causes of death among circulatory diseases. Lung cancer is the leading cause among the malignant neoplasms, and chronic obstructive pulmonary diseases among respiratory diseases. *Table 3* shows the leading causes of death, based on the best available estimates. Though quite a few deaths can be ascribed to infection, most of the leading causes of death just mentioned are related to long-term exposure to risk factors and to population ageing.

Table 3. Global health situation: leading causes of mortality, morbidity and disability, selected causes for which data are available, all ages, 1996 estimates[a]

Diseases/conditions[b] (based on ICD-10)	Deaths		Cases				Disabled persons	
	Rank	Number (000)	Rank	New (incidence) (000)	Rank	All (prevalence) (000)	Rank	Number (permanent and long-term) (000)
Ischaemic heart disease	1	7 200		...		...		...
Cerebrovascular disease	2	4 600		...		9 000		...
Acute lower respiratory infection	3	3 905	3	394 000		...		...
Tuberculosis	4	3 000		7 400		...		...
COPD	5	2 888		...	5	600 000		...
Diarrhoea (including dysentery)	6	2 473	1	4 002 000		...		...
Malaria	7	1 500-2 700	2	300 000-500 000		...		...
HIV/AIDS	8	1 500		3 100		22 600		...
Hepatitis B	9	1 156		...		...		...
Prematurity	10	1 150		...		...		...
Measles	11	1 010	12	42 000		...		...
Cancer of trachea, bronchus and lung	12	989		1 320		1 205		...
Trichomoniasis		...	4	170 000		113 000		...
Occupational diseases		...	5	160 000		...		...
Occupational injuries		225	6	125 000		...	10	12 500
Mood (affective) disorders		...	7	122 865	8	340 000	1	146 000
Chlamydial infections		...	8	89 000		85 000		...
Amoebiasis		70	11	48 000		...		...
Alcohol dependence syndrome		103	9	75 000		120 000		...
Gonococcal infection		...	10	62 000		23 000		...
Iron deficiency anaemia		...		...	1	1 788 600		...
Neck and back disorders		...		...	2	1 039 200		...
Goitre		...		...	3	760 000	4	76 000
Hypertensive disease		...		...	4	690 600		...
Anxiety disorders		...		...	6	400 000		...
Arthritis and arthrosis		...		...	7	354 500		...
Ascariasis (roundworm)		60		...	9	250 000		...
Malnutrition including PEM		372		...	10	200 000		...
Schistosomiasis		20		...	11	200 000		...
Hepatitis C		...		...	12	170 000		...
Hearing loss (41 or more decibels)		...		...		...	2	121 000
Lymphatic filariasis		...		...		119 100	3	119 100
Mental retardation (all types)		...		...		60 000	5	36 000
Cretinoids		...		...		...	6	33 600
Schizophrenic disorders		...		4 500		45 000	7	27 000
Cataract-related blindness		...		...		19 340	8	19 340
Dementia		200		2 610		29 000	9	15 950
Cretinism		...		...		...	11	11 200
Poliomyelitis, acute		7		20		...	12	10 600

[a] Source: Table 2.
[b] Chronic diseases given in italics.

Leading selected causes of mortality	Deaths Rank	Deaths Number (000)
Ischaemic heart disease	1	7 200
Cerebrovascular disease	2	4 600
Acute lower respiratory infection	3	3 905
Tuberculosis	4	3 000
COPD	5	2 888
Diarrhoea (including dysentery)	6	2 473
Malaria	7	1 500-2 700
HIV/AIDS	8	1 500
Hepatitis B	9	1 156
Prematurity	10	1 150
Measles	11	1 010
Cancer of trachea, bronchus and lung	12	989

Leading selected causes of morbidity	New cases annually (incidence)		Total cases (prevalence)	
	Rank	Number (000)	Rank	Number (000)
Diarrhoea (including dysentery)	1	4 002 000		...
Malaria	2	300 000-500 000		...
Acute lower respiratory infection	3	394 000		...
Trichomoniasis	4	170 000		113 000
Occupational diseases	5	160 000		...
Occupational injuries	6	125 000		...
Mood (affective) disorders	7	122 865	8	340 000
Chlamydial infections	8	89 000		85 000
Alcohol dependence syndrome	9	75 000		120 000
Gonococcal infection	10	62 000		23 000
Amoebiasis	11	48 000		...
Measles	12	42 000		...
Iron deficiency anaemia		...	1	1 788 600
Neck and back disorders		...	2	1 039 200
Goitre		...	3	760 000
Hypertensive disease		...	4	690 600
COPD		...	5	600 000
Anxiety disorders		...	6	400 000
Arthritis and arthrosis		...	7	354 500
Ascariasis (roundworm)		...	9	250 000
Malnutrition including PEM		...	10	200 000
Schistosomiasis		...	11	200 000
Hepatitis C		...	12	170 000

Leading selected causes of disability	Disabled persons (permanent and long-term) Rank	Number (000)
Mood (affective) disorders	1	146 000
Hearing loss (41 or more decibels)	2	121 000
Lymphatic filariasis	3	119 100
Goitre	4	76 000
Mental retardation (all types)	5	36 000
Cretinoids	6	33 600
Schizophrenic disorders	7	27 000
Cataract-related blindness	8	19 340
Dementia	9	15 950
Occupational injuries	10	12 500
Cretinism	11	11 200
Poliomyelitis, acute	12	10 600

Fig. 2. Global causes of death, 1996[a]

Distribution of deaths by cause and distribution of major noncommunicable diseases by level of development

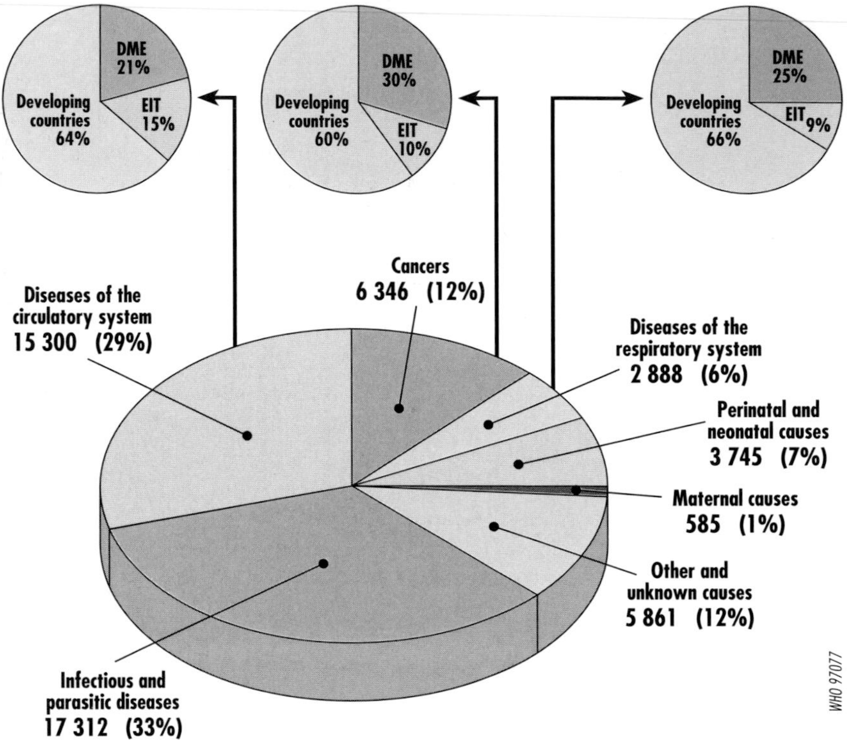

a – Deaths in thousands and percentages of total.
– Breakdown for the three major noncommunicable causes: developing countries (including least developed countries); DME=developed market economies; EIT=economies in transition.
– Infectious and parasitic diseases include acute lower respiratory infections and neonatal tetanus and are excluded from diseases of the circulatory system and perinatal and neonatal causes respectively.

Of the estimated 52 million deaths worldwide in 1996, about 40 million were in the developing world, including nearly 9 million in the least developed countries (LDCs); the developed world accounted for more than 12 million, of which 4.4 million in the economies in transition. When standardized for age and sex, the death rates per 100 000 population were 446 for developed market economies, 800 for economies in transition, 880 for developing countries excluding LDCs, and 1575 for LDCs (i.e. almost twice the rate of other developing countries). Out of a total of 11.2 million deaths in children under 5 in the developing world in 1995, around 5 million were due to neonatal and perinatal causes and at least 6 million to causes associated with malnutrition (*Fig. 3*).

Of the 40 million deaths in the developing world in 1996, more than 17 million were due to infectious and parasitic diseases, with about 10 million due to circulatory diseases, 4 million to cancers and 2 million to respiratory diseases (*Fig. 4*). Even though about 65% of deaths due to circulatory diseases, 60% of deaths due to cancers and more than 65% of deaths due to respiratory diseases occur in developing countries, the most important killer conditions in these countries as a group remain infectious and parasitic diseases. Recent studies indicate that these diseases continue to predominate among the disadvantaged, and distinguish the health situation in poor countries from that of the rich (*Box 4*). However, chronic diseases such as those mentioned above are emerging as major causes of premature death and disability in the developing world, accounting for almost 40% of all deaths.

As shown in *Table 3*, leading causes of ill-health due to noncommunicable chronic conditions (given in italics) are broadly: circulatory diseases, respiratory diseases, mental and behavioural disorders, iron deficiency disorders, occupational diseases and injuries, and visual disability and hearing loss. Of over 15 million deaths due to circulatory diseases, more than 7 million were due to ischaemic (or coronary) heart disease; for cancers, nearly 2 million deaths (of more than 6 million) were due to cancer at only three sites, all related to the digestive tract, namely stomach, colon-rectum and liver.

Health expectancy

The continuing decline in the human mortality rate has important consequences. Not only is it increasing life expectancy and the proportion of the population reaching advanced ages in many (especially developed) countries, but it is also modifying the average state of health of populations. In particular, the growing prevalence of chronic diseases and disabilities – which best reflects this change in the relation between mortality and morbidity – has focused attention on the increasing tension between the length of life on the one hand and the quality of the extra years lived on the other.

As traditional health indicators were not adequate to cover this new epidemiological transition, several indicators with various assumptions are being investigated to reflect the state of health: years of (potential) productive life lost (YPLL); disability-free life expectancy (DFLE); quality-adjusted life years (QALY); disability-adjusted life years (DALY) (*Box 5*). One interesting new indicator is "health expectancy". This indicator integrates information on mortality and morbidity, especially the consequences of diseases. The international network of researchers on health expectancy (REVES), which is working on this new indicator, has adopted the WHO International Classification of Impairments, Disabilities and Handicaps (ICIDH) as a framework.

Over the last decade calculations of health expectancies have been carried out in 37 countries. Analysis of all these studies by REVES allows important conclusions to be drawn concerning inequalities between the sexes, between regions and according to social status. Generally the inequalities found emphasize the differences which already exist in life expectancies. Women have greater life expectancies than men, but the proportion of life that they spend free of disability or handicap is slightly lower; health expectancy in more developed (urban) regions is longer than in less developed (rural) areas; and the poorest and least educated not only experience shorter lives but also a larger proportion of ill-health. The available chronological series show some general trends over a 30-year period: in most developed countries, concurrent with the increase in life expectancy, an equivalent increase in life expectancy free of severe disability is found. When all severity levels are combined, however, disability-free life expectancy seems to be stabilizing. Thus, contrary to widely held beliefs, on the basis of available evidence and this first analysis, years with severe handicap and/or disability are not increasing. While the results for all severity levels combined seem to favour the "expansion of morbidity" hypothesis, the evolution of severe disability and handicap appears to follow the equilibrium theory. Level of severity and reversibility will be important issues in future health expectancy studies.

Fig. 3. Main causes of death among children under age 5, developing world, 1995[a]

Total deaths: 11.2 million

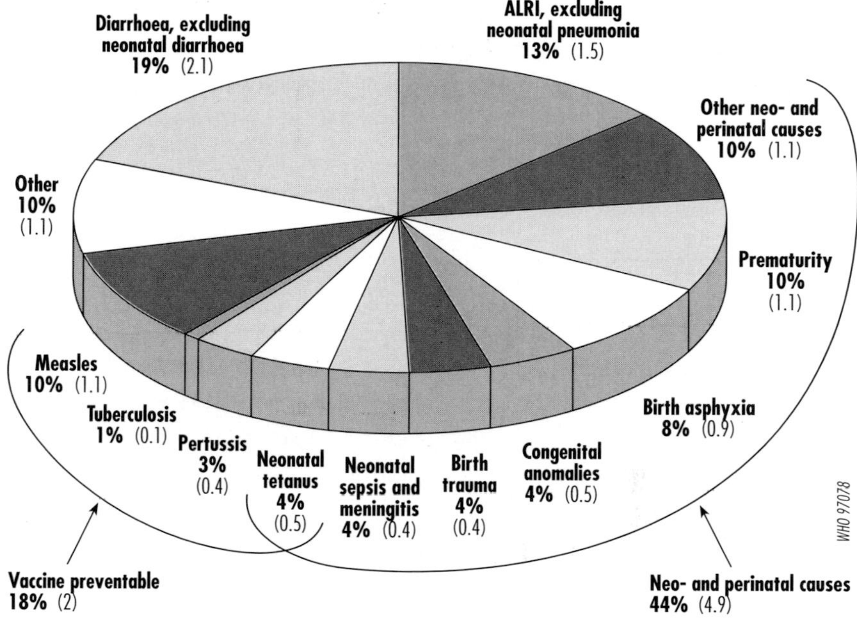

[a] Figures in brackets refer to the number of deaths in millions.

Fig. 4. Causes of death, developed and developing world, 1996[a]

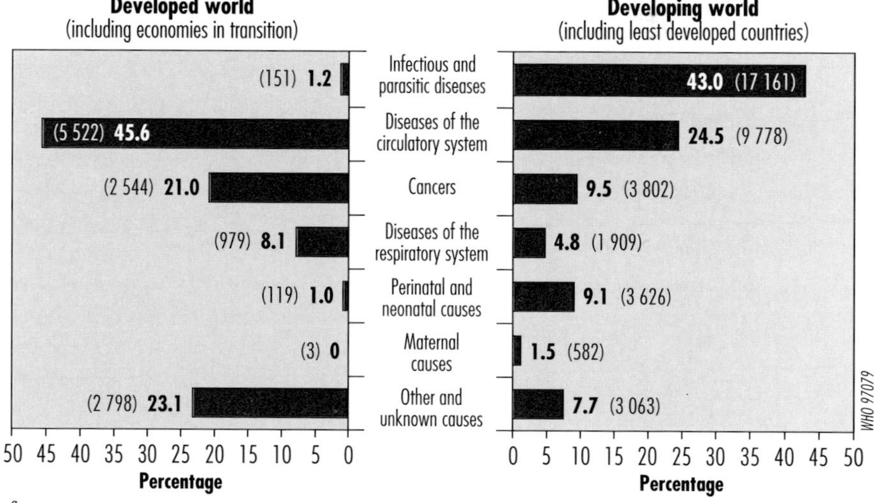

[a] Figures in brackets refer to the number of deaths in thousands.

Box 4. Reducing rich-poor health disparities

How can the health gaps between rich and poor be bridged effectively? One answer is to focus prime attention on the causes of death and disability that most afflict the world's disadvantaged – in other words, infectious and related diseases.

Globally, infectious diseases, maternal and perinatal conditions are killing seven times as many people among the world's poorest billion than the richest billion. Chronic diseases are responsible for 40% fewer deaths among the poorest billion than the richest. On the other hand, cancers kill twice as many among the richest billion, and cardiovascular diseases two-thirds more.

However, chronic diseases and accidents are quickly emerging as leading causes of death and disability worldwide. At present, they cause almost as much death and disability globally as infectious diseases – 41% compared to 44%. In the developing world alone, chronic diseases account for some 36% of total death and disability, and that proportion is expected to rise to more than 55% by the year 2020. Diseases are not distributed equally among social classes; for example, in the emerging middle and upper classes of the developing world, infectious diseases among infants and children are now increasingly coming under control.

Nevertheless, the fact remains that the poorer an individual is, the more likely it is that he or she will die of an infectious disease; while the richer an individual is, the more likely it is that he or she will suffer and die from a chronic condition. Furthermore, life expectancy comparisons show that the poor die sooner than the rich. The comparison holds good within countries as well as between them. Thus, the poor stand to benefit much more than the rich from a continued emphasis on infectious diseases.

If all continues to go well in the fight against these diseases, the time will come when chronic diseases will require higher priority in actions oriented towards the poor as well as the rich. In the meantime, it is important to carry on with recently-initiated efforts to develop less expensive, more effective ways of preventing and controlling those chronic conditions which are of greatest importance to the poor. But improving the health of the poor demands in addition a renewed determination to combat infectious diseases, especially among the young.

Achievement of adequate health for all remains the goal, rather than simply still better health for those whose health is already adequate.

Personal communication from Davidson R. Gwatkin, International Health Policy Program, The World Bank.

In the absence of an acceptable method that combines the quantitative and qualitative aspects of global health, and taking into account ethical, social and cultural considerations related to death and disability, this report discusses in the following sections a number of chronic diseases and conditions in terms of the three components – mortality, morbidity and long-term or severe disability – and ways of confronting them, with a focus on reducing suffering and enhancing quality of life.

Confronting chronic conditions

Cancer

The growing burden

More than 10 million people developed cancer in 1996, and at least 6 million others who already had the disease died from it. Globally, a clear trend is emerging: cancer is becoming a leading cause of death in old age. The explanation is simple: the gradual elimination of other fatal diseases, combined with rising life expectancy, means that the risks of developing cancer are steadily growing. Most cancers arise in adults and at an advanced age, and the risk increases exponentially with age. The burden of cancer is, therefore, much more important in populations with a long life expectancy, relative to other groups of diseases.

Probably more than any other single disease, cancer provokes fearful images of pain, disfigurement and inevitable death. Yet cancer is not one single disease; it exists in more than 100 forms and has many causes, from genetic factors to infections. Many types of cancer are both preventable and curable, all are treatable (even those which are not curable), and advances in pain relief have greatly reduced suffering.

The growing cancer burden calls for greater investment in health facilities specific to cancer treatment and for preventive strategies. However, rational planning of the use of resources depends on knowledge of the frequency and distribution of the disease in the population concerned. Unfortunately, good-quality data are still largely missing. In many developing countries, setting up reliable monitoring systems – at least to understand the magnitude of the problem – should be given high priority.

The eight leading cancer killers worldwide are also the eight most common in terms of incidence. Together, they account for about 60% of all cancer cases and deaths. An analysis of the risk factors involved in the development of these cancers shows that a few major factors dominate: diet, tobacco, alcohol, infections and hormones – all of which lend themselves to preventive actions.

Among men, the leading eight cancer killers are lung, stomach, liver, colon-rectum, oesophagus, mouth-pharynx, prostate and lymphoma. Among women, they are cancers of the breast, stomach, colon-rectum, cervix, lung, ovary, oesophagus and liver.

Cancers now account for about 20% of all deaths in developed regions and about 10% of all deaths in developing regions. In 1996 there were an estimated 17.9 million persons with cancer surviving up to five years after diagnosis. Of these, 10.5 million were women, 5.3 million of whom had cancer either of the breast, cervix or colon-rectum. Among men, prostate, colorectal and lung cancer were the most prevalent (*Fig.* 5).

Of more than 10 million cancer cases newly diagnosed in 1996 worldwide, 57% occurred in developing countries. For both developed and developing countries the most common cancer site in men was the lung. In developed regions it is followed by prostate cancer (289 000 new cases), colorectal cancer (273 000); and stomach cancer (226 000). In developing regions stomach cancer is second with 408 000 new cases per year, followed by cancer of the liver (309 000) and cancers of the mouth and pharynx (288 000) (*Fig.* 6).

In women, breast cancer is the most common in affluent populations with 494 000 cases followed by colon and rectum (282 000) and then by cancer of the lung (168 000) and of the stomach (147 000). In developing areas, cancer of the cervix is the most common (421 000 cases), but breast cancer is almost as common (416 000). Third is cancer of the stomach (231 000) and fourth is cancer of the lung (164 000).

The most remarkable changes in the ranking compared to 10 years ago are the steep upward trend of prostate cancer (partly due to the introduction of programmes for early detection), the increase in breast cancer (a site more common in high-income populations), and the increase in lung cancer in women worldwide.

Box 5. Measuring health

Because of the complexity of health and disease, there are severe practical difficulties in collecting, analysing and interpreting the data needed to express the full facts. Concepts such as "burden of disease" have been introduced for use as a guide to health status and as a basis for planning policies and actions for health improvement. In order to assess the scale of the burden of disease, and the need for intervention, indicators are needed that capture – and do not obscure – the important components contributing to it. The real determinants of health need to be identified so as to plan where interventions should be directed. In order to decide how to intervene, it is necessary to understand the effectiveness and consequences of various types of intervention. Formulating these issues illustrates the dimensions of the "health measurement" problem and underlines the need for fresh consideration.

As a measure of burden of disease, the disability adjusted life year (DALY) indicator has been proposed. This purports to represent, on a common footing, the years of healthy life lost either through premature death or as a result of life lived with a disability. Adding these two numbers produces a single measure: the DALY. The total number of DALYs in a population in any given year is supposed to indicate that population's disease burden for that year.

However, WHO's Advisory Committee on Health Research (ACHR) has serious reservations on the application of the DALY approach for decision-making and policy formulation. Pooling mortality and morbidity data masks facts that are known to be important to the economics of a given intervention, whether at family or community level; it obscures the socioeconomic circumstances and sociocultural environment of the sick within different communities, which both have an impact on the allocation of scarce resources. In addition, using a DALY-type approach does not take into consideration the multifactoral origins of diseases, their multiple manifestations nor, above all, the problem of inequity.

Determinants of health are not necessarily wholly biological: economic, sociocultural and behavioural elements are involved. However, methodologies to identify the fundamental determinants of health, in the health sector or elsewhere, are not yet available. Clearer insights into the determinants of health are required as a basis both for informed allocation of resources and for effectively targeted interventions. Methodological advances are needed, not only for identifying determinants but also for decision-making about interventions.

Recognizing these needs, in the face of a rapidly changing global demographic and epidemiological situation, and continuing pressure on resources for health improvement, the ACHR has established a subcommittee on measurement of health. It aims to identify new approaches to health measurement, new indicators, and methodologies usable for linking health to its underlying determinants, for establishing research priorities and for supporting decision-making about interventions.

Trends in cancer cases

In the United States, mortality from all cancers increased by 7% from 1973 to 1990 (both sexes combined) but all such increase occurs after the age of 65, while a decline of 4.5% has been recorded in younger age groups. In some European countries, e.g. Sweden and Finland, can-

Fig. 5. The burden of cancer, 1996

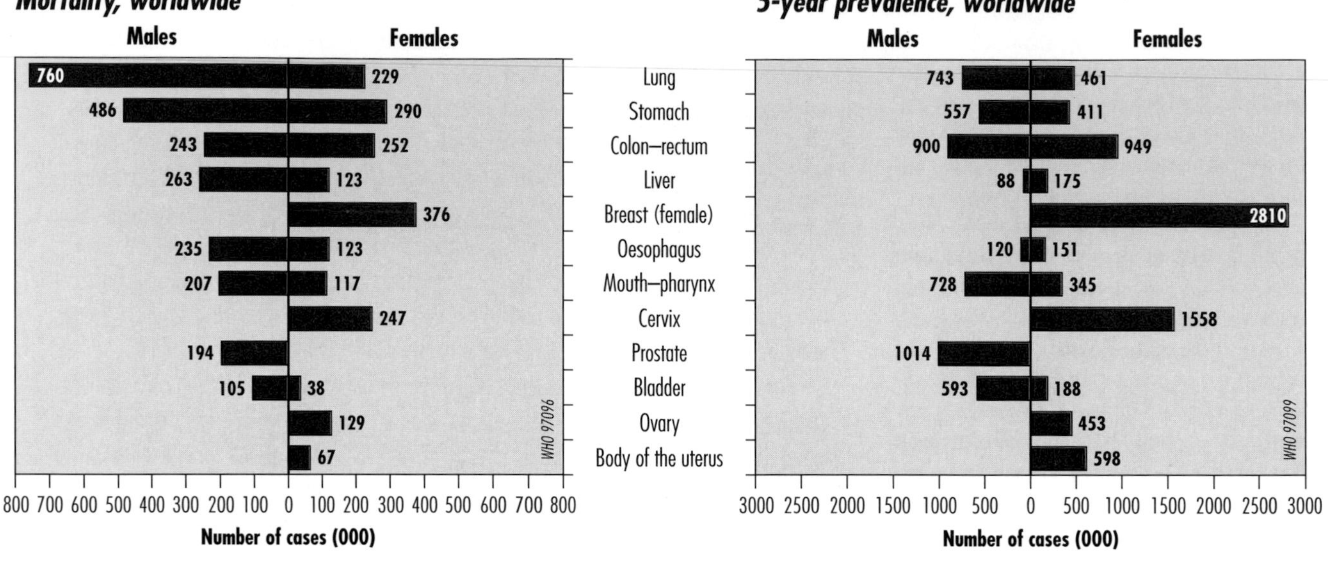

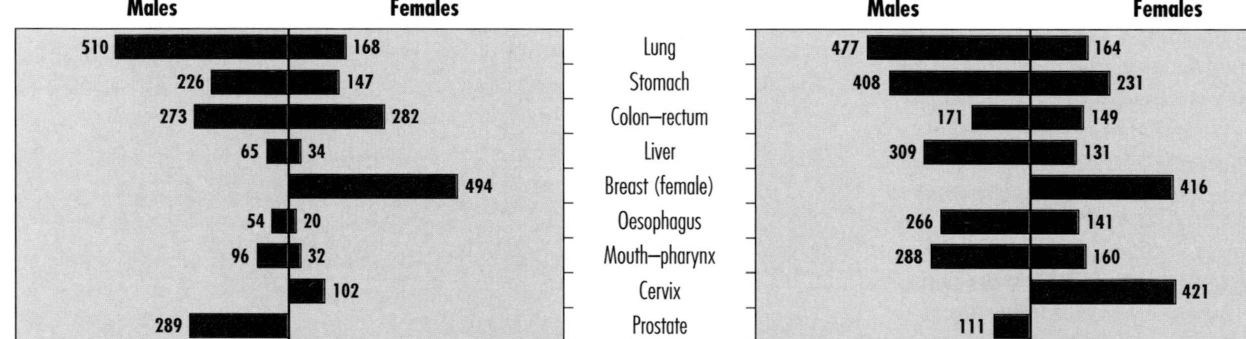

cer mortality is also declining in the population below age 75.

Much of the upward trend in the last few decades in rich countries is due to tobacco smoking, which became widespread during the first half of the century. Smoking is now declining in men in most of these countries and the effect of this – a reduction in deaths from lung cancer and heart disease – is already apparent in some populations. Conversely, the tobacco epidemic is now affecting women, particularly in southern Europe, and the effects of these changing habits will become apparent in some 10-20 years.

The risk of cancer unrelated to tobacco is not increasing dramatically in high-income countries in spite of the increasing number of cases observed. The diminished risk of dying from other causes such as cardiovascular disease leaves a greater proportion of the population, and for a longer period, exposed to the risk of developing cancer. Thus, effective interventions to prevent and treat other diseases contribute to the upward trend of the proportion of deaths

Fig. 6. Major cancers in men and women, 1996
Incidence (000)

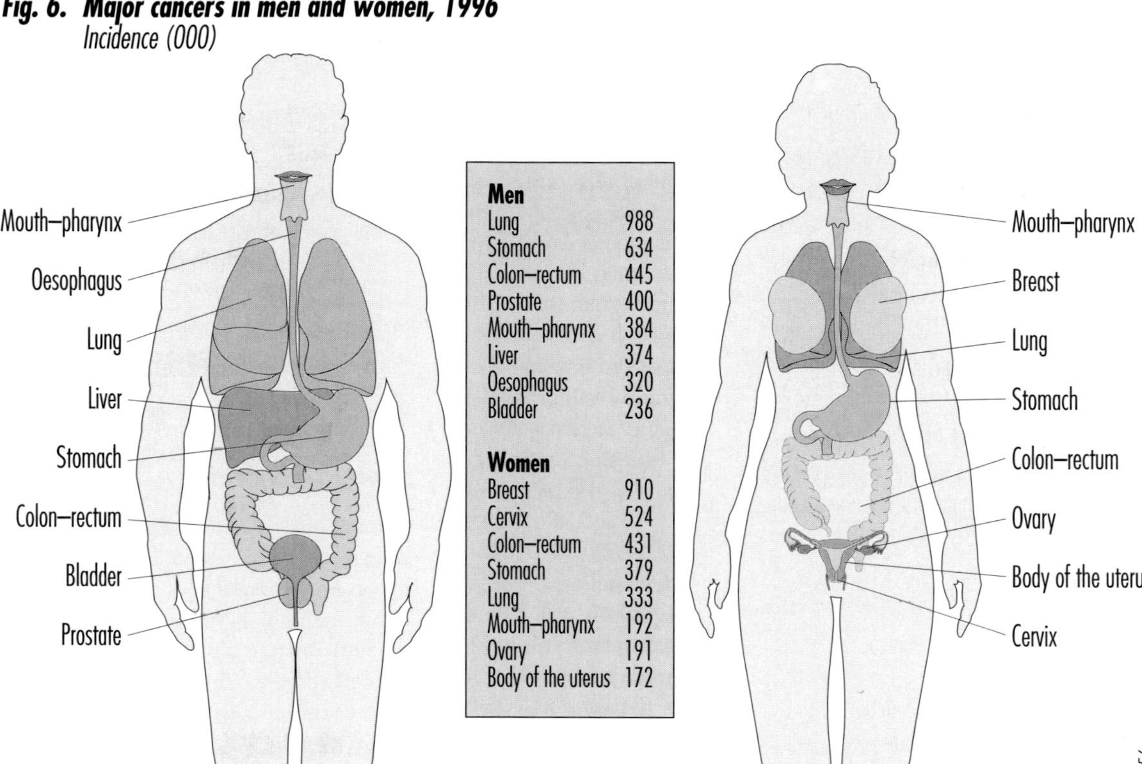

Men	
Lung	988
Stomach	634
Colon–rectum	445
Prostate	400
Mouth–pharynx	384
Liver	374
Oesophagus	320
Bladder	236
Women	
Breast	910
Cervix	524
Colon–rectum	431
Stomach	379
Lung	333
Mouth–pharynx	192
Ovary	191
Body of the uterus	172

attributed to cancer. Continuous efforts are therefore required to improve the understanding of the causes and mechanisms of cancer and to develop effective preventive and therapeutic protocols.

The weight of cancer relative to other diseases is increasing in countries currently undergoing rapid economic development. Developing countries succeeding in improving life expectancy often perceive the outbreak of a "cancer epidemic". Indeed any increase in the size of the population induces an increase in the *number* of cases and deaths observed, even if the *risk*, or rate, does not change. The risk of developing those cancers typical of higher socioeconomic groups (e.g. breast, colon and rectum) is expected to increase with economic development.

In the world's less developed regions the cancer problem still largely relates to those sites linked to infectious agents and tobacco smoking. In sub-Saharan Africa at least 38% of all cases can be attributed to some type of infection. Many of these cancers, namely those of the liver related to chronic infection with hepatitis B, are readily preventable by immunization in childhood. Vaccines to prevent infection with the papilloma viruses which cause cervical cancer are being developed and tested (*Box 6*).

Understanding cancer

In their healthy state, human cells reproduce and proliferate in an orderly, controlled way.

Cells normally contain a group of genes controlling cell growth called "oncogenes". Damage or mutations in these genes may interfere with the ability of oncogenes to regulate normal cell growth (*Box 7*). This is how abnormal cancer cells develop. These cells multiply in an uncontrolled way, and eventually invade surrounding tissues and distant organs. This invasion (metastasis) is characteristic of cancers, and is responsible for most of the treatment failures in this disease.

Box 6. Vaccines against cancer

In recent years, the link between some cancers and infectious agents – viruses, bacteria and parasites – has been firmly established, opening the way to producing vaccines against them. Leading researchers are hopeful that vaccines against several deadly cancers caused by infections can be developed in the near future. A more distant but still exciting prospect is that advances in molecular biology will lead to vaccines against other forms of cancer that are not connected to infections. They would work by inducing human T cells or other components of the immune system to seek out and attack malignant tissue.

There already is one extremely efficient vaccine in use – the *hepatitis B* vaccine, which protects against chronic hepatitis that leads to liver cancer. WHO estimates that globally there are about 540 000 new cases a year of liver cancer, of which 83%, or 448 000 cases, are attributable to infection with the hepatitis B virus.

The hepatitis vaccine became available in 1982 and has since been used to immunize almost 400 million people. Safe and effective, it can be given to people of any age, but is most effective when used as part of routine infant immunizations. This is now the case in about 75 countries. Dramatic cuts in the cost of the vaccine in developing countries are allowing it to be more widely available. WHO is recommending that general hepatitis B vaccination of newborns, children and adolescents should be implemented in 1997. Such use could reduce the number of liver cancers by up to 70% in areas such as sub-Saharan Africa and eastern Asia, including China (see *Box 9*).

There is also optimism that the number of cases of cancer of the cervix can ultimately be reduced by the introduction of a human papilloma virus vaccine. It is well known that sexually transmitted infection of the cervix with human papilloma viruses types 16 and 18 involves a very high risk of developing cervical cancer. The viruses are responsible for an estimated 436 000 cases of the disease a year – 83% of the annual total. Of all cases, 65% in industrialized countries and 87% in developing countries are due to these viruses. The viruses also cause 31 000 cases a year of vaginal cancer – 80% of the annual total. Vaccine research has been progressing for more than five years and several candidate vaccines have undergone trials. However, as and when a safe and effective vaccine does reach the market, its cost will be a crucial factor in determining the extent to which it will be available in developing countries.

A third potential vaccine under investigation is against *Helicobacter pylori*. About 550 000 cases a year of stomach cancer – 55% of the total – are attributed to infection with this bacterium. First identified in 1982, it has been shown to cause duodenal ulcers and gastritis. Although other factors must also be involved in the development of stomach cancer, the role of the bacterium is significant enough to justify research into a vaccine against it.

The major categories of cancer are:

- *Carcinomas*, which arise from epithelial cells lining the internal surfaces of the various organs (e.g. mouth, oesophagus, intestines, uterus) and from the skin epithelium.
- *Sarcomas*, which arise from mesodermal cells constituting the various connective tissues (e.g. fibrous tissue, fat and bone).
- *Lymphomas, myeloma and leukaemias* arising from the cells of bone marrow and immune systems.

The term "primary tumour" is used to denote cancer in the organ of origin, while "secondary tumour" denotes cancer that has spread to regional lymph nodes and distant organs. When cancer cells multiply and reach a critical size, the cancer is clinically evident as a lump or ulcer localized to the organ of origin in early stages. As the disease advances, symptoms and signs of invasion and distant metastases become clinically evident.

Cancer treatment

Surgery and radiotherapy are the main ways of treating cancer. Surgery usually involves the removal of the primary tumour with some surrounding tissue to prevent further spread. For many early cancers surgery alone is often enough to remove the tumour completely and cure the patient. Where the tumour has spread to nearby lymph nodes, these too must be removed surgically. Chemotherapy and hormone therapy are used to treat cancers which are too advanced locally for surgery or radiotherapy. A combined approach involving all of these methods provides the best results for many patients with moderately advanced disease but without distant spread, and is increasingly used to treat many forms of cancer.

At the outset, individual cancer patients are usually assessed to decide whether there is a possibility of cure or whether treatment should be palliative or symptomatic. This decision is based on the stage of tumour and the patient's age and general health. If the clinical evidence indicates a reasonable chance of cure, radical single or combined curative treatment is provided. However, if there is no chance of cure, palliative treatment is given, aimed at relieving symptoms and improving quality of life without inducing treatment-related toxicity or complications. Symptomatic measures such as pain relief with opioid and non-opioid analgesics are almost always used in advanced cancers. Due to considerable progress in this area in

Box 7. From laboratory to medical practice: the results and prospects of cancer research

Advances in molecular and cellular biology add substance to the fundamental ideas on the nature of cancer, which date back to the early years of this century, and even before. At their core is the notion that cancer is essentially a genetic disease at the cellular level, and that its initiation and progression is a form of somatic evolution. But now we are at the threshold of new opportunities for the application of the rapidly accumulating fundamental knowledge to new approaches for preventing, treating and curing cancer.

The most dramatic and worthwhile changes in the last two decades have been in the science, the new discoveries, the technology that comes with them and above all the exciting pointers to future developments which will have a major impact on cancer. Oncogenes and tumour suppressor genes with known functions have now been identified and there is a whole range of new knowledge concerning the mechanisms within cells which control growth, cell division and programmed cell death. Understanding of the immune system has been revolutionized so that cancer immunotherapy and even vaccination have become plausible targets.

Cells will only divide when they receive the appropriate stimulus from one or more external growth factors. Certain substances (neuropeptides and bombesin) could act as growth factors. This provides a rationale for the mechanism of oncogene mutations as facilitating the division of cancer cells, through their effects on growth factor production and other functions.

DNA repair mechanisms are essential for maintaining the integrity of genetic material. Their absence leads to a high incidence of mutations and therefore of cancers. Damage to the DNA induces relevant repair activity. Mutations in these repair genes explain a major subset of colorectal cancer families and also occur in sporadic colorectal tumours.

The complement of cell division is cell death, now realized to be an important and programmed part of the maintenance, differentiation and development of all living organisms. The process of tumour growth is a balance between division and differentiation or death. Cancer has often been described as a form of de-differentiation. Fundamental studies of differentiation and development should thus help in the understanding of the cancerous process.

Over the last 15 years, the combination of modern molecular and cellular biology and animal experimentation has made a fundamental contribution to our understanding of the immune system. Any changed protein, whether expressed inside or outside the cell, is a potential target for immunotherapy, or even vaccination. This new understanding opens up opportunities for developing immune therapies for cancer. Another important application of immunology is the use of monoclonal antibodies for *in vitro* and *in vivo* diagnosis and eventually the therapy of cancer. The first promising clinical results are in the treatment of colorectal and ovarian cancer. Most genes work through the proteins they specify. The study of protein structure is therefore a key part of understanding genetic functions and therefore of the functions of the changes that occur in cancer cells.

Now that the range of biological processes which underlie the initiation and progression of a cancer is better understood, we can envisage a basic framework for the carcinogenic process. In the case of tumours derived from epithelial cells (the carcinomas), which are still the most common cancers and the most difficult to treat or prevent, initiating a cancer most probably involves the facilitation of independent growth by loosening or abrogating the attachment of cells to each other and to their extracellular matrix substrates. The long lag periods, sometimes 20 years from initiation to final cancer, can be explained by a series of steps, each determined by a new mutation and each leading to a new plateau in growth until the next mutation occurs.

Many parts of the puzzle are still missing. The function of each step remains to be elucidated and reconstructed in the laboratory. The discoveries of the last two decades have, however, provided a striking new range of targets for the development of novel and more specific drugs for the treatment of cancers.

Computing is only one, though a major, example of the importance of techniques and equipment in modern cancer research. Genome analysis has stimulated the automation of laboratory procedures so that robots are now almost as common in laboratories as big centrifuges were 15 years ago. Enzymes and complicated procedures that used to be painstakingly put together in laboratories can now be elaborated using commercially available kits. New and more powerful techniques in the laboratory can be incorporated almost overnight into a developing experimental programme.

We have witnessed a golden age of discoveries about cancer. The future prospect is a golden age of new approaches to the prevention and treatment of cancers based on these fundamental discoveries. The challenge for the future is to develop more and better ways of translating the laboratory research into practice, whether in the clinic, the general practitioner's office or the population at large through the adoption of preventive strategies.

Even the full implementation of current best practice in the clinic could increase overall cancer survival by as much as 10%. Current trends in smoking cessation and the projected effects of breast cancer screening, adjuvant therapy and tamoxifen prevention, could reduce the overall mortality due to breast cancer by 50% of what it otherwise might be in 25 years' time. A similar effect could be seen for colorectal cancer if sigmoidoscopy screening turns out to be effective.

Many new drugs will be discovered by the new molecular and cell biology approaches. Forms of gene-based or DNA-based therapy will target a cancer in such a way that it becomes susceptible to a particular drug whereas normal tissue is not. However, all successful drug developments, and most applications of diagnostic procedures, depend on the involvement of the pharmaceutical industry.

The challenge is not only to maintain excellence in cancer research, but also to ensure a balance between basic and applied research. We have already seen the tremendous advances in the laboratory over the last two decades beginning to be translated into effective ways of improving the prevention, early diagnosis and treatment of cancer. In future years it may be possible to realize the promise of better understanding, and the reality of conquering cancer.

Personal communication from Sir Walter Bodmer, formerly Director of Research, Imperial Cancer Research Fund.

recent years, a painful death from cancer can most often be avoided.

Advances in cancer therapies

Increasing understanding of the natural history of cancers and advances in radiotherapeutic techniques and equipment, as well as in chemotherapy, have allowed less and less radical surgery to be performed for certain cancers (e.g. cancers of the breast, ovary, testis). This helps avoid complications arising from tissue loss, cosmetic problems and some loss of function.

Radiation can selectively destroy malignant cells while sparing normal cells. Radiotherapy involves radiation delivered from external radiotherapy machines or from sealed radioactive isotope sources placed in the tissues or body cavities. The total radiation dose required depends on the radiosensitivity of the tumour.

Cytotoxic chemotherapy involves the use of drugs that interfere with the ability of the cells to divide, and with synthesis of essential proteins. These drugs have their maximum effect on dividing cells. Spectacular improvement in survival and cure rates from childhood cancers and testicular cancers, and significant improvements in other cancers, are mainly due to advances in chemotherapy.

Hormone therapy is part of the management of tumours that occur in tissues under hormonal regulation, such as cancers of the breast, endometrium and prostate. Therapy is carried out either by removing or destroying the organs that produce hormones which promote tumour growth (e.g. removal of the ovaries in premenopausal patients with breast cancer) or by supplementing hormones that interfere with tumour growth.

Adjuvant therapy with chemotherapy or hormone therapy is used in situations where a cancer has been treated with surgery and/or radiotherapy but the risk of local or general recurrence is judged to be high. Examples include breast cancer with local lymph node involvement, some childhood cancers and ovarian cancer.

The eight most common cancers, with a combined total of over 6 million new cases a year, should be the main targets for prevention and cure.

Supportive care, to alleviate both the psychological and physical impact of cancer, has a distinct role that is likely to enhance the patient's ability to withstand the side-effects of treatment and to improve quality of survival. Palliative care aiming at relief of distressing symptoms is important in managing advanced incurable disease. Relief of cancer pain by radiotherapy, surgery, chemotherapy and/or opioid and non-opioid analgesics is an integral part of cancer care.

The main targets

The eight most common cancers, with a combined total of over 6 million new cases a year, should be the main targets for prevention and cure. Three account for more than 50% of these cases – lung cancer (1.3 million), stomach cancer (1 million) and breast cancer (0.9 million). All of them have one or more major risk factors which can be considered under five headings; tobacco-related; alcohol-related; infection-related; hormone-related. Some of these factors are common to several cancers. Each of these cancers is briefly described below in terms of its risk factors, clinical features, treatment, survival and prospects for prevention.

Lung cancer

Risk factor: tobacco

Lung cancer (including cancer of the trachea and bronchus) is the most common cancer in the world, with 51% of cases occurring in developed countries, and 75% occurring in men. Globally, 85% of cases in men and 46% in women are due to smoking. In developed countries the proportions are 91% for men and 62% for women, and in developing countries 76% for men and 24% for women. These patterns reflect the earlier adoption of smoking by men. Rates in men are increasing in most countries, although where the smoking epidemic began first, and has now passed its peak, the rates are beginning to fall (e.g. Finland, United Kingdom, United States). The highest national rates are currently found in eastern Europe.

In developing countries and regions the highest rates are seen where the smoking habit has been longest established – e.g. South Africa and Zimbabwe in Africa, China in the Western Pacific, and in the Eastern Mediterranean. Incidence rates in women are rising briskly in countries where female smoking is long established, and lung cancer is now the most common cause of death from cancer in women in the United States. In most developing countries, women rarely smoke, so rates there remain low.

Tobacco smoking is by far the most important risk factor. A lifetime smoker has a risk some 20-30 times that of a non-smoker. The risk increases with the amount smoked. Passive exposure to tobacco smoke is generally accepted as increasing risk by 30-50%. Genetic mechanisms define susceptibility to tobacco smoke.

Chinese women, although few of them smoke, have a modestly raised incidence of lung cancer, possibly because of exposure to environmental smoke, particularly cooking fumes, but they may be at genuinely higher risk too. Other factors known to increase risk of lung cancer are occupational exposures to asbestos, some metals (e.g. nickel, arsenic and cadmium), radon and ionizing radiation.

The disease usually presents with cough or breathlessness; the first signs may result from the spread of the disease to other parts of the body, as this occurs early in lung cancer. It is readily diagnosed by chest X-ray and bronchoscopy, or by examining cells taken from sputum.

About 20% of lung cancers (small-cell carcinoma) are treated with chemotherapy, while for non-small-cell carcinoma surgery and/or radiotherapy are used.

Overall, survival is poor (7-12% alive after five years). Although 50% of persons with small, localized tumours survive five years, such cases are rare.

Individuals can be convinced to give up smoking or persuaded not to start. But this is very difficult in the absence of reinforcing social pressures that make smoking unattractive, and a legislative framework that makes smoking expensive and difficult. The opposing pressures (from agricultural and finance ministries, tobacco companies) are enormous.

Tobacco consumption has been rising in most countries (at least in men), so that it is easy to predict a continuing evolution of the epidemic over the next 10-20 years.

Stomach cancer

Risk factors: diet, infection

Stomach cancer is the world's second most common cancer, with over 1 million new cases per year. Nearly two-thirds occur in developing countries. High-risk areas include Central and South America and eastern Asia, and also Japan. Incidence in men is nearly twice that in women. Cases have declined steadily in most affluent countries over the last 30 years. Similar trends are apparent in some less developed regions of the world. Most gastric cancers are adenocarcinomas. In contrast to the overall decreasing trend, there has recently been a rapid increase of cancers localized to the cardia (the upper part of the stomach). The reasons for this increase are not known.

The constant decline of stomach cancer in industrialized countries is linked to improved food preservation practices; better nutrition more rich in vitamins from fresh vegetables and fruits; and less consumption of preserved, cured and salted foods. Infection with the bacterium *Helicobacter pylori* contributes to the risk, probably by interacting with the other factors.

Symptoms are nonspecific, which explains why most of the cases are diagnosed when the disease is at an advanced-stage. Patients may complain of weight loss, fatigue or gastric discomfort. Diagnosis is performed by barium X-rays and with biopsy.

This cancer is treated by surgical removal of the tumour, with or without adjuvant chemotherapy.

Stomach cancer cases have a generally poor survival prognosis, averaging no more than 20% survival after five years. If the tumour is localized to the stomach, 60% of patients survive five

It is easy to predict a continuing evolution of the lung cancer epidemic over the next 10-20 years.

years or more. However, only 18% of all cases are diagnosed at this early stage.

Consumption of fresh vegetables and fruit and reduced intake of salty and cured foods decrease the risk. Screening by photofluoroscopy has been widespread in Japan since the late 1960s and mortality rates are declining. It is unclear whether this trend can be attributed to mass screening alone.

Despite declining rates in developed countries in the last 30 years, stomach cancer is still the second most common cancer worldwide, and is a highly lethal disease.

Breast cancer

Risk factors: hormones

The most common cancer in women, breast cancer, causes 376 000 deaths a year worldwide; about 900 000 women a year are diagnosed with the disease.

The most common cancer in women, breast cancer causes 376 000 deaths a year worldwide; about 900 000 women a year are diagnosed with the disease. More than half of these cases are in industrialized countries – about 220 000 in Europe and about 180 000 in North America, for example. The disease is not yet as common among women in developing countries but is increasing. The highest reported rates are for white or Hawaiian women in the United States. High rates are also found for North America in general and some parts of Europe. In contrast, low rates are found in Africa and Asia. Studies indicate that when women migrate from low-risk to high-risk regions, after two or three generations their descendants slowly acquire the rates of the host country, which illustrates the importance of lifestyle in addition to genetics. Breast cancer incidence is still increasing in most parts of the world, particularly in regions which previously had low rates.

The strongest risk factor is age, with more than half of the cases occurring after menopause. The risk is also linked to reproductive and hormonal factors. It is increased by early menarche, late age at first birth, never having given birth, and late menopause. All of these reflect a hormonal pattern. Other risk factors include obesity after menopause, exposure to ionizing radiation (especially at the time of breast development) and exogenous hormones such as oral contraceptives at an early age and estrogen replacement therapy at menopause.

Recently, genetic predisposition has been much better understood with the identification of at least two genes which carry a high risk of breast cancer, but in only 2-5% of cases.

The most common clinical sign is a lump in the breast. Diagnosis is confirmed by biopsy or fine-needle aspiration.

Depending on the stage of the tumour, treatment may include surgical removal of the tumour and surrounding tissue from the breast (lumpectomy); surgical removal of the whole breast (mastectomy); radiotherapy; chemotherapy. Combinations of surgery followed by chemotherapy, hormonal therapy and radiotherapy improve the chances of long-term survival.

At least half of all cases will survive for five years if treated adequately. Trends in survival show clear improvement over time. The main determinant of survival is the stage of the tumour, localized disease being associated with an excellent prognosis. In contrast, distant spread carries a high risk of death in the five years following diagnosis.

Currently, the only effective prevention strategy is mammography with routine breast examination, which can reduce by one-third the risk of death from breast cancer among women over 55. In the developing world, detection by breast examination may lead to a reduction of the disease.

Improved facilities for radiography and clinical diagnosis should be made available worldwide. General health promotion, including avoidance of obesity from childhood onwards, could also help. Chemoprevention (*Box 8*) is currently only a research exercise. No optimal strategy has yet been defined for women who are at a very high risk. Advances in the control of cancer pain, in palliative care and in psychological counselling for cancer sufferers are also needed.

Colorectal cancer

Risk factor: diet

This is one of the most common cancers worldwide, with about 870 000 new cases per year. It is more frequent in North America, Europe and Australia than in Africa, Asia and Central or South America, but the incidence is increasing in several populations previously at low risk. Cancer of the colon occurs with similar frequency in men and women, but cancer of the rectum is 20-50% more frequent in men than women in most populations. Migrant studies indicate that when populations move from a low-risk area (e.g. Japan) to a high-risk area (e.g. the United States) the incidence of colorectal cancer increases rapidly within the first generation of migrants.

Studies in both developed and developing countries consistently show a higher risk of colorectal cancer in people consuming a diet low in vegetables and in unrefined plant foods (i.e. whole cereals, legumes, etc.). Studies in developed countries have also found that frequent consumption of red meat (beef, lamb, etc.) increases the risk, while consumption of fish and poultry has been found to be either unrelated to risk or even associated with a slight reduction in risk. The mechanisms by which a diet rich in vegetables and whole plant foods and moderate in meat may protect against colorectal cancer are still unclear.

The disease usually presents with intestinal symptoms including pain, rectal bleeding, and/or alternating diarrhoea and constipation. Diagnosis can be made by means of endoscopy and/or X-ray.

For small tumours of limited extent a segment of the colon is removed by surgery. For larger tumours more extensive removal of the large bowel may be necessary. Radiotherapy and chemotherapy are used together with surgery, or if the tumour recurs.

Overall, five-year survival is about 50-60%. For localized cancers it is almost 90%, but when diagnosed at advanced stages with distant localization, it is only 3-8%.

Box 8. Cancer chemoprevention: trials and troubles

Chemoprevention is an attempt to use natural and synthetic compounds to intervene in the early stages of cancer development, before invasive disease actually begins. Such substances taken as pills or tablets, for example, could protect individuals at high risk of cancer.

Food is the source of some of the most promising chemopreventive compounds. Many vegetables, fruits and grains are known to offer protection against various cancers. However, such compounds must be nontoxic and relatively free of side-effects, because they are meant to be administered to healthy people for long periods of time. Isolating the effects of individual food constituents has proved difficult. For instance, while fruits and vegetables rich in betacarotene have reduced the risk for certain types of cancer – especially lung cancer – large-scale chemopreventive trials with betacarotene in pills have produced unexpected and even disappointing results.

Beginning in 1985, betacarotene was included in two such long-term trials, one conducted in Finland and the other in the United States. For several years, daily doses of betacarotene and either vitamin E or vitamin A were administered to tens of thousands of people at high risk of developing lung cancer, particularly cigarette smokers. Expectations were based largely on the results of dietary studies in which the daily intake of betacarotene was associated with a lower risk of lung cancer.

The hypothesis was that administering the nutrients would protect against the disease. Surprisingly, however, the rate of lung cancer in cigarette smokers taking betacarotene increased slightly in both trials, for reasons that are still to be explained. Possibly other substances found in fruits and vegetables are responsible for the protective effects. These disappointing results show some of the difficulties faced by chemoprevention researchers, and help explain why progress in cancer research is often painstakingly slow.

The "gold standard" of chemoprevention trials is still the large prospective study, which monitors future development of disease in either high-risk individuals or the general population. In these trials, the experimental agent may need to be administered for many years, after which another number of years will be needed to assess the effects fully.

To help speed up the results of such trials, researchers are now investigating the use of biomarkers as surrogate measures of a compound's success. Biomarkers are physiological manifestations of changes that may occur in the pathway to cancer. If an intervention reduces the incidence of these signs in a population, the chances are better that the agent will lower the incidence of the cancer itself.

As an example, current trials of chemoprevention agents for colon cancer will determine the efficacy of nonsteroidal anti-inflammatory drugs on the incidence of intestinal polyps, a benign precursor to colon cancer, rather than the incidence of the cancer itself. These drugs seem to protect the body against cancer, especially cancer of the colon, in a number of ways; but their prolonged use may cause gastrointestinal side-effects, such as bleeding or ulcers.

Difficulties and disappointments inevitably occur in cancer research. But with increasing knowledge of how cancer develops, chemoprevention will undoubtedly play a significant role in future cancer control.

Box 9. Chronic liver diseases and liver cancer – the Gambia Hepatitis Intervention Study

A population-based vaccination campaign against hepatitis B virus (HBV) was initiated in the Gambia in 1986 with the objective of evaluating the effectiveness of hepatitis B vaccination in the prevention of hepatitis B infection, chronic liver diseases and primary liver cancer in a population at high risk. The study comprises three overlapping phases:

Phase I Vaccination of approximately 60 000 children during the first five years, concluded in 1990;

Phase II Longitudinal and cross-sectional surveys of selected groups of vaccinated (Group 1) and unvaccinated (Group 2) children, up to 10 years of age, now in progress;

Phase III Long-term follow-up for 40 years.

Hepatitis B vaccine, which was approved by the World Health Organization, was integrated into the Gambian Expanded Programme on Immunization (EPI) in a phased manner over a four-year period. During this period, two groups of children were recruited, one comprising some 60 000 children who received all vaccines in the EPI schedule plus the hepatitis B vaccine, the other comprising a similar number of children who received the EPI vaccines but not the hepatitis B vaccine. These two cohorts are being followed up over a 30-40-year period in order to evaluate the effectiveness of hepatitis B vaccination in preventing liver cancer and chronic liver diseases. A population-based national cancer registry was also established in 1986 with the aim of improving the reporting of cancers in both public and private health sectors, so that the net effect of vaccination in preventing liver cancer can ultimately be assessed.

The study clearly shows that HBV vaccination can be effectively integrated in the EPI vaccination programme in developing countries. Phase II of the study is now approaching 10 years and serological markers of hepatitis B infection in two cohorts (1000 children each) of vaccinated and unvaccinated children show that vaccine efficacy in preventing primary infection and carrier state is 84% and 94%.

Other important outcomes from the study relevant to the implementation of HBV vaccination in other developing countries are: the evidence that dose interval is unimportant in immunogenicity; the evidence that infection in the family does not affect the response of the child; the relatively low contribution of hepatitis C to liver cancer in this population; and the high cost-effectiveness of the vaccination in prevention of the carrier state.

The Gambia Hepatitis Intervention Study is a project run by the International Agency for Research on Cancer, in collaboration with the Government of the Republic of The Gambia and the United Kingdom Medical Research Council laboratories in The Gambia. It is supported by the Direzione Generale per la Cooperazione allo Svilluppo of the Ministry of Foreign Affairs of Italy, the Regione Autonoma Valle d'Aosta, Italy, and the Medical Research Council of Sweden.

Epidemiological studies strongly suggest that a diet rich in vegetables and minimally refined plant food and moderate in meat can reduce the risk of colorectal cancer. Early detection of colorectal polyps and of localized cancers is possible by means of a laboratory test or endoscopic examination of the large bowel.

Oral cancer

Risk factors: tobacco, alcohol, diet

Oral and pharyngeal cancers are common in regions where tobacco use and alcohol consumption are popular. Each year, about 575 000 new cases and 320 000 deaths occur worldwide. Increases in cases and deaths have been reported in recent years in western, central and eastern Europe, Japan and Australasia, and among nonwhites in the United States.

Patients generally present with red lesions in the mouth. Those with pharyngeal cancers may complain of difficulty in swallowing or hoarseness, particularly at advanced stages. Cancers of the oral cavity are often preceded by restricted mouth opening and tongue mobility.

Treatment is by surgery and radiotherapy, alone or in combination. Advanced disease is generally treated with both, with or without chemotherapy.

Five-year survival approaches 70-80% in early stages and ranges from 5% to 20% in advanced disease.

Tobacco and alcohol control and a healthy diet can effectively prevent some cancers. Whether long-term chemopreventive therapy can prevent oral cancers is not known. Screening by visual inspection of the mouth has been shown to be feasible, although its effectiveness is not yet clear.

Liver cancer

Risk factors: infection, alcohol, diet

Liver cancer is a major problem of developing countries, where 82% of the world total (540 000 new cases per year) occur, with 55% of all cases in China. The risk in men is twice that in women.

83% of the cases worldwide are attributable to infection with the hepatitis B virus. The attributable fraction is 91% in developing countries and 52% in the more affluent areas of the world, where the majority of the remaining cases are explained by excessive consumption of alcohol. Exposure to aflatoxins, naturally occurring contaminants of grains, enhances the effect of chronic hepatitis B infection.

Map 1. Hepatitis C, 1997 estimates

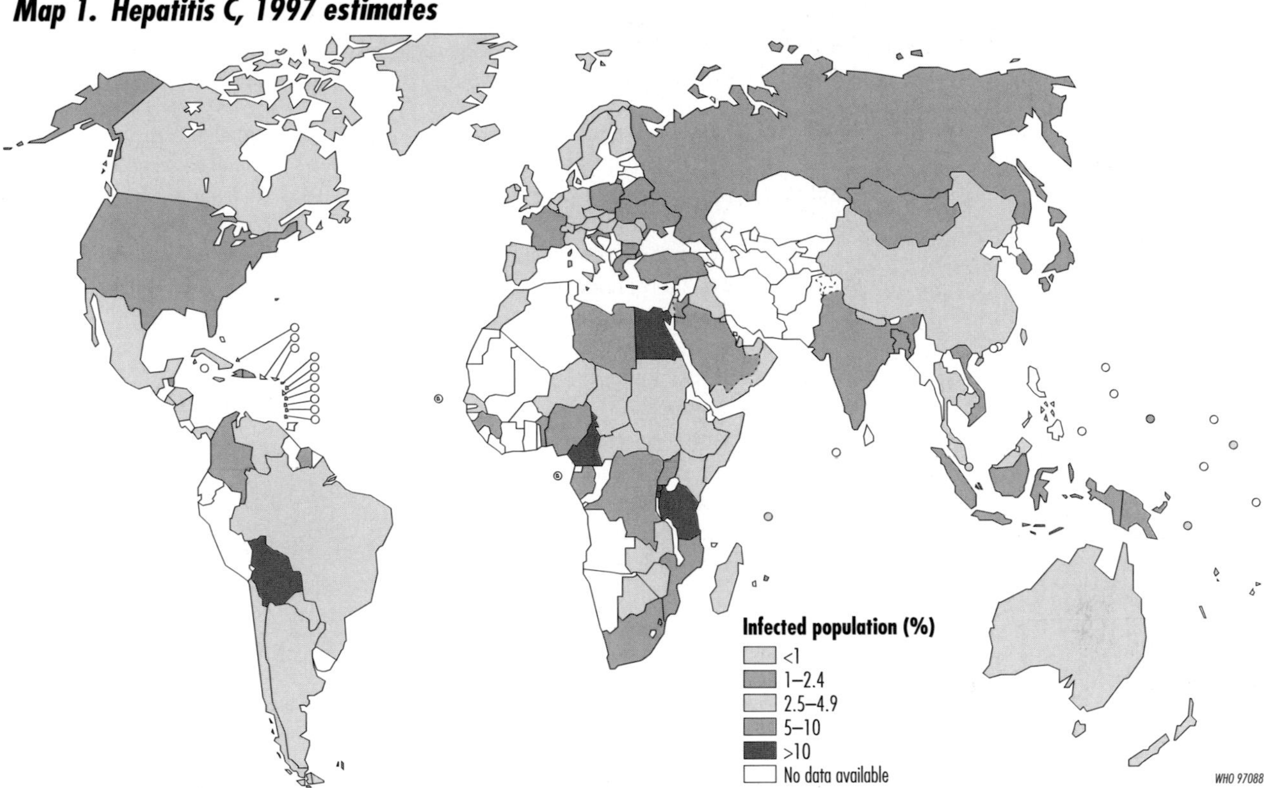

Common symptoms are abdominal pain, weight loss, fatigue, abdominal swelling, loss of appetite and jaundice. The majority of the cases can be diagnosed by ultrasonography.

There is no effective treatment. Only 6% of the cases survive at least five years in the United States and similar figures or worse are likely to apply in developing countries.

In developed areas, 30% and in developing areas 70% of cases could be prevented by the introduction of vaccination against hepatitis B virus into the primary immunization schedule for infants (*Box* 9). Screening programmes have not proved effective in reducing mortality.

Primary liver cancer is a highly lethal disease the burden of which could be substantially reduced by preventing hepatitis B and C infection (*Map 1*).

Cervical cancer

Risk factor: infection

This is the second most common cancer among women worldwide, with an estimated 524 000 new cases in 1995. Developing countries, where it is often the most common cancer among women, account for 80% of cases. Wide variations in incidence and mortality from the disease exist between countries: North America, western Europe and some countries in the Eastern Mediterranean have the lowest rates, and Latin America, sub-Saharan Africa and South-East Asia have the highest. Cases and deaths have declined markedly in the last 40 years in most industrialized countries, partly owing to a reduction in risk factors, but mainly as a result of extensive screening programmes. More limited improvements have been observed in developing countries, where persistently high rates tend to be the rule.

Early age at initiation of sexual activity, increasing number of sexual partners of females or their sexual partners, and other indicators of sexual behaviour have long implicated a sexually transmitted agent. Additional factors include number of pregnancies, and possibly exposure to oral contraceptives.

Recently, certain types of human papilloma virus (HPV) have been established as the sexually transmitted agents responsible for initiating the disease in the vast majority of cases. The virus is found in more than 95% of the cancers. Current evidence suggests that the virus is a necessary but not sufficient cause of the disease and researchers are now trying to define other cofactors.

The development of vaccines may help to reduce the incidence of cervical cancer in the future.

The initial infection with HPV is very common after initiation of sexual activity, and is usually latent and only detectable with laboratory methods. Infections usually regress spontaneously after variable periods of time, probably by immunological mechanisms. In a small minority of affected women, the condition progresses to invasive cancer, which usually appears more than a decade after the initial infection. The diagnosis can be made years before the initiation of cancer. When invasive disease is established, symptoms include vaginal bleeding or discharge, pelvic pain, and eventually rectal and urinary complications.

Treatment is by surgery or radiotherapy for early stages, and radiotherapy for more advanced disease. Results depend on the stage of the disease at the time when it is diagnosed.

Survival depends on the stage of the disease, with 90% of localized cases surviving five years, but less than 10% of cases with distant spread. Important differences in survival are related to age and ethnic or socioeconomic characteristics, probably because of variations in access to medical care.

Mass screening programmes covering large proportions of the female population and providing high-quality screening and treatment are the most effective secondary prevention method. These have proved effective in developed countries, but their potential impact is limited in developing areas, because of the extensive resources and organization required. Simpler, cheaper and more reproducible screening methods are needed. Increased use of condoms and the development of vaccines may help to reduce the incidence of disease in the future now that HPV has been recognized as the central cause of the disease.

Oesophageal cancer

Risk factors: tobacco, alcohol, diet

About 480 000 cases of cancer of the oesophagus occur worldwide each year, of which about 85% are in developing countries. The highest risk areas of the world are in the Asian "oesophageal cancer belt" (stretching from northern Islamic Republic of Iran through the central Asian republics to north-central China). High rates are also present in parts of East and South-East Africa, eastern South America and certain parts of western Europe.

Smoking accounts for 45% of cases in men, but only 11% of cases in women. Nutritional deficiency (especially of micronutrients) has long been suspected to be the major factor in Asian high-risk areas. Drinking home-brewed alcohol in Africa, and herb tea (maté) in South America, is also implicated. The combination of tobacco and alcohol is a significant risk.

Almost all patients complain of difficulty in swallowing, first liquids and later all foods, with accompanying weight loss. Diagnosis is by oesophagoscopy or barium swallow X-ray examination.

Treatment is by surgery, for instance, bypass operations pulling up the stomach or colon, to provide temporary relief from obstructed swallowing. Radiotherapy can palliate advanced cases.

About 75% of patients die within a year of diagnosis, and survival after five years is only 5-10%.

Prostate cancer

Risk factors: diet, hormones

Prostate cancer is much more frequent in Europe, North America and Australia than in other regions of the world. About 400 000 new cases are diagnosed yearly around the world. Black populations of African origin living in Central America, the Caribbean, and the United States have a particularly high risk. The incidence increases particularly after 60-70 years of age.

High consumption of meat and animal fat is a risk factor, and hormonal patterns may also be involved.

Depending on the stage of the condition, clinical characteristics and the age of the patient, different combinations of hormonal treatment, radiotherapy and surgery are used.

Five-year survival is generally quite high, of the order of 70-90%. Survival is lower for patients presenting with distant metastases (20-30% after five years).

Prevention is through dietary advice (moderate intake of meat and animal fat, avoidance of obesity), and early detection. The disadvantage of generalized early detection is that such screening detects cancers in elderly men who would otherwise have suffered no symptoms during their lifetime.

Bladder cancer

Risk factors: tobacco, infection (diet)

An estimated 236 000 new cases of bladder cases occur each year in men and 74 000 in women. Just over half the cases occur in industrialized countries. Incidence is particularly high in North America, Europe, northern Africa and in Chinese populations.

Cigarette smoking is the single most important risk factor and is responsible for 37% of cases in men and 14% in women. Carcinogens that affect the bladder occur in certain populations; for instance, there is an increased risk among rubber workers. Chronic infection with *Schistosoma haematobium* is an important risk factor, where infection with this parasite is still endemic. A diet rich in fruits and vegetables is associated with lower risk.

Treatment is by surgical removal of the tumour; surgical removal of the whole bladder (cystectomy); chemotherapy and radiotherapy.

For localized tumours, five-year survival is over 90%, but is 50% or less for more advanced stages.

This cancer can be prevented by control of tobacco smoking, occupational carcinogens and *S. haematobium* infection. Occupational screening has been ineffective but the control of occupational carcinogens has taken place in many countries. Screening procedures are being developed.

Ovarian cancer

Risk factors: hormones, diet

About 190 000 cases occur each year, with slightly more in developing than in developed countries. Recent trends are decreases in countries which previously had high rates, and increases in countries previously at low risk.

Cancer of the ovary is influenced by hormones and reproductive factors. Risk is slightly increased in women who have never given birth and those with a personal history of breast cancer or a family history of breast or ovarian cancer. A clearly decreased risk is found in those who have used oral contraceptives, and the degree of protective effect is proportional to the length of treatment. In contrast, treatment for infertility entails a clearly increased risk, whereas treatment of the menopause is only associated with a small risk. Diet plays a role, with increased risk linked to obesity and height, as well as some nutritional factors. Recently, genetic factors have been shown to play an important role, particularly in young women.

Small tumours are generally clinically silent and symptoms appear late. The use of endovaginal echography can lead to a diagnosis, which has to be confirmed by biopsy.

Surgery is used in early disease; radiotherapy and chemotherapy for more advanced stages.

Chronic infection with Schistosoma haematobium *is an important risk factor for bladder cancer, where infection with this parasite is still endemic.*

The five-year survival rate is less than 30% in most countries, and is highly dependent on the stage of disease.

No screening has been shown to be effective in reducing incidence or mortality. The only factor linked to a reduced risk of ovarian cancer is use of oral contraceptives.

Effective forms of therapy have still to be found for advanced forms of the disease. Better understanding of the genetics of ovarian cancer will help to define better strategies for research and treatment.

Cancer of the body of the uterus

Risk factors: hormones, diet

About 170 000 cases of cancer of the uterus occur worldwide each year, with slightly more than 100 000 in developed countries. Africa and Asia have low rates; the highest are in the United States and Canada, where a clear decline in cases and deaths has occurred, particularly among young women. Most cancers appear after the age of menopause.

Cancer of the endometrium, the internal lining of the uterus, is linked to reproductive life, with increased risk among women who have never given birth and women undergoing late menopause. It is clearly associated with obesity, diabetes and hypertension. Unopposed estrogen therapy for menopause, without the use of progestins, increases the risk whereas combined oral contraceptives lower it.

Surgery is the main treatment, although chemotherapy and hormone therapy may be used.

Survival is usually good, in particular for localized disease. Poor prognosis is associated with distant spread, and some types may be more aggressive.

So far screening has not shown any real benefit. The only recommendation may be general good health including the avoidance of obesity and of treatment with unopposed estrogens.

In order to evaluate changes in incidence, there is a need to have detailed population statistics on hysterectomy rates. In the United States, up to 40% of women undergo hysterectomy after the age of menopause, which means that most analyses of trends in the incidence of uterine cancer can only be tentative.

A rapid increase in incidence of testicular cancer has been observed in most countries.

Testicular cancer

Risk factors: hormones

The highest incidence of testicular cancer is recorded in Denmark and Germany and in general in white populations of high-income countries. The maximum risk is during the third and fourth decades of life and declines after age 50. A rapid increase in incidence has been observed in most countries, for reasons that are not well understood. Deaths have markedly declined since the introduction of effective chemotherapy in the mid-1970s.

Hormonal and genetic factors are likely to be important but their role is currently unclear. In general, testicular cancer is more common in higher social classes.

Treatment is by surgery combined with chemotherapy.

Above 95% survive after five years except for the small fraction of patients in whom the condition is at an advanced stage. Survival in developing countries is only 40-60%, indicating limited access to appropriate therapy.

No effective preventive strategies exist. Therapeutic improvement has reduced deaths, but the causes of this cancer remain largely unknown, so that there is little scope for preventive action.

Laryngeal cancer

Risk factors: tobacco, alcohol, diet

About 190 000 new cases of cancer of the larynx occurred worldwide in 1995, of which more than 60% were in developing countries. High-risk countries are found in Latin Europe (France, Italy, Spain) and Latin America (Brazil, Uruguay); India is an intermediate risk country. The disease is much more frequent in males than in females.

Tobacco smoking and alcohol consumption, which have a synergistic effect, are the main risk factors. Studies show a protective effect of a diet rich in fruit. This cancer may be induced by exposure to asbestos.

The early symptoms are hoarseness, difficulty in swallowing or pain in the throat, depending on the exact site of the tumour. Diagnosis is carried out by laryngoscopy and biopsy.

Cryotherapy or laser treatment is used for the less advanced lesions; for more advanced lesions, surgery and radiotherapy are the more frequent treatment. Overall, 50-60% of patients survive five years.

Leukaemias

Risk factor: radiation

Incidence rates for all types of leukaemia together vary from 2 to 12 per 100 000 population. These cancers constitute 3% of all new cancers worldwide. Occurrence in North America, western Europe, Australia, Israel, Japan, and New Zealand is high. Most leukaemias in children are acute lymphoblastic leukaemia (ALL), with a distinct peak of occurrence at 1-4 years of age. Death rates, particularly in childhood, have fallen substantially, thanks to therapeutic advances which improve survival. At other ages, broad categories of leukaemia are: acute non-lymphoblastic or myeloid (AML – young adulthood); chronic myeloid (CML – usually age 30-50); and chronic lymphocytic (CLL – rare before the age of 50).

Risk factors include ionizing radiations, certain drugs and chemicals (e.g. benzene) and industrial exposure to hydrocarbons. A high risk is observed among long-term survivors of cancer treated with chemotherapy and radiotherapy. However, all these factors are unlikely to account for a large proportion of leukaemias. Genetic conditions, such as Down syndrome and chromosomal anomalies, are also associated with increased risk. Viral infections are suspected of playing a role.

Patients with acute leukaemias (ALL and AML) present with anaemia, pallor, features of infection, and bleeding which are of rapid onset; enlargement of liver and spleen are common. Patients with ALL in addition present with bone and joint pain and multiple lymph node enlargements (lymphadenopathy). Patients with CML present with slow onset of symptoms of anaemia and weight loss, and massive enlargement of spleen. CLL develops gradually and presents with multiple lymph node enlargement, with or without splenic enlargement. As the disease progresses anaemia sets in slowly.

Combinations of chemotherapy and steroids, with intensive supportive care, are used for treatment. Prophylactic treatment is mandatory in the management of ALL against a possible involvement or relapse in the central nervous system. Bone marrow transplantation is one form of therapy for inducing remission in young patients with AML when other treatment fails. Relapse is still a major problem in acute leukaemias; treatment is essentially palliative in chronic leukaemias.

60-70% of complete responders in ALL, and 20-30% of complete responders in AML survive in excess of five years. 30-50% of the patients diagnosed with chronic leukaemias survive five years.

Leukaemia death rates, particularly in childhood, have fallen substantially, thanks to therapeutic advances which improve survival.

Lymphomas

Risk factor: infection

There are two major groups: Hodgkin and non-Hodgkin lymphomas. An estimated 229 000 new cases of lymphoma occur each year in men, and 164 000 in women. In both sexes, 65% of all lymphomas are non-Hodgkin lymphoma with about 60% of all lymphomas occurring in developing countries. Incidence rates are highest in Europe and North America. Specific types of lymphoma have distinct geographical patterns, such as Burkitt lymphoma, which is endemic in certain areas of Africa and Oceania and affects children.

Infection with Epstein-Barr virus, a common herpes virus, has been linked with Burkitt lymphoma and Hodgkin lymphoma. Infection with HIV is another risk factor. However, these explain only a small percentage of all the cases. Exposure to herbicides and dioxins is suspected. Lymphomas tend to occur in families.

Cancer update

After this report was completed, the International Agency for Research on Cancer provided revised estimates of cancer mortality worldwide. The revised number of deaths for 1996 is 7.1 million, distributed as follows (in thousands):

- lung 1160
- stomach 835
- liver 536
- colon and rectum 510
- oesophagus 456
- breast 390
- mouth and pharynx 366
- cervix 242
- other cancers 2616

Superficial lymph node enlargement is the most common clinical feature of lymphomas. General symptoms, such as fever and weight loss, are more common in patients with Hodgkin lymphoma. Involvement of tissues other than lymph nodes is common in non-Hodgkin lymphomas, resulting in a variety of clinical pictures. Diagnosis is based on biopsy complemented by laparotomy and radiological examinations to determine the extent of the disease.

Control of known risk factors, such as HIV infection, is likely to prevent only a small fraction of lymphomas. Effective screening methods are not available.

Treatment is by combinations of chemotherapy and radiotherapy, and in advanced disease, options include bone marrow transplantation.

Survival of Hodgkin lymphoma patients after five years is between 70% and 80% in North America and Europe, but only 30-55% in developing countries. Survival for non-Hodgkin lymphoma patients in developed countries is 50%.

Malignant lymphomas are an important group of cancers showing an increase in incidence. Their etiology is mostly unknown, making it difficult to develop effective preventive strategies.

Myeloma

Risk factor: radiation

Multiple myeloma, a malignant tumour of the plasma cells in the bone marrow, is very rare in persons under 40 years of age. A slow increase in cases and deaths is being seen in most regions of the world.

Ionizing radiation is the only well-established risk factor. An increased risk is observed among survivors of atomic bomb explosions in Japan, women irradiated for cervical cancer, and in radiologists and nuclear industry workers. Chemicals, such as benzene and carbon monoxide, and occupational exposures in farming and in the wood, rubber and petroleum industries are associated with an increased risk.

Patients with multiple myeloma present with bone pain, anaemia, and symptoms and signs of infections. As the disease progresses bone and soft tissue tumours, fractures, features of kidney failure and neurological dysfunctions including partial paralysis become clinically evident. The proliferation of plasm cells within the bone marrow leads to skeletal destruction of the skull, spine, ribs, pelvis and long bones.

Treatment is by chemotherapy with or without steroids, to which 50-60% of the patients respond. Radiotherapy effectively relieves bone pain and other symptoms. Opioids are effective in controlling generalized bone pain and neuropathy in advanced disease. The five-year survival rate is 15-25%. Control of ionizing radiation exposures in related occupations and applications is the only preventive measure available.

Malignant melanoma

Risk factor: ultraviolet radiation

Of 115 000 cases worldwide each year, 70% are in Australasia, Europe, and North America. Rapid increases in incidence and mortality are observed in both sexes in many countries, even where rates were formerly low, such as Japan. In the Nordic countries, for example, this increase has averaged some 30% every five years.

Malignant melanoma of the skin is a tumour of the white-skinned races (Caucasians), when they are exposed to strong ultraviolet irradiation at low latitudes. Early signs – benign naevi, believed to be precursors of melanoma – are induced by ultraviolet irradiation, particularly in childhood. The tumour eventually presents as a pigmented mole that increases in size and colour, developing into a nodule that often bleeds.

While ultraviolet radiation is the main risk factor, the risk is determined by susceptibility, related to skin type. Fair-skinned individuals who sunburn readily are at highest risk. Intermittent exposure to strong sunlight – e.g. recreational (sunbathing) – is more dangerous than chronic exposure (e.g. in outdoor occupations).

Melanomas are divided into three histological types; most melanomas in white populations are superficial spreading and nodular melanomas. These are proportionately most common on the back and face in men, and on the legs in women. Lentigo malignant melanoma occurs later in life and on sun-exposed sites. Acral lentiginous melanoma is proportionately more common in populations in eastern Asia.

Treatment is by surgery, with excision of the regional lymph nodes only when these are obviously involved. Malignant melanoma is generally resistant to radiotherapy. Chemotherapy for metastatic melanoma has not been successful.

Survival depends on the stage of disease. In localised melanoma, some 90-95% cases survive five years. Females have better survival rates than males.

White-skinned populations should take precautions to limit the exposure of their skin to ultraviolet radiation (avoid direct sunlight, use of hats, appropriate clothing, sun screens). Awareness of melanoma risk in susceptible populations can lead to earlier presentation.

Increased ultraviolet exposure (due to thinning of the ozone layer) may lead to an increase in the risk of melanoma. However, the potential for prevention is good; recent data suggest that mortality rates in young persons (recent generations) are no longer rising in several high-risk countries, and in some (e.g. Canada, Denmark, United States) are actually decreasing.

Cancer in childhood

Cancer is rather rare in children; about 2 children in every 1000 develop a cancer before their 15th birthday. However, the importance of cancer in children depends on two other factors. The first is the age structure of the population – in some developing countries, children comprise 40-50% of the population, so that some 3% of cancers occur in this age group, compared with 0.9% in developed countries. Secondly, other competing illnesses are important. Thus, although cancer accounts for some 4-5% of childhood deaths in developed countries, only some 0.7% of deaths are due to cancer in developing countries, where infectious diseases play a much more important role.

Acute leukaemia, especially in early childhood, is the most common cancer in children in most countries, although in tropical Africa, lymphomas are more common. Brain tumours generally account for one-fifth to one-quarter of childhood cancers. Many of the other solid tumours are the so-called "embryonal cell" cancers (arising in primitive cells found in the human embryo); they occur in the first years of life in the kidney, eye, adrenal gland and liver. The sarcomas of bones and soft tissue are also much more common in children, accounting for over 10% of cancers, compared with 1-2% in adults.

Little is known about the causes of childhood cancer. As might be expected in cancers occurring so early in life, exposure to environmental factors, either *in utero* or after birth, seem to play a very small part. A few cases are the result of genetic defects passed on to children by their parents – for example, a sizeable proportion of retinoblastomas (eye tumours) are inherited.

Circulatory diseases

Circulatory diseases such as heart attacks and stroke are among the world's most feared diseases, and kill more people than any other disease, accounting for at least 15 million deaths, or 30% of the annual total, every year. Many millions more are disabled by them.

Diseases of the heart and circulation – cardiovascular and cerebrovascular – are for most people the biggest risks to life. Many who die of circulatory diseases are under the age of 65, and given today's increased life span, these deaths are premature. They cause grief in families and are a loss of valuable talent that many countries need for economic development.

Perhaps the greatest tragedy is that many of these deaths are preventable or avoidable – occurring prematurely despite a wealth of knowledge on how to reduce the risks of contracting these diseases. Political commitment, combined with government and individual

Circulatory diseases such as heart attacks and stroke kill more people than any other disease, accounting for at least 15 million deaths every year.

action, could prevent about half of the annual deaths from circulatory diseases.

In the past, circulatory diseases were thought of as affecting exclusively industrialized nations since they were regarded largely as lifestyle diseases because the risk of developing them was increased by smoking, obesity, unhealthy diet and heavy alcohol consumption. Now, as developing countries modernize, they are gradually controlling infectious diseases, and the life expectancy of their populations is increasing. Unfortunately, the risks of circulatory diseases are also increasing, partly because of the adoption of lifestyles similar to those common in industrialized countries, and these diseases now account for about 25% of all deaths in developing countries – 10 out of 40 million. In developed countries almost half of all deaths – more than 5 out of 12 million – are attributable to these same diseases.

More than twice as many deaths from stroke occur in developing countries as in developed countries.

The most important circulatory diseases are high blood pressure (hypertension), coronary heart disease, cerebrovascular disease, and cardiomyopathies (diseases affecting the heart muscle). Worldwide, there are more deaths from coronary heart disease (7.2 million) than stroke (4.6 million), although their relative importance varies considerably from country to country. For example, more than twice as many deaths from stroke occur in developing countries as in developed countries.

Developing countries, however, also still suffer from other heart conditions such as rheumatic heart disease, which is linked to poverty, and from cardiac damage related to Chagas disease, a parasitic illness afflicting about 17 million people in Latin America. About 30% of those who develop chronic Chagas disease become incapacitated because of heart damage that may also lead to sudden death. Rheumatic fever is the commonest cause of heart disease in young people worldwide, accounting for about one-third of all deaths from cardiovascular diseases.

Circulatory diseases, like other noncommunicable conditions, are emerging rapidly as a major public health concern in most developing countries, which are already heavily burdened with infectious diseases. In all countries, the costs of caring for patients with circulatory diseases are rapidly rising. In developed countries, they already account for about 10% of direct health care costs, equal to between 0.5% and 1% of a country's gross national product.

Because of their prevalence and importance, circulatory diseases have been the subject of intensive research in recent decades. It has become clear that their incidence and impact can be reduced substantially through a range of well-established measures.

Cardiovascular diseases

The two main cardiovascular diseases examined in this section are coronary heart disease and rheumatic heart disease. Whereas in coronary heart disease, lifestyle and socioeconomic factors play a major role, the main underlying cause of rheumatic heart disease is bacterial infection, against a background of poverty, leading to rheumatic fever.

Coronary heart disease (CHD), accounted for more than 7 million deaths worldwide in 1996. Although these deaths are only 14% of the global total, they are responsible for about one-third of all deaths in industrialized countries.

Most cases of CHD result from narrowing of the arteries due to fatty deposits called plaques (atherosclerosis). When a coronary artery is completely blocked, usually by the formation of a blood clot on top of a plaque, the result is a heart attack (myocardial infarction) or disturbed heart rate (cardiac arrhythmia), either of which may cause sudden death.

Atherosclerosis, together with its complications, underlies most cases of coronary heart disease, including clinical manifestations such as angina pectoris, congestive heart failure, and other major disturbances of cardiac function. The atherosclerotic process in major arteries, including the coronary arteries, has its origin early in life. Its initial stages often occur in children and young people and it tends to progress silently and without symptoms from the beginning of the second decade of life onwards until illness strikes.

In a large proportion of cases, the first manifestation is sudden death. A substantial majority of CHD deaths occur outside hospital because the time between onset of the event and death is too short to permit effective emergency care and hospitalization. These problems persist, despite significant recent advances in many countries in emergency services and acute and long-term care. Possibilities for rehabilitation of survivors are limited.

The CHD epidemic began in North America, Europe and Australasia in the early decades of this century. In many industrialized countries death rates peaked in the 1960s and early 1970s and have since declined dramatically. In Australia, New Zealand and the United States, for example, CHD deaths have fallen by over 50% since the mid-1960s. But CHD is now increasing in developing countries as their populations age and adopt unhealthy habits and behaviours. The mortality rates in eastern and central Europe are now the world's highest, and they are still rising in countries such as Bulgaria and Hungary, in both men and women.

Decades of research have shown conclusively that a number of determinants – most of them associated with lifestyle – operating from early childhood onwards, are responsible for coronary heart disease. The term "risk factor" was first used for CHD. Some risk factors facilitate the development of atherosclerosis, while others sustain or accelerate the formation of plaques, producing the clinical manifestations. CHD and all cardiovascular diseases are multifactorial in origin.

The major risk factors for CHD are high blood pressure, cigarette smoking, dietary habits (particularly excessive intake of saturated fat), elevated blood cholesterol levels, lack of physical activity, obesity and diabetes. The role of dietary fat and blood cholesterol in the production of atherosclerosis is complex; it is necessary to consider the whole diet, rather than any single nutrient, since some dietary components have a protective effect and others cause damage.

High blood pressure (hypertension) is a significant risk factor for CHD The primary prevention of hypertension is critically important in the prevention of premature death from CHD.

Cigarette smoking is the most readily preventable risk factor for coronary heart disease and all other cardiovascular diseases. It causes around 15% of all CHD deaths, mostly in people over 65, and accounts for one-quarter of all CHD morbidity in people under 45. Restrictions on smoking in public places, economic incentives and disincentives and health education are effective in helping to decrease smoking.

High blood cholesterol levels are a major risk factor, contributing to CHD deaths more commonly among women than men (*Box 10*). The causes can be genetic, but are more commonly related to a diet rich in animal fats. Cholesterol levels can be reduced by dietary change or by medicines.

Lack of physical activity is also increasingly recognized as a major risk factor for CHD; it is the most prevalent modifiable risk factor in many industrialized countries.

Obesity which itself is related to inappropriate nutrition and inactivity, and diabetes mellitus, are two other important risk factors. In diabetes, the relative risk is higher in women than in men. Diabetics are at increased risk because the increased levels of glucose in their blood damages blood vessels. Premenopausal women are normally less liable to heart disease than older women or than men, but they lose this protection if they suffer from diabetes.

Genetic factors interact with environmental factors to produce variations in individual risk factor levels. Differences between populations in genetic make-up have been shown to play only a minor role at most in large inter-population differences in morbidity and mortality from CHD, for which other factors are mainly responsible.

Coronary heart disease is now increasing in developing countries as their populations age and adopt unhealthy habits and behaviours.

Box 10. Women – neglected victims of heart disease?

Coronary heart disease (CHD) is often regarded, both by doctors and the general public, as primarily a man's disease. This is partly because it kills fewer younger women than their male contemporaries. Also, heart attacks are usually seen as striking men who have a combination of stressful occupations and unhealthy lifestyles – the workaholic executive who smokes and drinks too much, has a heavy-fat diet and takes too little exercise has become a stereotype for the heart attack candidate.

This is a dangerously misleading picture – dangerous, most of all, for women. It has bred a certain complacency among doctors and health professionals, and among women themselves, who in many countries have become a neglected group as far as both the prevention and treatment of heart disease are concerned. Much of the research on causes, prevention and treatment has focused on men. Symptoms of heart disease in women are often not recognized, or even suspected, as early as they are in men. As a consequence, many women with the condition are diagnosed too late, and some studies have shown that they are treated less promptly and less efficiently than men.

The fact is that in many parts of the world, CHD is the single most common cause of death among women, even among those under 65 years of age. While women on average live longer than men, their extra years are often years of disability, in which the impact of heart disease plays a large part. With an increasingly ageing population worldwide, together with evidence that women are going to be at increased risk of heart disease, and given that much heart disease is eminently preventable, there are major implications for health and social services.

The major risk factors for CHD are the same for women as men – smoking, high blood pressure and high blood cholesterol levels. But there are good reasons why women should receive special attention. For example:

- Teenage girls are now more likely to smoke than boys, and fewer women smokers stop than men – fear of weight gain being one reason. The epidemic of smoking-related heart disease in women will become more evident in the years ahead.
- Women taking oral contraceptives who also smoke have an increased risk of heart disease.
- Blood cholesterol levels among women increase with age. After the menopause, women's cholesterol levels are on average higher than those of men about the same age.
- After the age of 45, women's blood pressure is also on average higher than men's.
- Obesity is linked to heart disease in women, and the number of overweight, obese women is increasing in many countries.
- Middle-aged women have particularly low levels of exercise, which again increases their risk.
- Although hormone replacement therapy for post-menopausal women reduces their risk of suffering from heart disease, there are new concerns about the increased risk of cancer of the endometrium as a result of the therapy.

These facts underline the need for more attention to be focused on women and heart disease. Women need to be better informed of their risks of CHD in order to respond better to preventive health advice and to recognize symptoms in themselves. At the same time, health professionals need to improve diagnosis, referral and treatment of women with CHD symptoms.

Based on: *Coronary heart disease: are women special?* United Kingdom National Forum for Coronary Heart Disease Prevention, 1994.

The widespread adoption of cigarette smoking and a reduction in regular physical activity may also have played a part in the emergence of the epidemic, together with the ageing of the population due to the decline in deaths from infectious diseases.

It appears that primary preventive efforts – such as encouragement to give up smoking or to change the diet – have made a major contribution to the recent decline in mortality, although medical and surgical treatment have also contributed. It is likely that the relative contribution of prevention and treatment has varied between countries and also over time.

Premature CHD is preventable and the disease can be treated at all ages. Furthermore, it appears that the epidemic of CHD is being substantially prevented in at least some industrialized countries. The most likely major contributor to the dramatic decline in death rates in North America, Australasia and some European countries is the control of major risk factors as a result of the preventive strategies mentioned above.

It therefore seems likely that at least half and perhaps as much as two-thirds of the burden of CHD is preventable. Prevention and treatment among elderly people, which have hitherto generally been given a low priority, require greater attention. Age in itself should not be a barrier to promoting health and preventing or postponing disease and disability, but there has been little enthusiasm in many countries for preventive approaches to heart disease in the elderly.

The treatment of established CHD involves both medical and surgical interventions. Low-cost, effective medical interventions have been identified such as the prescription of aspirin and "clot buster" drugs such as streptokinase which are simple to administer.

Surgery for CHD is widely practised in industrialized countries and is gradually becoming established in developing countries, although it is obviously relatively expensive for them. The cost-effectiveness of surgical interventions depends on the risk status of the patient.

Both the physical and mental health of people recovering from a heart attack, other heart conditions or cardiac surgery can be greatly improved by a combination of exercise, health education and counselling. The main components of cardiac rehabilitative care can be applied even in societies with minimal medical personnel and equipment resources. The goals of rehabilitation are to improve functional capacity, alleviate or lessen activity-related symptoms, reduce unwarranted invalidism, and enable the cardiac patient to return to a useful and personally satisfying role in society.

Rheumatic fever/rheumatic heart disease (RF/RHD) is the most common cardiovascular disease in children and young adults. Now very rare in developed countries, it remains a major public health issue in developing countries.

At least 12 million people are estimated to be currently affected by RF/RHD. More than 2 million require repeated hospital admission, and 1 million will need heart surgery in the next 5-20 years.

There are 500 000 deaths annually, and hundreds of thousands of people disabled, mainly children and young adults, who have no access to the expensive medical and surgical care that their condition demands. Thus, RF/RHD is both a biological and a social problem. It is very costly because of repeated hospitalizations, and causes much suffering to patients and their relatives.

A devastating childhood disease in developed countries in the 19th century, RF began to decline in incidence in these countries slowly but steadily after 1900, and much more emphatically after the 1940s. A really dramatic decline occurred in the late 1960s, due to steady improvement in standards of living, and the benefits of improved medical care, especially the introduction of antibiotics.

The condition now rarely occurs in developed countries, although small outbreaks of RF which occurred in the mid-1980s in the United States and other countries show that the risk still remains. In contrast, since the 1940s RF/RHD has become a significant health problem in tropical and subtropical countries – often with very severe effects similar to those observed in Europe a century ago. In some developing countries, the RHD mortality rate varies from almost 1 to 8 per 100 000 population. The prevalence in schoolchildren ranges from 1 to 10 per 1000 and incidence ranges from 10 to 100 per 100 000, with a high rate of recurrence.

Rheumatic fever results from bacterial (streptococcal) infections of the upper respiratory tract, and has a marked tendency to recur. It affects mainly the large joints and the heart, and less frequently the brain, skin and underlying tissues. The effect on the heart (rheumatic heart disease) is the only one that may cause death or disability.

RF/RHD often results in significant, chronic morbidity for children and young adults, with two important features. Firstly, frequent outpatient and inpatient care is a drain on already limited family resources, and involves work absenteeism for the family members who accompany the patient to hospital or visit the patient in hospital. Secondly, educational opportunities are lost (as many as 60% of children debilitated by RHD drop out of school in some areas).

Medical treatment for RF/RHD is not curative and usually has to be continued indefinitely. The costs progressively increase, further adversely affecting the cost-benefit balance in favour of prevention. Surgical treatment is even more expensive and often unaffordable or unattainable.

Climate and socioeconomic factors linked to low income, poverty, overcrowding, poor housing conditions and inadequate health services appear to influence the occurrence of RF/RHD. Those aged 5-19 years are at greatest risk.

Although there is, as yet, no available safe and effective antirheumatic streptococcal vaccine or genetic marker to identify people at high risk of developing RF, there are proven, cost-effective methods for the secondary and primary prevention of RF/RHD. Effective methods also exist for the diagno-

Both the physical and mental health of people recovering from a heart attack, other heart conditions or cardiac surgery can be greatly improved.

Even modest blood pressure reduction in hypertensive people could reduce half of the stroke events worldwide.

sis and treatment of acute attacks of RF, as do clinical and surgical methods for the palliative care of RHD and for its rehabilitation.

Although RF/RHD has been declining in some developing countries recently, the decline is slowing, because few of these countries are implementing prevention and control strategies that would help raise living standards and access to effective medical care. In contrast, prevention programmes which have been implemented in several countries achieved reductions in the mortality, prevalence, incidence, hospital admissions and severity of RF/RHD.

RF/RHD is a chronic disease for which an eminently feasible and cost-effective prevention strategy exists.

Primary prevention consists in early detection and correct treatment of streptococcal sore throat or pharyngitis whenever feasible (to prevent the first attack of acute RF). The initial acute attack can be avoided if such conditions are correctly treated.

Secondary prevention consists in early detection, diagnosis and long-term secondary prophylaxis with oral penicillin for all patients with RF/RHD (to prevent a recurrence of acute RF attack and more severe RHD). When secondary prophylaxis is applied, more than 75% of RF/RHD patients recover completely.

Cerebrovascular diseases

Among circulatory diseases, stroke and other cerebrovascular diseases are the second most common cause of death, accounting for more than 4.6 million deaths worldwide, one-third in industrialized countries, and the rest in developing countries. As is the case with CHD, there is considerable geographical variation, and morbidity and mortality occur mainly in the over-65 age group.

Cerebrovascular diseases are diseases of the central nervous system of vascular origin. They include transient cerebral ischaemia, stroke and vascular dementia, all involving disturbance of blood circulation in the brain. In a large proportion of cases, the first manifestation of cerebrovascular disease is stroke. As with CHD, atherosclerosis is the underlying determinant in most cases.

Stroke is a sudden neurological impairment, due to a cerebrovascular disorder. It can take the form of bleeding from a blood vessel in the brain (haemorrhagic stroke) or of an obstruction of a brain blood vessel (ischaemic or thrombotic stroke). About one-third of stroke patients die within six months of the event; most of these deaths occur in the first month. Survivors may be severely disabled, with partial paralysis or other physical disability, loss of speech, loss of memory and damage to other intellectual functions.

High blood pressure is the most important risk factor for both ischaemic and haemorrhagic stroke. Even modest blood pressure reduction in hypertensive people could reduce half of the stroke events worldwide.

Other major risk factors mentioned above in the context of CHD are equally important for cerebrovascular disease, in particular smoking. Alcohol consumption also increases the risk.

In developed countries, there has been a consistent decline in stroke mortality over the last 40 years, with an acceleration of this decline in the mid-1970s. The fall in stroke deaths has been greater than that in CHD deaths. For example, in Canada, Japan, Switzerland and the United States stroke mortality has declined by more than 50% in men and women aged 65-74 years since the 1970s. Although the reasons for this decline are not fully understood, the limited evidence available suggests that a decline in case-fatality may be related to decreased severity of the disease, with the acute event becoming more mild, probably as a result of prevention efforts. Improved management in the acute phase may also have contributed.

Control of hypertension and smoking cessation are of the utmost importance for stroke prevention. Other approaches, as described for CHD, should also be considered since many strokes occur in people who do not have high blood pressure. As regards other modifiable risk factors, antithrombotic therapy for chronic atrial fibrillation has been found to be useful for primary prevention. Control of hypertension may also be a key factor in reducing vascular dementia.

A WHO study published in 1996 on the risk of haemorrhagic stroke associated with the use of oral contraceptive pills showed that the pill does not increase the risk in women below 35 years, who form the great majority of pill users worldwide. In current users over 35, however, the study found a small increase in risk. This was also found in relation to ischaemic stroke in current pill users, but was lower in women under 35, in non-smokers and in those who did not have high blood pressure. For both types of stroke, the study found no increased risk in women who had used the pill in the past. Women's risks of stroke can be reduced by avoiding using the pill if they have high blood pressure, and for users of the pill, by avoiding smoking.

Hypertension

Hypertension, or high blood pressure, is the most common cardiovascular disorder, affecting about 20% of the adult population, both in the developed and developing world, and is an important public health problem of global dimensions. It affects an estimated 50 million people in the United States alone, costing 29 million working days and $2 billion per year in lost earnings.

Although it is virtually symptomless, except in its severe form, high blood pressure is considered both as a disease category and as one of the major risk factors for heart disease, stroke and kidney disease.

In most populations, average blood pressure increases with age and elevated blood pressure is particularly common in elderly men and women. The risk of cardiovascular events is substantially increased by the presence and levels of other risk factors such as smoking, elevated serum cholesterol and diabetes. Equal blood pressure levels therefore carry different risks when associated with different combinations of risk factors.

A number of determinants – many of them associated with lifestyle – are directly linked with the development of hypertension. While some risk factors and predictors of high blood pressure such as heredity, age and genetic factors are not modifiable, others can be modified in a variety of ways.

The major risk factors for hypertension are overweight, poor dietary habits – in particular, excessive intake of salt (sodium chloride) and alcohol – and inadequate physical activity. Studies suggest that taking less salt every day could result in smaller rises in blood pressure so that by the age of 55 there could be a 16% reduction in mortality for CHD, 23% for stroke and 13% for deaths from all causes. In contrast, potassium, found in some fruits and other foods, is considered to be a protective factor.

Both acute and chronic effects of alcohol on blood pressure have been noted. Regular aerobic physical activity, adequate to achieve at least a moderate level of physical fitness, has been shown to be beneficial for both prevention and control of hypertension.

A family history of elevated blood pressure is one of the strongest predictors for future development of hypertension. Several genetic factors have been identified as determinants of high blood pressure.

A number of aggravating factors contribute to variations of blood pressure within countries. In developed countries, higher prevalence of hypertension has been noted in groups with lower socioeconomic status (education, income, occupation). However, in developing countries, higher levels of blood pressure are found in upper socioeconomic groups. Generally, this corresponds to emerging middle-class populations; and it probably represents the initial stage of the epidemic of cardiovascular disease. Major geographical and ethnic variations also occur within countries.

In developing countries, higher levels of blood pressure are found in the emerging middle-class populations, and probably represent the initial stage of the epidemic of cardiovascular disease.

Chronic nonspecific lung diseases

Chronic nonspecific lung diseases include asthma, chronic bronchitis and emphysema. Together they kill almost 3 million people every year, representing around 6% of deaths globally. Chronic bronchitis and emphysema are usually grouped as chronic obstructive pulmonary disease (COPD), which is especially prevalent in older age groups. Deaths from COPD worldwide are expected to increase significantly with the rise in smoking prevalence and environmental pollution.

Asthma and COPD have common characteristics such as obstruction of the airways (respiratory passages). However, the airway obstruction in asthma is variable and reversible whilst in COPD it is poorly reversible and usually progressive. There is a large overlap between asthma and COPD, and asthma can evolve into COPD.

Studies clearly suggest a true increase in asthma prevalence in the past two to three decades in both children and young adults.

The asthma epidemic

Asthma is a chronic inflammatory disorder of the airways which causes recurrent episodes of wheezing, breathlessness, chest tightness and cough, particularly at night and/or in the early morning. These symptoms are usually associated with widespread but variable airflow limitation that is at least partly reversible either spontaneously or with treatment. The disease is also characterized by recurrent exacerbations often provoked by factors such as allergens, irritants, exercise and virus infections.

Asthma occurs in all races, and its highest prevalence is found in Australia. While genetic factors are of major importance as predisposing factors in the development of atopy (increased allergic response) and probably asthma, present evidence (especially regarding the increasing prevalence of asthma in developing countries all over the world) suggests that environmental rather than racial factors are important in the onset and persistence of asthma. Studies clearly suggest a true increase in asthma prevalence in the past two to three decades in both children and young adults. In children, there is evidence of increased prevalence worldwide. In adults the data are more controversial.

Asthma is more prevalent in children, causes a high morbidity and can be fatal even in young people. The reasons are poorly understood. It may be due to changes in the indoor or outdoor environment and may involve allergens in the air, especially domestic mites and occupational allergens. Climate is of importance because it directly affects the amount of allergen present in the environment, for example, a damp and warm climate favours the growth of mites and moulds. Possibly the increased prevalence of allergy and asthma is due to the synergistic action of air pollution or tobacco smoking with allergic sensitization. Passive smoking has also been involved in the allergic sensitization of children, boys especially, to common allergens in the air. Links with urbanization in some parts of the world have been suggested, as have housing environments, and dietary factors. Socioeconomic status within countries may also be involved because of related problems in obtaining appropriate medical care.

COPD and smoking

The two main symptoms of COPD are breathlessness and cough, sometimes accompanied by wheezing or sputum production. Breathlessness develops gradually over many years and eventually limits daily activities. The chronic cough is very frequently associated with sputum production. The coughing and expectoration of sputum is usually worst in the morning. In contrast with asthma, most patients with COPD do not have nocturnal symptoms. The symptoms and signs of COPD, more frequent in winter, may be worsened by viral or bacterial infection, increased air pollution, cigarette smoking and changes in weather conditions. In COPD, lung function is characterized by progressive airflow limitation.

The prevalence of COPD largely depends on the prevalence of its most important risk factor – cigarette smoking. The disease is highly prevalent in affluent and partly affluent populations worldwide. At least 15% of middle-aged smokers have abnormal lung function, and a chronic cough with phlegm. Evidence suggests only about 25% of cases of COPD are diagnosed. The disease is more common in men than in women, even for the same degree of smoking, but the trend towards increased smoking in women will undoubtedly increase the prevalence of COPD among them.

Respiratory diseases rank among the three principal causes of lost workdays and COPD is responsible for the majority of these. It leads to substantial disability, loss of productivity and reduced quality of life. The disease is almost always progressive, with frequent exacerbations and respiratory failure, resulting in frequent hospitalizations and sometimes death.

Most deaths due to COPD occur in individuals over the age of 65, and rates vary from country to country: in Europe, for example, from 2-41 deaths per 100 000 males per year. Smoking cessation is not associated with any decrease in mortality until at least 10 years after stopping.

Economic and social costs

Chronic nonspecific lung diseases have a high economic and social cost due to their high prevalence, substantial morbidity and mortality and chronicity. It is estimated that asthma is responsible for about 2% of the health care costs in affluent populations. About half of the costs are direct costs including those for long-term treatment of the disease and for hospital care of patients with exacerbations of asthma. The remaining half are indirect costs to society such as loss of productivity in the case of the asthma patient and of relatives who have to care for the patient. The increasing prevalence of the disease and the increasing cost of asthma medications will necessitate the development of national strategies aimed at reducing morbidity and mortality due to asthma in a cost-effective way.

The social and economic burdens of COPD are greater than those of asthma due to its high prevalence and significant morbidity, disability and mortality. The direct cost of managing COPD, which frequently results in hospitalization, is high. The treatment of complications such as respiratory failure (chronic oxygen therapy) is expensive. COPD occurs typically in middle-age and results in loss of productivity either intermittently during exacerbations or permanently because of disability.

Early detection of COPD may increase the success of secondary prevention, including the possibility of pharmacological prevention.

Metabolic disorders

Diabetes mellitus

Diabetes mellitus is one of the most daunting challenges posed today by chronic diseases. Recent data show that approximately 135 million people suffer from diabetes mellitus worldwide, and that this number will rise to almost 300 million by the year 2025. This more than twofold rise is projected to occur because of population ageing, unhealthy diets, obesity and a sedentary lifestyle. While the rise will be of the order of 45% in developed countries, it will be almost 200% in developing countries (*Fig. 7*).

Fig. 7. Diabetes mellitus, regional estimates, 1995–2025

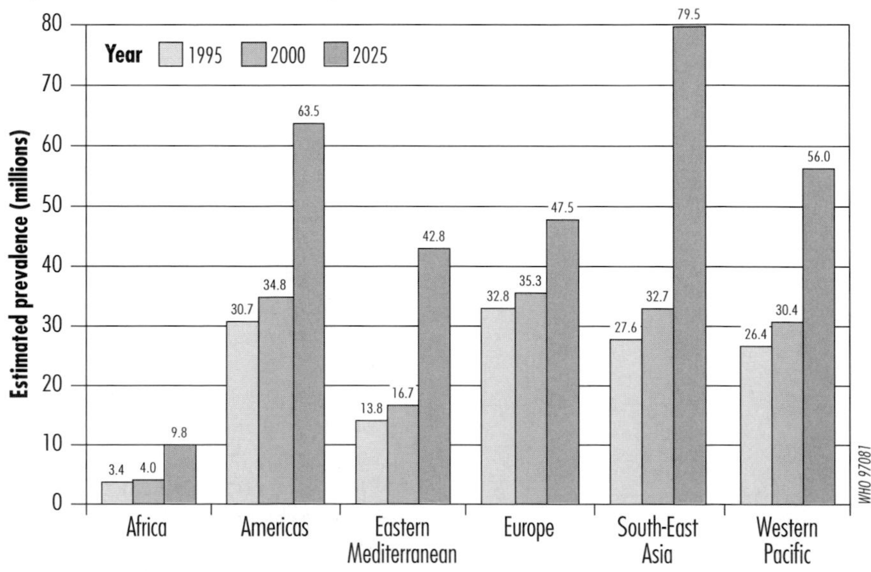

Box 11. The cost of diabetes

Because of its chronic nature, the severity of its complications and the means required to control them, diabetes is a particularly costly disease for the health care services, the affected individual and society. However, costs vary enormously, depending on social, economic and health service factors. A meeting convened by the International Diabetes Federation in December 1996 and cosponsored by WHO reviewed these variations and some of the factors responsible for them. The main purpose of the meeting was to prepare a detailed report on the current situation for the benefit of health planners, programme managers, clinicians and teachers.

Recent estimates suggest that the annual per capita health care cost for persons with diabetes was $13 in Bangladesh (1988), $103 in the United Republic of Tanzania (1990), $104 in Mexico (1992), and as much as $8500 in the United States (1992). These are "cost of illness" estimates, but in order to understand the potential for improvement, and the efficiency of interventions, the cost-effectiveness of alternative prevention and control strategies in different health systems and physical environments should be estimated.

Evidence has accumulated in recent years that improved blood glucose control substantially reduces both the development and progression of some of the more important diabetic complications such as retinopathy, neuropathy and nephropathy. These are major contributors to the morbidity and premature mortality of people with diabetes. Measures which improve blood glucose control are therefore likely to have far-reaching economic benefits in both the short and long term. The cost-effectiveness of such improvements is likely to be greatest in countries which have the least developed health care systems.

Attention has also focused on the involvement of people with diabetes in the management of their own disease and thus on the benefits of patient education, in addition to adequate treatment. National diabetes programmes dealing with these issues (a number of which already exist in all WHO regions) have a central role to play. Such programmes may also form the basis for developing an integrated approach to the control of other chronic diseases.

Because of the relationship between diabetes and increased risk of other diseases, its prevention and treatment are priority issues. Diabetes is closely linked with heart disease, kidney failure and blindness; it adversely affects the outcome of pregnancy and can lead to male impotence. Peripheral vascular disease and neuropathy can give rise to foot lesions which may progress to gangrene and limb amputations, entailing high costs to individuals and to health services (*Box 11*).

Diabetes mellitus is a chronic disease caused by inherited and/or acquired deficiency in the production of insulin by the pancreas, or by ineffectiveness of the insulin produced. Such a deficiency results in increased concentrations of glucose in the blood, and this in turn results in damage to many parts of the body's systems, especially the blood vessels and nerves.

Diabetes mellitus is a hereditary disease. Certain genetic markers are known to increase the risk of developing insulin-dependent diabetes. Such markers have not been described for non-insulin-dependent diabetes, though this form is strongly familial.

There are basically two major forms of diabetes: the insulin-dependent (IDDM) and non-insulin-dependent (NIDDM) forms (these terms are currently under review). In IDDM, the pancreas fails to produce the insulin which is essential for survival. This form develops most frequently in children and adolescents, but is being increasingly recognized later in life.

NIDDM is much more common and accounts for up to 90% of all diabetes cases worldwide. It occurs principally in adults and results from the body's inability to respond properly to the action of insulin produced by the pancreas.

Malnutrition-related diabetes has also been described in some developing countries. It is found in undernourished individuals in some tropical countries. The cause and distribution of this form are still not clearly understood.

The symptoms of diabetes may be pronounced or subdued. In IDDM the classic symptoms are excessive secretion of urine (polyuria), thirst (polydipsia), weight loss and a feeling of lassitude. These symptoms may be less marked in NIDDM; it can also happen that no early symptoms appear in this form and the disease is only diagnosed several years after its onset, when complications are already present.

Insulin was discovered in 1921 and revolutionized the treatment of diabetes and prevention of its complications. It transformed IDDM from a fatal into a treatable disease. Diet, physical exercise and oral hypoglycaemic agents are other important components of treatment.

People with IDDM are totally dependent on daily insulin injections, which for them is a life-saving medication. Although most people suffering from diabetes have the non-insulin-dependent form, up to 30% of them may use insulin injections, some or all of the time to control their condition.

The price of insulin (without syringes and necessary equipment for monitoring blood glucose levels) varies widely internationally, ranging from only a few dollars per vial in some countries to the equivalent of a month's salary in many African countries.

Recent research provides clear evidence of the potential for adequate treatment to delay or even prevent the long-term complications of diabetes, including blindness, kidney failure, heart attacks, and gangrene and amputation of the limbs.

Diabetic retinopathy, which is caused by damage to the small blood vessels in the retina, is the leading cause of blindness and visual disability in adults in economically developed societies. After 15 years of diabetes, approximately 2% of people become blind and about 10% develop severe visual handicap. Loss of vision due to certain types of glaucoma and cataract may also be more common in people with diabetes than in those without the disease.

Loss of vision and blindness in persons with diabetes can be prevented by early detection and treatment of vision-threatening retinopathy: regular eye examinations and timely intervention with laser treatment; or surgery in cases of advanced retinopathy. A recent study has demonstrated that good metabolic control can also delay the onset and progression of diabetic retinopathy. There is evidence that, even in developed countries, many of those in need are not receiving such care due to lack of public and professional awareness. In developing countries, in most of which diabetes is now epidemic, the majority of the population does not have access to such care.

Diabetes is a leading cause of renal failure, the frequency of which varies in different populations and is related to the severity and duration of the disease. Measures to slow down the progress of renal damage include control of hyperglycaemia and of hypertension. Screening and early detection of diabetic kidney disease are an important means of prevention.

Heart disease accounts for 75% of all deaths among people of European origin with diabetes. Risk factors for

Box 12. Diabetes in New Zealand

Studies suggest that diabetes affects 2-5% of all New Zealanders, 5-10% of Maori and 4-8% of Pacific Islands people. The higher prevalence of diabetes in Maori has been known for several decades. A recent survey in South Auckland found the diabetes rate in Maori to be 2.5 times higher than in European New Zealanders. For Pacific Islands people the figure was 1.6. Other studies have yielded similar results. Non-insulin-dependent diabetes mellitus is relatively more common in Maori and Pacific Islands people than in New Zealanders of European origin, while Pacific Islands people appear to have a generally low rate of insulin-dependent diabetes mellitus.

Maori are thus disproportionately affected by diabetes, which is one of many factors contributing to their low health status. A strategy for reducing the impact of diabetes on Maori must be set within the context of making general improvements in their health. Maori health services recognize the importance of family support for the diabetic person. Conversely, the direct threat of diabetes can lead to behaviour changes for the family as well as the individual concerned (healthy food, smoking cessation, exercise and freedom from drugs). Thus, diabetic patients can also be effective educators.

The national organization of Maori diabetes workers is developing a family approach to diabetes care, as well as ensuring that diabetes services are appropriate and safe for Maori. The good relationship between diabetes educators and the community has been one of the most significant factors in achieving long-term changes in the Maori diet .

In New Zealand, diabetes is among the leading causes of hospitalization and death among Pacific Islands people, especially in the age group 44-64. Those affected have high rates of obesity, poor blood glucose control, inadequate knowledge of their condition, inadequate blood glucose monitoring, and poor blood lipid control. They are the least physically active ethnic group and an estimated 75% are overweight. Genetic predisposition and diet are major risk factors. Diabetes is more prevalent in Polynesians than Melanesians, and in those living a modern rather than traditional lifestyle. Dietary changes and physical inactivity have contributed to the rise in diabetes prevalence amongst Pacific Islands people over the last 30 years, both in New Zealand and in the Pacific. In some communities the degree of fat or richness in certain foods is associated with status and prestige, as is large body size. Preventing some modifiable risk factors is thus more difficult.

Maori and Pacific Islands people suffer more diabetic complications than Europeans, including end-stage renal failure, proteinuria, blindness, severe retinopathy, cataracts and foot amputations. Intervention programmes for the prevention of diabetes and its complications must address specific needs of ethnic groups within the population. Similar initiatives with migrant populations overseas have been shown to be effective. Some progress is already being made through local diabetes intervention programmes. Expertise gained from these initiatives, such as the South Auckland Diabetes Project, should be made available to other regions.

heart disease in people with diabetes include cigarette smoking, hypertension, raised blood cholesterol and obesity. Recognition and management of these factors may delay or prevent heart disease in people with diabetes. Premenopausal women with diabetes are more prone to heart disease than those without diabetes.

Diabetic neuropathy, leading to sensory loss and damage to the limbs, is probably the most common complication of diabetes. Studies suggest that at least 50% of people with diabetes are affected to some degree. It is also a major cause of impotence in diabetic men. Major risk factors are the level and duration of hyperglycaemia. Foot care is an important means of reducing the impact of diabetic neuropathy; foot ulceration and amputation is one of the most costly complications of diabetes, resulting from both vascular and neurological disease processes. Diabetes is the most common cause of nontraumatic amputation of the lower limb, which may be prevented by regular inspection and good care of the feet.

Developing countries will bear the brunt of the diabetes epidemics in the 21st century.

Overall, a parallel approach is recommended in strategies for diabetes prevention. Short-term gains may be made by improving health services and the availability of essential medications, blood glucose monitoring and patient education (*Box 12*). An integrated approach to the primary prevention of diabetes and other common, noncommunicable diseases by lifestyle modification and risk factor reduction should be developed as a long-term strategy for containment.

Developing countries will bear the brunt of the diabetes epidemics in the 21st century. National plans and policies for prevention and control will be needed, together with improved availability of essential drugs and materials. Many countries have already begun to move in this direction.

Nutrition-related disorders

Adequate food and nutrition are essential for proper growth and physical development from conception to adulthood, to ensure optimal work capacity and normal reproductive performance, and also to ensure the adequacy of immune mechanisms and resistance to infections.

An inadequate diet produces two main types of metabolic nutritional disorder: protein-energy malnutrition (PEM), and micronutrient disorders (mainly deficiencies).

Nutritional disorders, besides being disease entities, are underlying factors in chronic diseases. Thus, an appropriate diet is also essential to avoid a number of diet-related noncommunicable diseases such as cardiovascular disease, diabetes mellitus, certain forms of cancer and liver disease, and dental caries.

Chronic undernutrition occurs when long-term food consumption is insufficient to cover the requirements for daily energy expenditure. It is usually assessed in terms of body measurements: in adults, thinness; in children, stunting. Acute malnutrition (wasting) occurs when food consumption is suddenly severely reduced.

The causes of chronic undernutrition are multiple and include chronically insufficient food availability or access to food, recurrent infection, and inadequate care, especially of children and mothers. All these factors are common in poorer countries, and in some poor communities in industrialized countries. Poverty and low levels of education are often but not always present. Acute malnutrition occurs particularly, but not exclusively, in emergency conditions, such as warfare or prolonged drought.

The consequences include diminution of body size and work capacity and performance, and enhanced severity of and mortality from infections. Malnutrition has been found to underlie more than half of deaths among children in developing countries.

Global data show no change in overall PEM prevalence in children aged under 5 from 1990 to 1995; but in South Asia and sub-Saharan Africa, there were large increases in the numbers of malnourished children.

Various types of ***micronutrient malnutrition*** are important causes of disability in themselves and often underlie other types of morbidity as outlined below. Their prevalence is even more widespread than that of protein-energy malnutrition.

Anaemia is clinically defined on the basis of the haemoglobin level in the blood. Iron deficiency is present when body iron stores are depleted; this is usually assessed on the basis of serum ferritin levels. Anaemia is a late sign of iron deficiency; about twice as many persons are affected by iron deficiency as are anaemic.

In addition to nutritional anaemias, there are haemolytic, genetically-determined and other types of anaemia. While iron is the nutrient that is usually deficient, deficiencies of folic acid, ascorbic acid, riboflavin and various minerals can contribute to anaemia. Iron deficiency is usually due to inadequate iron intake or absorption. Concurrent factors which may often play a role, particularly in developing countries, include: blood loss (menstruation, childbirth, hookworm disease, schistosomiasis), and haemolysis due to malaria.

Mainly women of reproductive age and children aged under 5 years are affected by iron deficiency, with prevalences of 40-50% in developing countries (over 50% in pregnant women). In industrialized countries about 10% of women, and 17% of pregnant women, are anaemic, and twice as many are iron-deficient. The prevalences are highest in South Asia (80% in some countries). Globally nearly 2 billion people are estimated to be anaemic and 3.6 billion iron-deficient.

In infants and young children even mild anaemia can impair intellectual as well as physical development. In older children and adults it reduces work capacity and output, and also is associated with increased incidence of absenteeism and of accidents at work. Maternal anaemia aggravates the effects of haemorrhage and sepsis during childbirth and is a major contributing cause of maternal mortality; it also increases the incidence of low birth weight, anaemia and protein-energy malnutrition in infants.

Iron deficiency usually is best alleviated by a combination of several approaches, including dietary improvement, iron fortification of food and iron supplementation.

Iodine deficiency disorders (IDD) occur when iodine intakes are less than physiological requirements (about 150 μg daily per person) over a long period, sufficient to produce goitre or other consequences.

The cause of iodine deficiency is usually a chronically inadequate dietary intake because of low iodine content of the soil, common foods and water in a geographical zone. Only sea foods are rich in iodine.

The consequences include goitre (or enlargement of the thyroid gland), and brain damage in the fetus and infant. Iodine deficiency is the most common cause of preventable mental retardation. In severe cases it causes cretinism with severe mental defect, and other problems. It leads to increased rates of abortion, stillbirth, congenital abnormalities, low birth weight and infant mortality. Moderate IDD in early childhood lowers the intelligence quotient by about 10-15 points.

Some 1.5 billion people live in iodine-deficient areas. About 760 million people in 118 countries are affected with goitre, 11 million with cretinism and 43 million with some degree of mental impairment. The highest prevalences are in Africa and the Eastern Mediterranean, but the highest numbers affected are in South-East Asia and the Western Pacific. About 10% of Europeans are also affected (*Map 2*).

Iodine-fortification of salt has been adopted in 110 IDD-affected countries as the major preventive measure, although it is often not yet countrywide or at an adequate level. Remaining actions needed are promoting the iodization of all food-grade salt in countries where this is not already done; ensuring appropriate legislation/regulations for salt iodization in all countries at risk of IDD; constant and systematic monitoring of salt iodine content at the produc-

In infants and young children even mild anaemia can impair intellectual as well as physical development.

Map 2. Iodine deficiency disorders, 1996

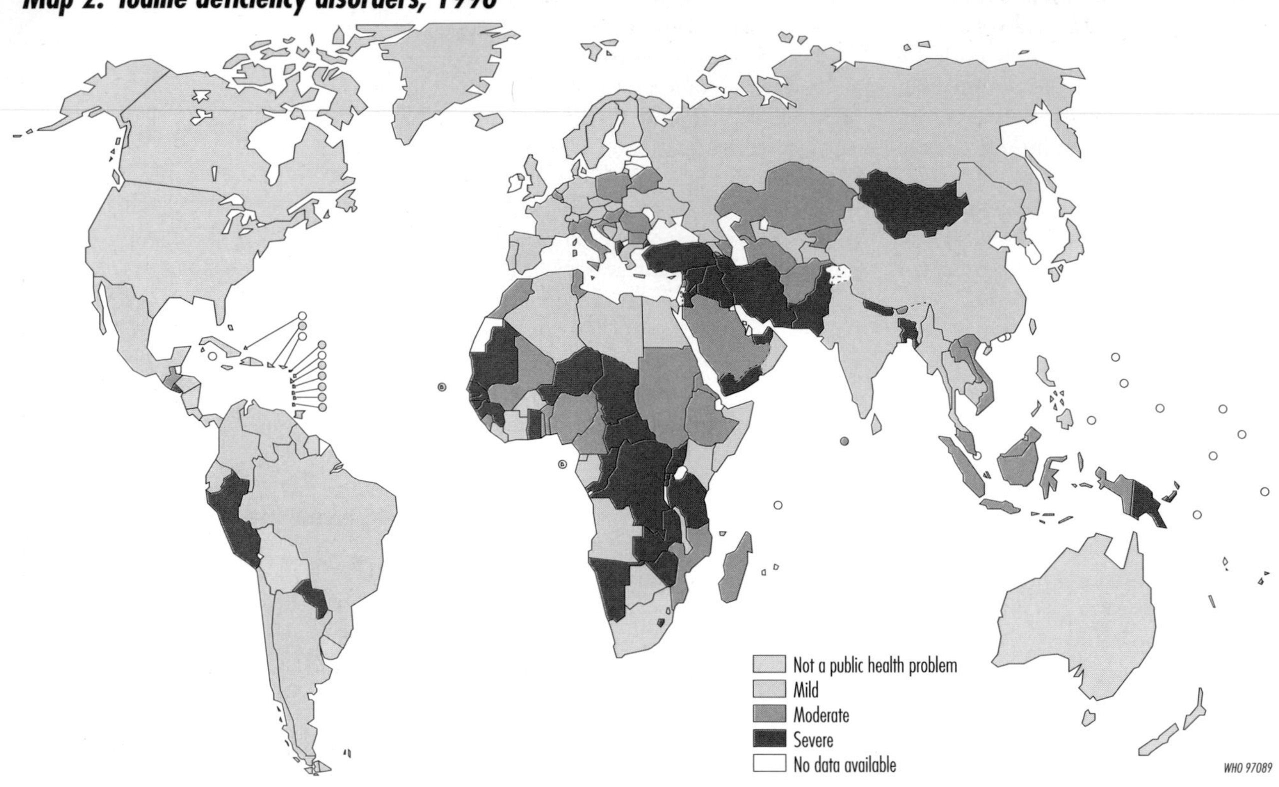

tion, importation, retail-distribution and household levels; regular monitoring of iodine status; and verification of the sustainable elimination of IDD.

The sustainable elimination of IDD as a public health problem by means of this approach may, through current efforts, be attained by the year 2000.

Vitamin A deficiency (VAD) occurs when body stores are depleted to the extent that the physiological functions are impaired.

Depletion occurs when the diet contains, over a long time, too little vitamin A to replace the amount used by tissues or for breast-feeding. Intakes are low when the intake of foods of animal origin is low, and particularly when the consumption of dark green leafy vegetables and orange-coloured vegetables and fruits (the main vegetable sources) is low.

The consequences include night blindness and eventual blinding conditions. VAD is the most common cause of blindness in young children, and can raise young-child mortality rates by 20-30%. It is known that 76 countries have a VAD problem. An estimated 2.8 million children aged under 5 years are clinically affected, and 258 million are subclinically affected. The highest prevalence and numbers are in South-East Asia.

As with iron deficiency, usually a variety of strategies may be needed, including: dietary improvement; fortification of fats or sugar; and supplementation with large doses of vitamin A.

The elimination of this deficiency by the year 2000 was adopted as a goal of the World Declaration on Nutrition.

Vitamin D deficiency and inadequate exposure to sunlight result in rickets in young children, and osteomalacia in adults, which are still widespread in parts of northern Africa and Asia.

Scurvy, beriberi and pellagra occur mainly in emergency conditions, due to deficiencies of ascorbic acid, thiamine and niacin respectively.

Human genetics, hereditary diseases and birth defects

Recent progress in medical research, particularly in molecular genetics, has shown that inherited predisposition plays an important role not merely in well-recognized congenital defects or in hereditary diseases such as haemophilia, but also in common diseases of later life, such as coronary heart disease, high blood pressure, diabetes, some cancers and some musculoskeletal and mental disorders. (*Box 13*). This section deals with some major genetic disorders and congenital abnormalities.

The term "birth defect" is defined as any structural, functional or biochemical abnormality present at birth, whether detected at that time or not, and includes the overlapping categories of genetic disorders and congenital abnormalities. Accurate prevalence data are difficult to collect because of the great diversity of the conditions, and because many that cause early death remain undiagnosed in the absence of specialist services. In typical developed societies, congenital and genetic disorders are the second most common cause of infant death after perinatal factors and of death in children aged 1-4, after accidents.

Although the causes of all birth defects are not known, some can be prevented by making use of past knowledge and recent research breakthroughs. Women can increase their chances of having a healthy baby by taking steps that include the following: adequate nutrition throughout the childbearing years (e.g. rich in vitamins and iodine); avoiding sexually transmitted diseases; being vaccinated against rubella and hepatitis; seeking advice early from qualified health workers; getting early and adequate prenatal care; and during pregnancy, avoiding alcohol and tobacco, and certain medicines (e.g. thalidomide).

Some of these disorders are hereditary diseases. They include ***haemoglobin disorders*** also known as hereditary anaemias, such as thalassaemias and sickle cell disorder. Each year about 300 000 infants are born with major haemoglobin disorders. Almost 70% of cases of sickle cell disorder occur in sub-Saharan Africa. Increasing global migration has introduced the disorder into many areas where it was not originally

Box 13. Chronic diseases: discovering the genetic links

Although the limits of intelligence, physical ability and longevity are genetically determined, external and environmental influences such as infections, malnutrition and war have long been the main determinants of health and survival. Now, with increased control of the environment, genetic make-up is becoming an ever-more important determinant of individual health. Genetic predisposition may lead to the premature onset of common diseases of adult life such as cancer, coronary heart disease, diabetes, hypertension and mental disorders.

The Human Genome Project is an international research venture that aims to draw up a complete map of the sequence of DNA. This research will eventually lead to the identification of every gene linked to susceptibility or resistance to disease.

Cancer. It is not yet certain whether most cancers are hereditary. But a genetic predisposition may be involved in as many as 10-25% of cases of cancer of the breast or colon. Numerous genes are being identified that may affect susceptibility to tumour development. This may lead to a general improvement in the diagnosis and treatment of cancer. For example, a DNA screening test for breast cancer could soon be available. Advice could be offered on the chemoprevention of cancers, tailored for families with different types of cancer risk.

Coronary heart disease. Until recently, it was generally believed that environmental factors alone cause coronary heart disease. But investigating family histories often uncovers genetic risk. Mapping the human genome will make the genetic predisposition to CHD much easier. High blood pressure and high blood cholesterol levels, major risk factors in CHD, are also genetically influenced. A combination of risk detection and lifestyle counselling, with drug treatment, might cut the incidence of heart attacks to the low levels of two or three generations ago.

Diabetes. Evidence for a genetic element in insulin-dependent diabetes mellitus has emerged from studies showing a higher concordance in identical twins (25-30%) than in non-identical twins (5-10%). About 85% of cases of diabetes in developed countries are of the non-insulin-dependent form of the disease, which has a particularly strong familial tendency. Diabetes of all types is an important candidate for future treatments such as gene therapy or pancreatic tissue transplantation.

Mental disorders. Evidence from family and twin studies demonstrates the existence of genetic predisposition to some common mental diseases. Alzheimer disease, the most common form of senile dementia, has a strong familial tendency and is known to be caused by at least four different genes. Research may lead to the development of drugs useful in preventing or delaying the onset of the disease.

Enough is already known about the genetics of common diseases to introduce a family-oriented approach into basic as well as specialist medical practice. A major effort will be made in the foreseeable future to study the genetic factors involved, develop appropriate therapies, and determine how these approaches can best be applied in practice.

Control of hereditary diseases: report of a WHO scientific group. Geneva, WHO, 1996 (Technical report series No. 865).

Among more than 140 million births each year, about 3 million fetuses and infants are born with major congenital malformations.

endemic. In the United States, for example, 10% of the population is at risk.

Haemoglobin disorders can be prevented by testing and counselling. Comprehensive control programmes that combine optimal treatment with a community-based approach to intervention exist in many countries and are successful. In the case of thalassaemia, practically no new births of thalassaemic children now occur in Cyprus or Sardinia, where it used to be a problem. In Greece and mainland Italy, the rate of such births is falling.

Cystic fibrosis is a genetic disease occurring worldwide which affects the respiratory and gastrointestinal tracts and the sweat glands. Incidence ranges from 2.5 to 5 per 10 000 live births in most European populations. The condition is less common in blacks and rare in orientals.

Until a few years ago, life expectancy of children with the disease was below 5 years of age. Now that it is recognized and treated earlier and more effectively, life expectancy in developed countries is about 30 years, and projections for young children alive with cystic fibrosis now suggest that they may live for 40 years or more, even without the development of new treatments. However, up to 95% of cases in Latin America are never diagnosed, and the life expectancy of those that are is only about 10 years.

The gene defect in cystic fibrosis was identified in 1989, since when there has been unprecedented progress in understanding the disease, leading to new approaches to drug treatment and hopes for gene therapy. Such treatments are expected to be available within the lifetime of most current patients, with a corresponding anticipated improvement in outlook.

Haemophilia is a hereditary bleeding disorder affecting 15-20 of every 100 000 males born, with equal incidence in all ethnic groups and geographical areas that have been surveyed. Prevalence, which depends on survival, varies according to available medical care. There are an estimated 420 000 people with haemophilia worldwide.

There are different forms of haemophilia. While the disorder affects males, it is carried by females, who are only occasionally affected, usually mildly. The disorder concerns the absence, decrease or deficient function in sufferers of blood coagulating factors, leading to excessive, prolonged or delayed bleeding. In severe cases it most commonly occurs in the large joints of the limbs.

Unless such bleeding is controlled promptly by infusion of the deficient factor, there is progressive joint disease and muscle atrophy, leading to serious physical, psychological and social handicaps. Until recently, the foremost cause of death was haemorrhage, especially in the skull.

In countries with highly developed haemophilia care programmes, therapy with plasma derivatives has reduced mortality. In the past decade, the main causes of death have stemmed from infections as the side-effects of treatment, including AIDS and liver disease secondary to hepatitis. Survival in patients without these infections is almost the same as that of the general population.

Improvement in haemophilia care worldwide depends on persistence in and support for proven methods of care, on continued research into possible means of cure, such as gene therapy, and on expansion of care to areas of the world where it is inadequate. Whenever possible, the mechanism for providing haemophilia care should be linked with that for sickle cell disease or thalassaemia. This will not only strengthen the control and prevention of these disorders, but will also improve health services generally, including public health, blood transfusion and laboratory services.

Among more than 140 million births each year, about 3 million fetuses and infants are born with major ***congenital malformations***. In recent years, these have become a relatively more important cause of death and morbidity in children as well as the reasons for hospitalization and causes of disability. Despite their significance, however, little progress has been made in determining their cause: the causes of about 70% are still unknown.

Supplements of folic acid before and during pregnancy have been shown to reduce neural tube defects, including spina bifida. Women with chronic diseases which also increase the risk of congenital malformations, such as diabetes, multiple sclerosis and epilepsy, should be under the care of a physician or other adequately trained health care provider.

Outlook

Current trends in the management of genetic diseases are strongly linked with the progress of international human genome research. Genetic technology may soon be used to identify people with genetic risk factors for common diseases. More needs to be known about the bioethical and social implications of genetic testing and the potential for gene therapy.

Musculoskeletal diseases

Musculoskeletal diseases, also often referred to as chronic rheumatic diseases, include about 200 conditions affecting joints, bones, soft tissues and muscles. Together they amount to a huge burden in pain and often crippling disability, and consequently, huge costs in terms of both health care and lost productivity.

Most chronic rheumatic diseases involve all organs and tissues of the body and require expert diagnosis. Well-established, standardized epidemiological criteria for use in the study of their global prevalence are lacking. Only a few of these diseases have been thoroughly investigated.

The most prevalent of these conditions are inflammatory joint diseases – rheumatoid arthritis and ankylosing spondylitis; gout; osteoarthritis; connective tissue disease; non-articular disorders, such as back pain and soft tissue rheumatism; and bone disease, particularly osteoporosis. This section concentrates on osteoarthritis, rheumatoid arthritis, osteoporosis and low back pain.

The prevalence of major rheumatic diseases in adults ranges from 24% in China and Indonesia to 45% in Chile. Although prevalence is best documented in industrialized countries, it is likely to be the same or even higher in developing countries. For example, these diseases are the most common cause of disability in the United Kingdom, accounting for 44% of all such disability in the elderly; and are estimated to cost $60 billion a year in the United States, where about a third of all adults are affected.

Osteoarthritis, also known as osteoarthrosis or degenerative joint disease, is the oldest disease known to have affected humans, and has emerged as the most common and important form of joint disease in almost all populations studied. It is strongly age-related. With ageing populations, severe osteoarthritis of the hip and knee joints has become an increasingly important burden on health services. It is rare in the knee before age 35 years, but 20-40% of people over the age of 70 years are affected; the hip is less commonly affected than the knee.

Osteoarthritis of the knee is predominantly a disease of women and is strongly related to age and associated with previous trauma. The other main risk factor is obesity. Osteoarthritis of the hip predominantly affects men. Some congenital/developmental bone and joint disorders lead to osteoarthritis of the hip in later life. Prior inflammatory joint disease could also be a risk factor; others may include joint usage, diabetes mellitus, and hysterectomy.

Medical management aims to reduce pain and maintain optimum function. Surgery is used to treat joints that are grossly damaged and causing severe pain. Hip replacement is well established as the best treatment for a badly damaged hip joint. Knee surgery includes osteotomy, which can promote healing, as well as joint replacement. Almost 80% of osteoarthritis patients have some form of limitation of movement, and a quarter cannot perform the activities of daily living.

Rheumatoid arthritis usually starts in early adulthood or middle age, but can also develop in children, and affects two to three times more women than men.

Genetic technology may soon be used to identify people with genetic risk factors for common diseases.

Given that osteoporotic fractures are most common in the elderly, the influence of increasing life expectancy on the number and regional distribution of hip fractures will be dramatic.

It is an autoimmune disorder, that is, body tissues are attacked by their own immune system, which has been disturbed in some way. The condition causes painful inflammation or even destruction of joints. So-called rheumatoid juvenile arthritis is a major cause of disability in children and is more common in girls than boys; seven forms of this disease have been classified.

Treatment for rheumatoid arthritis includes nonsteroidal anti-inflammatory drugs, immunosuppressant drugs, physiotherapy and surgery.

Osteoporosis and associated fractures are a major cause of death, illness and disability, and a cause of huge medical expense worldwide. Bone fractures are the main complication of osteoporosis. The lifetime risks for osteoporotic fractures in women are at least 30% and probably closer to 40%. In men the risk is 13%. The incidence is higher in women than men and higher in Caucasian populations than others. Even among white populations, however, rates vary by geographical region – hip fracture rates are higher in the Nordic countries, for example, than in North America or Oceania, and lower in the countries of southern Europe.

The reason for these regional differences is unclear. The race and sex differences are partly explained by the heritability of skeletal size. Bone mass is greatest in those of African heritage, who have the lowest fracture rate, and is least in Caucasian women of northern European extraction, who have the highest fracture rate. Differences in bone mass might also relate to regional patterns of diet and exercise.

Given that osteoporotic fractures are most common in the elderly, the influence of increasing life expectancy on the number and regional distribution of hip fractures will be dramatic. Worldwide, it is estimated that the number of hip fractures could rise from 1.7 million in 1990 to 6.3 million by 2050.

Lifestyle factors are also associated with the development of osteoporosis (diet, physical activity, smoking), opening a perspective for primary prevention.

The primary aim is to prevent fractures: this may be achieved by increasing bone mass at maturity, by preventing subsequent bone loss or by restoring the bone mineral. Lifestyle modifications could be of great importance. To prevent osteoporosis, hormone therapy is used generally, especially in women at the menopause.

Low back pain blights the lives of many millions, and afflicts almost everyone at least once. It accounts for much absenteeism from work and impaired quality of life. It is self-limiting regardless of therapeutic approach, and no specific therapy has been satisfactorily validated.

Mental and neurological disorders

In recent decades, scientific research has considerably extended knowledge of the functions of the human brain, and of mental and neurological illnesses. Many disorders whose origins were mysterious can now be investigated, using painless, noninvasive methods. Some of these conditions can now be treated either with well-tested and effective drugs (e.g. drugs for anxiety, depression, schizophrenia or epilepsy) or with a wide range of other psychiatric and psychological tools.

Nevertheless, mental and neurological illnesses continue to account for a significant proportion of disability due to disease – larger, for instance, than hypertension, arthritis and diabetes combined. They impose a heavy burden of human suffering on individuals and their families, and have enormous direct and indirect financial costs.

Their impact on society is likely to become more and more profound in future years. Already, many hundreds of millions of people worldwide are affected by some form of mental disorder, from the relatively minor to the incurable and life-threatening; many individuals suffer from several simultaneously.

There are an estimated 400 million cases of anxiety disorders and 340 million of mood disorders. Estimates of people with mental retardation range as high as 60 million; there may be as many as 29 million people with dementia, and 45 million with schizophrenia. One of the most common neurological disorders is epilepsy (40 million). In addition stroke, which should be regarded as a neurological as well as a circulatory condition, kills more than 4.6 million people a year and disables many millions more.

Different types of substance abuse have a major impact on both mental health and public health in general. About 120 million people are dependent on alcohol. Most of the world's 1.1 billion smokers are probably dependent on nicotine. There are an estimated 28 million drug users.

The serious challenges ahead include improving mental health care at the primary level, including neuropsychiatric care, essential drugs and essential psychosocial interventions.

Community participation and support need to be promoted in providing non-institutional care, especially for the elderly. The psychological causes of violence and suicide need to be better understood and dealt with. The healthy growth and development of children, particularly as regards brain functions, should be encouraged. A set of global activities should be developed for the prevention of mental disorders, and the improvement of mental health care, focusing on reducing both individual suffering and the overall prevalence of mental disorders. The best and most widespread use must be made of the knowledge and technology currently available for dealing with schizophrenia, depression, sleep disorders, epilepsy, dementia, mental retardation and substance abuse. Good practice and ethical standards should be promoted in this area which fully take into account the rights of people with mental disorders.

Schizophrenia

It is estimated that approximately 45 million people are affected by schizophrenia worldwide. An increase in its prevalence is expected, largely as a result of demographic changes, with an increase in the proportion of the population moving into the age range at risk. Relatively greater numbers of the population will be in their twenties and beyond.

Schizophrenia is a disorder affecting mostly young people around the age of 20. It is characterized by distorted thinking, perception and judgement. In approximately a quarter to a third of cases, the outcome is complete recovery from an episode which may last just a few months. In the majority of cases however, the disease becomes chronic, lasting for the rest of the person's life, either being continuous or with episodes between which the person may be less affected or even normal. The sexes are almost equally affected but the onset tends to be a little later in women. The condition is very disabling and it is difficult for those affected to lead a normal life.

Given the chronic nature of schizophrenia, in addition to its frequently disturbing symptoms, the disease represents a burden not only for the sufferers, but also for their families. Social rejection and discrimination often reinforce a spontaneous tendency to withdraw, which is observed in most people affected by schizophrenia.

The causes of schizophrenia are not known, probably because this label covers a group of related disorders, each having a different, specific cause. Vulnerability to schizophrenia may be partly inherited. Scientific advances in recent decades have led to a much better understanding of the way that the brain is affected in schizophrenia, and it is now known that some kind of disturbance associated with one of the natural chemical transmitters in the brain (dopamine) is linked to the disorder.

The introduction of neuroleptics (e.g. chlorpromazine) in the early 1950s was a major breakthrough in the treatment of schizophrenia. These medicines, if taken every day, greatly reduce the symptoms, often allowing the patient to function well in the community, with many fewer episodes of disorder. In view of the great family involvement and disruption that schizophrenia

Estimates of people with mental retardation range as high as 60 million; there may be as many as 29 million people with dementia, and 22 million with schizophrenia.

Many people with schizophrenia unnecessarily remain in or return to mental hospitals, with a great deal of personal suffering and at huge costs to health budgets.

involves, psychoeducational interventions aimed at patients' families have been proposed and implemented and have been shown to reduce relapse rates, when combined with the appropriate pharmacological management.

Despite the affordability, simplicity and cost-effectiveness of the pharmacological and psychoeducational approach, it is not, unfortunately, widely practised. In many developing countries the supply of essential drugs (including medications for schizophrenia) cannot always be maintained. The introduction of psychoeducational programmes alongside the pharmacological one as a routine procedure for the management of schizophrenia has been very slow even in developed countries.

As a consequence, many people with schizophrenia unnecessarily remain in or return to mental hospitals, with a great deal of personal suffering and at huge costs to health budgets. This situation could be reversed, in the short term, with appropriate supplies of essential drugs for the treatment of schizophrenia and with the widespread introduction of psychoeducational programmes for families affected by schizophrenia. There is good evidence that this approach is feasible within the primary health care strategy.

Dementia

The ageing of the global population will inevitably result in huge increases in the number of cases of dementia, of which the incurable Alzheimer disease is the most common form. The other major type of dementia is cerebrovascular dementia, which is related to stroke. Less commonly, dementia occurs in other brain diseases such as Parkinson disease, Creutzfeldt-Jakob disease and AIDS. Already, around 29 million people worldwide are estimated to suffer from dementia, and the risk of developing the condition rises steeply with age in people over 60 years, to as much as 25% in people aged 90 or over. Alzheimer disease is likely to become one of the leading causes of disability in the elderly worldwide. Africa, Asia and Latin America between them could have more than 80 million people with senile dementia in the year 2025.

For some diseases causing dementia (Alzheimer disease, for instance) a genetic factor has been identified as contributing to its cause, whereas for others (such as vascular dementia) characteristics of lifestyle (such as excessive alcohol use or a diet which contributes to hypertension) are major predisposing factors.

Alzheimer disease is a brain disorder characterized by a progressive dementia that occurs later in life, but occasionally occurs earlier. It involves the decline of memory and other cognitive functions such as comprehension, learning capacity, language and judgement, as well as the ability to think and calculate. Forgetfulness, a symptom in the early stages, and often a part of normal ageing, is overtaken gradually by severe memory loss, especially of recent events, confusion about time and place, and mood and personality changes.

The possibilities for prevention of Alzheimer disease are extremely limited because the major determinants – age and family history – cannot be modified. Vascular dementias are, however, amenable to prevention through the modification of factors associated with vascular disease in general, for example, control of hypertension.

Electroencephalograms reveal slowing of the electrical impulses in the brain, and other types of hospital scanning show evidence of reduced brain size.

Most cases are diagnosed from an examination of the patient's mental state. The disease can be definitely diagnosed by biopsy – removal of a sample of brain tissue for microscopic analysis – or by postmortem examination.

Some important advances have occurred in recent decades in understanding the brain changes that take place in dementia. However, an effective treatment for Alzheimer disease has yet to be found. Vascular dementia, on the other hand, can be prevented or slowed down by treatments that reduce the risk of stroke. Research is continuing into drug treatment to restore brain chemicals, particularly acetylcholine, which are depleted in Alzheimer disease, and important advances are being made, but such treatments only temporarily improve symptoms and do not stop the progress of the disease.

The management of dementia is based on long-term care, preferably at home, with support from a community-based health care team, which also provides continuity of care. Admission to hospital or a special home should be envisaged only when the disease is so advanced that specialized care is necessary on a more or less continuous basis, or when family care cannot be provided.

The objectives of treatment for people with dementia include general attention to their health, improving quality of life, minimizing disability and preserving autonomy. Too often, an elderly person's mental deterioration is considered to be part of an inevitable decline. In many cases, however, it is due to, or at least aggravated by, a treatable physical or mental disease or the inappropriate use of drugs, especially sedatives and tranquillizers. Proper treatment sometimes leads to a dramatic restoration of function in people who were considered "lost".

Living with and caring for a person with dementia can be very burdensome and caregivers are at a high risk of becoming exhausted (i.e. of suffering from "burn-out"). The needs of these carers should be kept in mind when planning services for people with dementia.

Depending on their general health, their age at the onset of the disease and the quality of the care that they receive, Alzheimer sufferers may survive for 10 years or more.

The biological complexity of the disease and restricted understanding of its causes limits hopes that drugs specifically designed to treat it will be forthcoming in the near future, and the best prospect may be treatments that delay its onset.

More women than men suffer from Alzheimer disease, given that in general they outlive men. Women account for more than 70% of the chronically mentally ill in nursing homes, where those exist, and these women are likely to be widowed. Compared with some other groups, elderly women in general have a greater need for health care, social welfare and economic support; this is especially true of those with Alzheimer disease.

Mood disorders

Mood disorders are estimated to affect some 340 million people in the world at any given time. At least 10% of people using primary health care services suffer from depression at the time of the visit. However, the main complaint may not immediately be perceived as related to depression or indeed may not be related to depression. In 1990, depression was estimated to rank fourth in terms of the burden caused by diseases in developing countries. It is likely to be first by the year 2020. In the United States alone, the yearly cost of depression is estimated at $44 billion, equal to the total cost of all cardiovascular diseases.

The fundamental disturbance in mood disorders is usually towards depression (with or without anxiety) and/or occasionally towards elation. This mood change is normally accompanied by a change in the person's level of activity, and in depression there is often a loss of interest and enjoyment, reduced energy, ideas of guilt and unworthiness, a bleak and pessimistic view of the future, and disturbed sleep and appetite. Suicide is an ever-present risk. Most of these disorders tend to be recurrent and the onset of individual episodes is often related to stressful events or situations. They affect all age groups, including children and adolescents. About twice as many women as men are affected by depression.

Effective drugs to treat depression have been developed over the last 40 years, as have useful psychotherapeutic approaches over the last 20 years. These treatments can be implemented within primary health care settings, but unfortunately are not always available to people in need, particularly in developing countries. This is mainly due to the

Living with and caring for a person with dementia can be very burdensome and caregivers are at a high risk of becoming exhausted.

absence of a regular supply of essential drugs and to a lack of appropriate training for health personnel.

With appropriate training of health personnel (particularly general physicians and other general health care staff) and the availability of essential drugs, individual suffering and social and economic losses due to depression can be dramatically reduced.

Anxiety disorders

As many as 400 million people at any one time are affected by one form or another of anxiety disorders, a group of mental disorders which can produce a considerable degree of disability. Among them are generalized anxiety disorder, obsessive-compulsive disorder, phobic disorders, panic disorder, acute stress reaction, dissociative disorders and somatoform disorders. Although they differ in their symptoms, their common trait is an abnormally high level of anxiety. Unless appropriately treated, they have a tendency to run a chronic course and in some instances can be disabling and can last a lifetime. Not uncommonly, these disorders occur in association with depressive disorders.

Although the potential for prevention of anxiety disorders is low, there are a few very effective treatment approaches for them, including psychotherapy, pharmacological treatments and psychosocial interventions. These approaches can considerably shorten the duration of these otherwise long-lasting disorders.

Epilepsy

More than 40 million people worldwide suffer from different types of epilepsy.

It is a recurrent condition characterized by fits (seizures) during which there are usually loss of consciousness and convulsions, or brief movements or sensations that start suddenly and stop abruptly with or without loss of consciousness. Some of these movements may look like bizarre behaviour. Although each fit lasts for only a few minutes, fits occur repeatedly, sometimes more than once a day, but sometimes as infrequently as once a month or less.

Epilepsy may be caused by genetic factors, infectious diseases in the prenatal period, by birth asphyxia and brain injury during labour, and in the postnatal period by infections (e.g. meningitis, encephalitis), parasitic diseases (e.g. malaria, schistosomiasis) or brain damage induced by alcohol, trauma or toxic substances (e.g. lead, pesticides).

People affected by epilepsy are frequently highly stigmatized, often because the condition is wrongly perceived as a contagious disease or as a result of sins and the misdeeds of the affected person or of his or her ancestors. Not infrequently, the affected people and their relatives are shunned to the point of isolation. Children with the disease are often kept away from school for absolutely no medical reason.

Some epilepsy can be prevented using simple methods such as proper prenatal care, safe delivery, control of fever in children, reduction of brain injury and control of infectious and parasitic diseases (e.g. through sanitation, immunization and appropriate treatment).

More than 80% of newly diagnosed cases of epilepsy can now be successfully treated and controlled with antiepileptic drugs.

More than 80% of newly diagnosed cases of epilepsy can now be successfully treated and controlled with antiepileptic drugs. These need to be taken every day, sometimes for life. Where the medication is effective the person can lead a normal life. In many cases, medication which can be provided even at the primary health care level is very effective for as many as 50% of sufferers and need cost only $6 per patient per year. Unfortunately, in many countries, a large proportion of those affected are improperly treated or not treated at all, mainly because of the unavailability of essential drugs, inadequate training of health personnel and misinformation of the general public.

While an occasional fit need not be markedly disabling, the stigma and consequent handicap of being known to be "an epileptic" imposes an enormous burden. Showing that fits are reduced (or even disappear altogether) with medication, coupled with public information to destigmatize the condition, can lead to a marked improvement in the lives of those affected.

Post-traumatic stress disorder

Post-traumatic stress disorder occurs after a catastrophic or other severely disturbing experience and persists long after that event, and can interfere with day-to-day functioning. Typical symptoms include flashbacks and disturbing dreams of the traumatic event, and efforts to avoid activities and situations that can reawaken painful memories.

The disorder is common among victims of man-made and natural disasters, military activities affecting both service personnel and civilians, violence, ethnic cleansing, rape, genocide, torture and repression.

Until fairly recently, most health sector attention was focused on the physical injuries and illnesses resulting from such traumatic incidents. There is now increasing recognition of the psychological harm that is also suffered, and psychological counselling for sufferers of post-traumatic stress disorders has been established in a number of countries.

Tobacco, alcohol and psychoactive drug dependence

The use of alcohol, illicit drugs and other psychoactive substances causes at least 123 000 deaths annually. Each year tobacco causes about 3 million deaths, mainly from lung cancer and circulatory diseases.

Alcohol-dependence syndrome is estimated to affect 120 million people. Alcohol is also implicated in a range of social problems including crime, violence (particularly against women and children), marital breakdown and major losses in industrial productivity.

The global trend among those dependent on drugs is towards the use of multiple ***psychoactive substances*** , with people moving from one substance to another, and using drugs in various combinations. Amfetamines or other psychostimulant drugs are increasingly used in every region of the world (*Box 14*). In many countries the use of amfetamine is more widespread than that of cocaine and heroin combined. It is likely that public health consequences, particularly intoxication, poisoning and overdoses will increase as these new combinations of substances are used.

Box 14. Substance abuse: the example of amfetamines

Amfetamines and other similar psychostimulants are used in every region of the world, and pose serious health and social problems. In many countries, amfetamine abuse, particularly among young people, is already more widespread than cocaine and heroin abuse combined. To make matters worse, the rate of spread is outpacing scientific knowledge of the health risks and of other associated problems. These may include psychiatric and neurological disorders (irritability, anxiety and apprehension), cardiac arrhythmias (rapid or irregular heartbeats), high blood pressure, liver damage and fatal overdose. When these drugs are injected, there is a risk of transmitting HIV and other viruses, such as the viruses of hepatitis B and C. Gaps in knowledge are a major obstacle to prevention, treatment and policy responses.

These drugs often have longer-lasting effects than, for example, cocaine. Because they increase endurance and delay sleep, and give a sense of added energy or euphoria, the consumption of some of them, such as MDMA ("ecstasy"), has become an established part of the all-night parties of youth culture in many countries. They and other drugs are also consumed by some groups of workers, such as long-distance truck drivers and others who work through the night or seek greater alertness.

Globally, the production and trafficking of illicit psychostimulants have increased dramatically over the last 20 years. Their production is relatively simple, and the chemicals used in their manufacture are cheap and freely available in most countries. The "licit" market for amfetamine-type stimulants is also significant, although it accounts for less than 1% of the world pharmaceutical market. In the United States alone, such a market is worth over $100 million a year. The legitimate medical use of amfetamines has declined in recent years, but overprescribing of them continues in many countries.

Some psychostimulants are of particular concern in certain countries. Methamfetamine, sometimes known as "ice", poses a significant public health threat in Japan, the Philippines, the Republic of Korea, Thailand and the United States. In some cities of the United States its use is believed to result in more deaths than the use of heroin or cocaine. Previously rare in Europe, its manufacture and use are now increasing in some central and eastern European countries, such as the Czech Republic.

To tackle the problem and help governments formulate policy responses, WHO convened in November 1996 the first-ever global scientific meeting on the health and social implications of amfetamine abuse. This meeting, attended by experts from 14 countries and observers from 11 international organizations, produced a state-of-the-art review of the nature, extent, context and public health consequences of psychostimulant use.

This is being followed by specific studies that will help identify and test policy approaches based on promising prevention and treatment initiatives in different cultural settings.

The identification of genetic markers for alcohol dependence could have a major impact on prevention and treatment.

In many countries drug injection is becoming increasingly common, and associated with this is the sharing of injecting equipment, which carries the risk of spreading of HIV/AIDS, hepatitis B and C, and other bloodborne infections. At least 28 million people worldwide incur a significant risk to their health as a result of using psychoactive substances other than alcohol, tobacco and volatile solvents. It is estimated that about one-third of them inject drugs.

In both developed and developing countries, the intentional inhalation of volatile solvents is an increasing problem, especially in marginalized groups such as street children and indigenous young people. These substances may cause neurological and psychological dysfunction, liver and kidney damage and sudden death.

Public health responses to psychoactive substance abuse need to reflect the fact that these substances present different grades of health risk. Levels of harm can be minimized through primary prevention including educational approaches. Persons whose problems related to drug use have been diagnosed at an early stage may be susceptible to brief interventions for reducing their individual risk and the potential risk to others.

The seriousness of health problems caused by ***tobacco*** warrants serious attention if the current epidemic of tobacco-related mortality and morbidity is to be reduced. While the health implications of tobacco use are largely individual and physical, the ramifications of premature mortality and morbidity are felt by families, communities and society at large.

Benefits to the individual patient with alcohol-related problems will also serve the health and welfare of family, friends, workmates and innocent bystanders who suffer third-party injury as a consequence of ***alcohol*** misuse. The cost of alcohol-related harm is estimated to account for 2-3% of GNP in many European countries.

Genetic traits may lead some individuals to experience alcohol in a different way, or render them more susceptible to dependence. The identification of genetic markers could have a major impact on prevention and treatment, and may also predict an individual's likelihood of suffering various physical consequences such as hepatic cirrhosis. The relationship between alcohol dependence and other psychiatric conditions such as depression, anxiety and eating disorders is currently being studied. New techniques of neuroscience investigation are improving understanding of the effect of alcohol on neurotransmitter and receptor systems in the brain, and research into drugs which will influence this process is under way. Although in many parts of the world, women either abstain from alcohol or drink very little, this situation is changing rapidly, and the consequences of increasing consumption by women need to be investigated.

Detection of hazardous drinking in primary care and early intervention have proved both effective and low-cost, in both developing and developed countries, and this is one of the most promising areas for secondary prevention of alcohol-related problems, although such simple interventions are insufficient for those patients who are more damaged, or have an established dependence. A recent study has shown the importance of the attitude and skill of the individual therapist, and has revealed that most patients with alcohol problems can be helped on an outpatient basis, with residential care needed for only a minority of the most affected individuals. Self-help groups are very effective in facilitating recovery from alcohol problems, but they need to be introduced in a way that is culturally appropriate. Most individuals who are physically dependent can be detoxified at home provided suitable supervision is available, with family involvement enhancing outcome.

Educational interventions directed towards children and the general population have been of unproven benefit, and the search for more effective methods continues, for example by focusing on particular at-risk groups such as pregnant women. Other approaches include local community action aimed at creating environments which reduce the demand for alcohol and promoting alternatives to alcohol as a focus for leisure pursuits, particularly for young people. Reducing the drink-driving limit and the introduction of random breath testing can be beneficial, with the likelihood of detection being a key factor in determining efficacy. Introducing successful alcohol control policies is a major challenge in developing countries and eastern Europe, where the commercialization of alcohol production and expanding international trade are important influences.

Living with risk and associated ill-health

Even in the absence of disease, human life is frequently put at risk, whether by accident or design. Wars, conflicts and violence between individuals date as far back in history as the oldest recorded diseases, and are at least as difficult to eradicate, if not more so. Technological advances, particularly in industry and transport, bring with them new dangers to human health, both in the workplace and in transport systems.

This section covers violence, including homicide and suicide. It also examines occupational health hazards, in terms of both injury and disease.

Violence

Violence in all its forms has increased dramatically worldwide in recent decades. Apart from civil conflict and war, violence can be interpersonal, self-directed, physical, sexual and mental, and its burden is disproportionately borne by young people and women. During 1993, at least 4 million deaths (8% of the total) resulted from unintentional or intentional injury, including 300 000 murders. Of the violent deaths, some 3 million were in the developing world.

Like other diseases, violence has its own risk factors. These include serious family problems, shortcomings in education, academic failure, idleness, alcohol and drug abuse, which predispose people to violence. Poverty, insecure living conditions, weakness and physical or mental handicap are among the factors which mark out the victims.

Target groups of violence can be grouped in the following ways:

By sex. Almost everywhere, women are the victims of violence ranging from sexual abuse to social and economic disadvantage.

By age. Children (and girls more than boys); adolescents, who are often the agents and the victims of their own risk-taking; and old people, especially elderly women living alone.

By social position. The homeless, the unemployed, the underclass, whether they be street children, adults of no fixed abode, groups regarded as deviant (e.g. homosexuals), migrants, refugees or members of ethnic minorities.

By state of health. The chronically ill, the physically and mentally disabled.

For economic and/or political reasons. Victims of war, the wounded and displaced; the poor and the indigent.

Homicide

In many developing and developed countries, 20-40% of deaths in males aged 15-34 are from homicide or suicide. In some countries, the figure can be over 70%, and the homicide rates in the 15-34 age group have more than doubled in the last five years.

In Latin America and the Caribbean, violence has become endemic. In 1993, 456 000 violent deaths were recorded, averaging 1250 a day. In half the countries of the region, homicide is the second leading cause of death in people aged 15-24.

In the United States, an average of 65 people are killed each day and over 6000 wounded in acts of interpersonal violence. During the 1980s in that country, more than 200 000 people died as a result of violence, and 20 million more suffered nonfatal injuries. The lifetime chance of becoming a homicide victim in the United States is approximately 1 in 240 for whites and 1 in 45 for blacks and other ethnic minorities. Homicide is the leading cause of death among

Technological advances, particularly in industry and transport, bring with them new dangers to human health, both in the workplace and in transport systems.

African American males aged 15-34. The death rate due to murder for all ages increased in the United States by 44% between 1968 and 1985.

Suicide

Suicide is an act, deliberately initiated and performed by an individual in the knowledge or expectation that it will result in a fatal outcome. It should be differentiated from a suicide attempt, or parasuicide, which is an act of deliberate self-harm, not necessarily intended to result in death.

In addition to the more than 800 000 deaths from suicide recorded every year around the world, an unknown number are not recorded for religious, cultural or other reasons. Experts believe that many deaths attributed to accidents are, in reality, disguised suicides. Nevertheless, it is likely that certain cultural pressures strongly influence the rate of suicide, with the highest rates being some 10 times the lowest.

Suicide is more frequent among men and increases in direct relationship with age. Thus the group at highest risk is men above the age of 65 years who live alone. Recently, however, an increase in suicide rates of young people (both men and women) has been observed. Suicide is closely associated with some mental disorders, particularly depression, personality disorders, substance abuse and schizophrenia.

Suicide rates can be considerably reduced by appropriate preventive measures. A few interventions have demonstrated their efficacy, among which are treatment of psychiatric patients at risk, gun-possession control, detoxification of domestic gas and of car emissions, control of toxic substances and the toning down of reports on suicide in the press. Concerted action involving many sectors, in addition to the health sector, is needed.

Violence against children

Violence against children can be in the form of physical abuse, sexual abuse, emotional abuse and neglect. These are worldwide problems, the dimensions and consequences of which are only beginning to be understood. There is a lack of epidemiological data. Studies suggest that the rate of presumed child abuse and neglect in children under 5 years could be between 13 and 20 per 100 000 live births. Child abuse deaths are considered rare events; studies estimate the presumed child abuse mortality rates for infants in most countries at around 6 per 100 000 live births. Surveys of adults in several industrialized countries suggest that 10-15% of children are victims of sexual abuse. The majority are girls.

In some countries, domestic violence is the leading cause of injury among women of childbearing age.

Violence against women

Gender violence is a universal plague, grossly underreported. In some countries, domestic violence is the leading cause of injury among women of child-bearing age; up to 35% of women's visits to emergency treatment centres are for that reason. Studies in selected countries indicate that violence against women is an important cause of morbidity and mortality throughout their life span.

Such violence takes numerous forms, only a few of which are sexual abuse, rape, physical assault and genital mutilation. Women are exposed to violence in the home, where the assailant is either related or known to them; in outside settings where they may be victims of random violence by people unknown to them; they are vulnerable to large-scale systematic violence in situations of conflict and mass movements of people. Studies show that the prevalence of violence against pregnant women ranges from 7% to 20%, and that such violence is more common than many other conditions routinely screened for during pregnancy.

Occupational risks

The figures seem like the casualties of a major war: over 200 000 killed, over 120 million injured. However, these losses occur not on a battlefield but in the workplace. They represent the annual number of occupational deaths and injuries worldwide. Even so, they are only part of the much wider impact of health hazards at work. To a large extent these are involuntarily imposed risks which the worker simply has to face in order to make a living.

Occupational risks become evident in two main ways. First, there may be an association of a particular occupation with a disease which appears among its workers to an extent greater than would normally be expected, when allowance has been made for age and other non-work factors. Second, a worker is exposed to some risk of injury from the unexpected release of energy (mechanical, chemical, electrical, radioactive and so on), which accounts for "accidents".

For an occupational injury to occur, a hazard has to exist in association with a particular pattern of worker behaviour. A worker whose performance is impaired by fatigue, alcohol or inexperience is more likely to be injured. Overall, injury rates are highest among males in their late teens and lowest in the middle years. They tend to rise again among older workers. Female employees generally have lower rates of death and injury than their male counterparts, although the differences are small in some industries.

Estimates suggest that there are up to 160 million cases a year of occupational diseases, of which 30-40% may lead to chronic disease, and about 10% to permanent work disability. These are largely "silent" epidemics, as most occupational diseases and injuries go undiagnosed and unreported.

The many hazards of the work environment include exposure to chemical and biological agents, and adverse factors which can be ergonomic, psychological or psychosocial. Workers in the chemical industry are exposed to a rather special set of risks, and injurious events often manifest themselves in the form of an illness a long time after exposure.

About 100 000 different ***chemicals*** are in use in modern work environments, and the number is growing constantly. They often affect the immune system, leading to dermal and respiratory allergies, and may increase susceptibility to cancers and to infections such as those of the gastrointestinal, urinary and female genital tracts, and of the respiratory system. Other known consequences include metal (e.g. lead) and pesticide poisoning, solvent damage to the central nervous system and liver, and reproductive disorders. Around 850 chemicals used in industry, agriculture and forestry are neurotoxic.

Some 200 ***biological agents*** present in the workplace include viruses, bacteria, parasites, fungi, moulds and organic dusts. They are estimated to be a risk for 15% of workers in industrialized countries. Hepatitis B and C and tuberculosis infections (particularly among health care workers), asthmas (among persons exposed to organic dusts) and chronic parasitic diseases (particularly among agricultural and forestry workers) are the most common occupational diseases resulting from such exposures.

There are about 3000 allergenic factors in our environment, most of them occurring as workplace exposures. Allergic dermatoses are among the most prevalent occupational diseases, with the respiratory tract, followed by the skin surface, being the most important route for hazardous agents to enter the body.

Physical factors such as noise, vibration, ionizing and non-ionizing radiation and microclimatic conditions affect up to 40% of the workforce in industrialized countries and up to 80% in developing and newly industrialized ones. Noise-induced hearing loss has been found to be one of the most prevalent occupational diseases in both developing and industrialized countries. Computers and other video display terminals are now an integral part of many workers' lives. Research into their potentially harmful effects remains inconclusive.

In many industrialized countries musculoskeletal disorders are the main causes of both short-term and permanent work disability. It is estimated that 10-30% of the workforce in industrialized countries, and 50-70% in developing countries, may be exposed to a heavy

10-30% of the workforce in industrialized countries, and 50-70% in developing countries, may be exposed to a heavy physical workload and unergonomic working conditions.

physical workload, and ***unergonomic working conditions*** such as lifting, moving heavy objects or repetitive manual tasks. The main consequences of these hazards are damage to the cardiorespiratory or musculoskeletal systems and traumatic injuries.

Recent surveys show increasing exposure to ***psychological stress*** and overload at work, particularly in industrialized countries. Apart from the loss of health and working capacity which may result, these human factors have been associated with sleep disturbances, burn-out syndrome, depression, and increased risk of cardiovascular disorders, particularly coronary heart disease and hypertension.

Machinery and work tools are often designed to be physically suitable only for men, although female workers use such equipment.

Women at special risk

Growing attention is being paid to reproductive health risks at work. Some 200-300 chemicals known to be mutagenic or carcinogenic tend to have adverse effects on reproduction (including infertility in both sexes, spontaneous abortions, fetal deaths, fetal cancer, or retarded development of the fetus or the newborn). Numerous organic solvents and toxic metals are associated with adverse effects on reproductive health. Many biological agents and heavy physical work are also associated with an increased risk of reproductive disorders. The reproductive health hazards caused by ionizing radiations have been well established, while hazards from non-ionizing radiations are still under intensive study. Both male and female workers may be affected by occupational hazards but women of fertile age and during pregnancy in particular need to be protected. In addition to the conventional preventive activities of occupational health and hygiene services, special arrangements have been made in some countries to remove pregnant women from exposure that may be hazardous to the health of the mother or fetus. Exposure at work should not be allowed for women who have recently given birth or are breast-feeding.

The special occupational health problems of working women are recognized in both developing and industrialized countries. In the former, heavy physical work, the double work burden of job and family, less developed working methods and traditional social roles increase the burden of female workers. In industrialized countries, where women also have the double work burden, lower-paid manual jobs are often left to female workers. In addition, machinery and work tools are often designed to be physically suitable only for men, although female workers use such equipment. In many service occupations the female workers may be exposed to the threat of violence from clients or to sexual harassment from fellow workers.

Prevention of occupational diseases

As explained above, a wide variety of occupational risks can lead to chronic diseases ranging from cancer to mental disorders, yet because of lack of properly trained human resources in occupational health, the majority of occupational diseases are not recognized, particularly in developing countries. Only 5-10% of workers in developing countries, and 20-50% in industrialized countries, have access to adequate occupational health services.

Estimates suggest that the total cost to society of work-related illnesses and accidents varies from about 3% of GNP, when the total sickness absence costs are considered, up to 20% where direct and indirect losses are taken into account. The majority of these illnesses, if not all, are easily preventable, for two reasons: first, their causal agents can be identified, measured and controlled; second, the populations at risk are usually easily accessible and can be regularly supervised and treated. Furthermore, the initial changes are often reversible if treated promptly. The early detection of occupational diseases is consequently of prime importance.

Medical intervention in the form of preplacement and periodic health examinations is essential for the early detection and management of occupational diseases, taking account of individual risk factors such as age, sex and individual susceptibility.

Workers should be informed about the principles and practice of occupational health and the nature of potential health hazards in the workplace, and should be encouraged to adopt practices that reduce health risks.

Other risks

Risks at home

Falls kill more people from unintentional injury than anything except traffic accidents, and most falls occur at home. Most deaths from burning happen at home. In addition, the air inside the home may be far more polluted than the air outside. Most injuries at home are sustained by children under 5 and elderly women, particularly those aged 75 and over. Others at high risk are those affected by alcohol or by ill-health. After falls, the most common cause of death from accidents in the home is fire (*Box 15*), with the elderly again over-represented. Poisoning comes next, followed by suffocation, usually from inhaling food. Stairs are the most common source of injury, followed by glass doors, windows and fences, and baths.

With improved insulation and sealing of windows and doors, the air exchange rate in many houses may be as slow as once in every 10 hours. The effect of this is that an enormous range of pollutants can gather in the household air, many of which have been linked to respiratory disorders, allergies and cancer.

Risks in transport

The measurable outcomes of road crashes include the number of deaths, the number of injuries and the number of crashes. Deaths are counted reliably and quite accurately. Serious injuries are counted fairly accurately, but a large number of minor injuries are not counted at all, and definitions of the various categories of injury tend to be inconsistent. A very high proportion of all crashes that do not result in injury go unreported. Those at highest risk are motorcycle riders, with the major cause

Box 15. Burn injuries

There is no international system for reporting and recording burn injuries or even deaths from burns. However, data collected in several countries, both developed and developing, indicate that annually around 300 individuals per million population sustain burns which require care in hospital because of extent, associated injury or other conditions related to the burns.

The rate of fire and burn deaths in the United States and Japan ranges from 0.2 to 3.8 per 100 000 population. Factors influencing the occurrence of burn injury include poverty, season of the year, tobacco smoking, type of building construction and occupation. The majority of fire deaths occur in residential fires (40% in Japan and 73% in the United States). Fire, typically that caused by ignition of flammable liquids, is the most common cause of burn injury in adults, and hot liquid scalding is the most common cause of burns in children. Recent studies suggest that the incidence of burn injury has decreased in developed countries. This has been attributed to improved construction, better quality of appliances, increased use of smoke and fire detectors, the use of flame retardant sleepwear for children, and effective prevention programmes.

The mortality and morbidity caused by burn injury have been significantly reduced by improvements in the management of burn patients. The prompt administration of adequate volumes of resuscitation fluid has essentially eliminated acute renal failure as an early post-burn complication. The use of fiberoptic bronchoscopy to diagnose smoke inhalation injury (the most important related condition in burn patients) has significantly reduced the occurrence of bronchopneumonia. Effective topical antimicrobial chemotherapy and surgical excision of the burned tissue in the early post-burn period have led to a substantial decrease in the incidence of invasive burn wound infection and facilitated early closure of the wound in all but those patients with very extensive burn injury. Recently, culture-derived tissue has been utilized with variable success to achieve permanent wound closure in patients with massive burns.

Effective regimens of dietary support have been used to minimize erosion of lean body mass, and hormonal interventions have been identified to improve the effectiveness of nutritional support regimens, hasten wound closure and accelerate convalescence. Lastly, new techniques of tissue expansion and tissue transfer have led to improved reconstruction capability, and current rehabilitation programmes facilitate the re-entry of extensively burned patients into society.

Prevention programmes should focus on the common causes of burn injury as the most effective means of reducing its consequences. Research should place emphasis on identifying pharmacological agents to reduce and reverse oedema formation, on developing improved means of mechanical ventilation to reduce barotrauma, and on elaborating techniques to quantify the severity of inhalation injury. Other important research areas include improved topical chemotherapeutic agents, non-antigenic culture-derived composite tissue, nutritional support regimens tailored to meet the specific metabolic needs of patients with sepsis and infection, and growth factor therapy to enhance wound healing.

Personal communication from the President, International Society of Burn Injuries.

An estimated 180 million people worldwide are visually disabled, of whom nearly 45 million are blind.

of death and permanent disability from crashes being head injury, the risk of which can be markedly reduced through the use of crash helmets.

Age is closely related to crash rate, with a peak in the late teens and early twenties and a steady decline thereafter. The first factor that can be modified to reduce the risk of death and injury from traffic accidents is the use of alcohol by road users. Another potent factor determining the risk of injury among those who have crashed in motor vehicles is the use of seat belts.

In contrast to road travellers, the risk to passengers travelling in a railway train is exceedingly low in developed countries. The picture is different in the less developed parts of the world, where unprotected railways run close to densely populated urban areas and where familiarity with risk can lead to complacency.

Aviation can be divided into two categories, the first being passenger-carrying "commercial" aviation, and the other being so-called "general" aviation, mostly using smaller aircraft in operations including pleasure flying, executive travel, crop spraying and land surveying. The picture of pleasure flying is generally very similar to the picture of recreational car or boat use, with operators getting into trouble because they exceed their capabilities, a problem often compounded by the use of alcohol. In a crash at equivalent speed, the passengers of a small aeroplane are at far higher risk of injury and death than those in a modern small car. Over the last decade, crashes involving modern wide-bodied jets have resulted in approximately three times fewer fatalities per number of passengers than was the case for piston-engined aircraft, although at least part of the reason for this is the present use of much better emergency services and hospital facilities near airports.

Recreational risks

As lifestyles have steadily changed over the years, an increasing proportion of the population is at risk from injury and death during recreational activities, especially in developed countries. Team sports involving violent body contact result in the highest risk of nonfatal injury, while mountaineering, motor racing, sport parachuting and hang gliding have lower injury rates overall, but much higher death rates. Boxing is particularly dangerous, as repeated blows to the head cause progressive and irreversible brain damage.

The state of physical conditioning is an influential risk factor for most sports, as well as the degree of natural talent and extent of experience and learned skill, and the equipment used. Typical injuries include drowning (which affects children most, and has been found in adults to be linked to alcohol use); impact injuries suffered from striking hard surfaces while diving (with alcohol again implicated as a risk factor); fractures and head injuries from skiing and riding; and heat stroke from long-distance running. Considering the whole spectrum of risks to participants in sporting and recreational activities, remarkably little systematic information is currently gathered on injury-producing events and on the risk that injury will be suffered. The epidemiology of this group of injuries is one of the major unstudied fields in risk assessment and injury control.

Other issues

Blindness

An estimated 180 million people worldwide are visually disabled, of whom nearly 45 million are blind, four out of five of them living in developing countries. About 80% of blindness is avoidable (treatable or potentially preventable). However, a large proportion of those affected remain blind for want of access to affordable eye care. Blindness leads not only to reduced economic and social status but may also result in premature death. The major causes of blindness and their estimated prevalence are cataract (19 million); glaucoma (6.4 million); trachoma (5.6

million); childhood blindness (more than 1.5 million); onchocerciasis (0.29 million); other causes (10 million).

Prevalence varies dramatically between countries, from 0.2% or less in developed countries to more than 1% in some sub-Saharan countries. About 32% of the world's blind are aged 45-59 but the large majority, 58%, are over 60 years old.

Cataract is the loss of transparency of the lens of the eye, leading to progressive loss of clarity and detail of images. It is generally ageing-related, but congenital cataract may result from maternal infection in pregnancy or from genetic conditions. Direct injury to the eye could also result in cataract. The condition is painless and causes only visual symptoms.

Intensive cataract surgical programmes, which have reached millions of persons blind from cataract in many countries worldwide, restore sight to the afflicted who usually do not have ready access to cataract surgical services. These programmes need to be expanded and sustained in the next 20 years if the backlog of cataract-related blindness is to be reduced and new cases are to be effectively managed. The development of affordable intraocular lens implantation procedures has improved the quality of life for those patients following surgery.

Trachoma is a major preventable cause of blindness. Apart from the 5.6 million presently blind, another 147 million, most of them in Africa and Asia, have an active form of the disease. The cause is an infectious microorganism, *Chlamydia trachomatis*, which spreads through contact with eye discharge from the infected person, for example via fingers, handkerchiefs or towels, and is also spread by eye-seeking flies. After years of repeated infections, the inside of the eyelids becomes severely scarred with the eyelashes rubbing on the eyeball.

Trachoma mainly affects women and children in the poorest communities in the developing world. A worldwide programme to target the elimination of trachoma as a blinding disease began in 1996. It is a coordinated effort to provide surgery, antibiotic treatment and improved environmental conditions to populations at risk, largely in Africa.

Glaucoma is a condition generally caused by excessive pressure of fluid in the eye leading to damage of the optic nerve and gradual, irreversible loss of vision. The fluid pressure rises because of a gradually increasing blockage of the outflow channels in the eye. The condition is uncommon below the age of 40 and commonly occurs over the age of 60. However congenital glaucoma may also occur. Chronic glaucoma often has no symptoms until late in the disease, because of its gradual onset and slow progression. However an acute form may present with dull severe pain in and above the eye. Diagnosis is by routine and specialized eye examination. Drugs administered as eye drops or laser treatment to lower the eye pressure could control the condition, but in advanced cases surgery is required to open new outflow channels.

Childhood blindness is largely caused by vitamin A deficiency, corneal blindness and cataract. The goal of the World Summit for Children in 1990 was to eliminate vitamin A deficiency as a cause of blindness by the year 2000; in many countries this is being achieved.

Onchocerciasis is a blinding parasitic disease found mainly in Africa, transmitted by blackflies. The disease has been targeted for control with distribution of the drug ivermectin, following the successful Onchocerciasis Control Programme which used vector control methods to eliminate the disease from a large area of West Africa. A new programme is targeting the remaining countries where the disease occurs.

Hearing impairment

Some 121 million people are estimated to have a disabling hearing impairment. There is an urgent need for more, accurate population-based data on the prevalence and causes of hearing impairment, so that countries may set priorities and determine needs. As more countries

Some 121 million people are estimated to have a disabling hearing impairment.

Map 3. Oral health status, 1996

A. At age 12

Decayed, missing, filled permanent teeth
Very low: <1.2
Low: 1.2–2.6
Moderate: 2.7–4.4
High: >4.4
No data available
WHO 97090

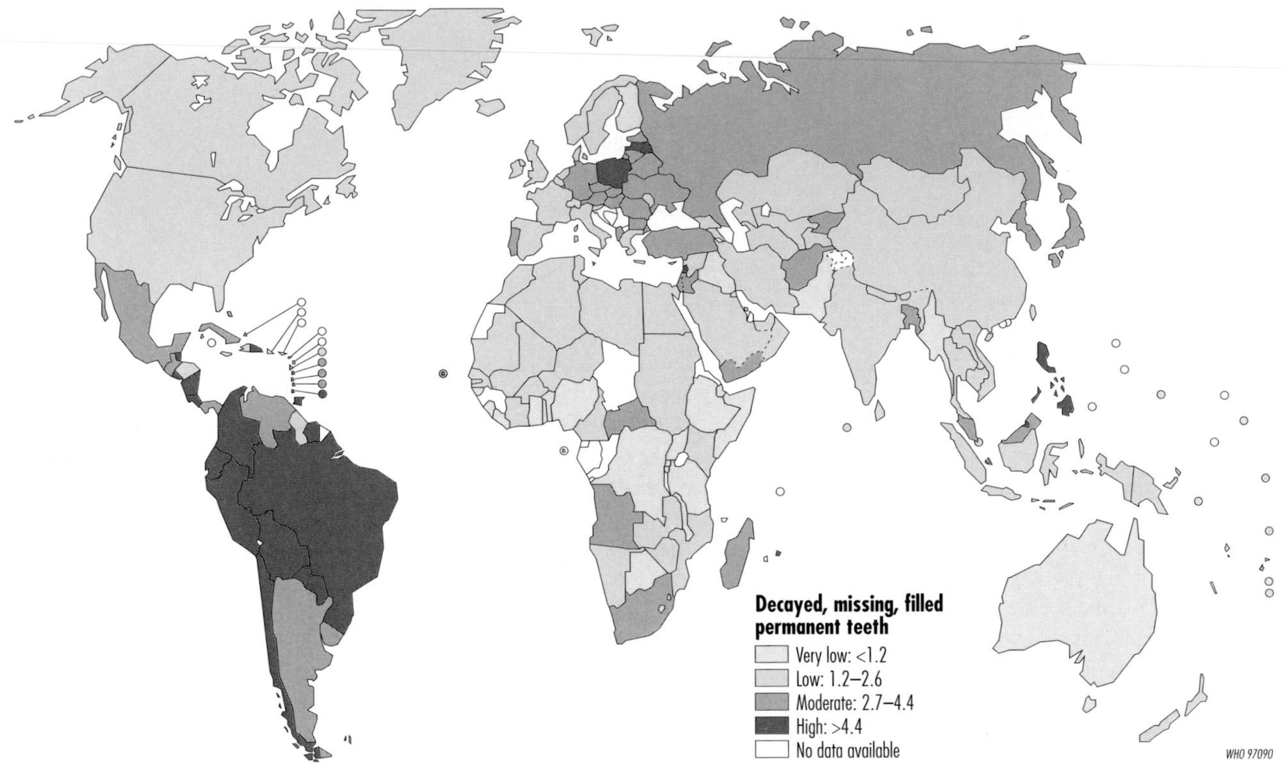

B. At ages 35–44

Decayed, missing, filled permanent teeth
Very low: <5.0
Low: 5.0–8.9
Moderate: 9.0–13.9
High: >13.9
No data available
WHO 97091

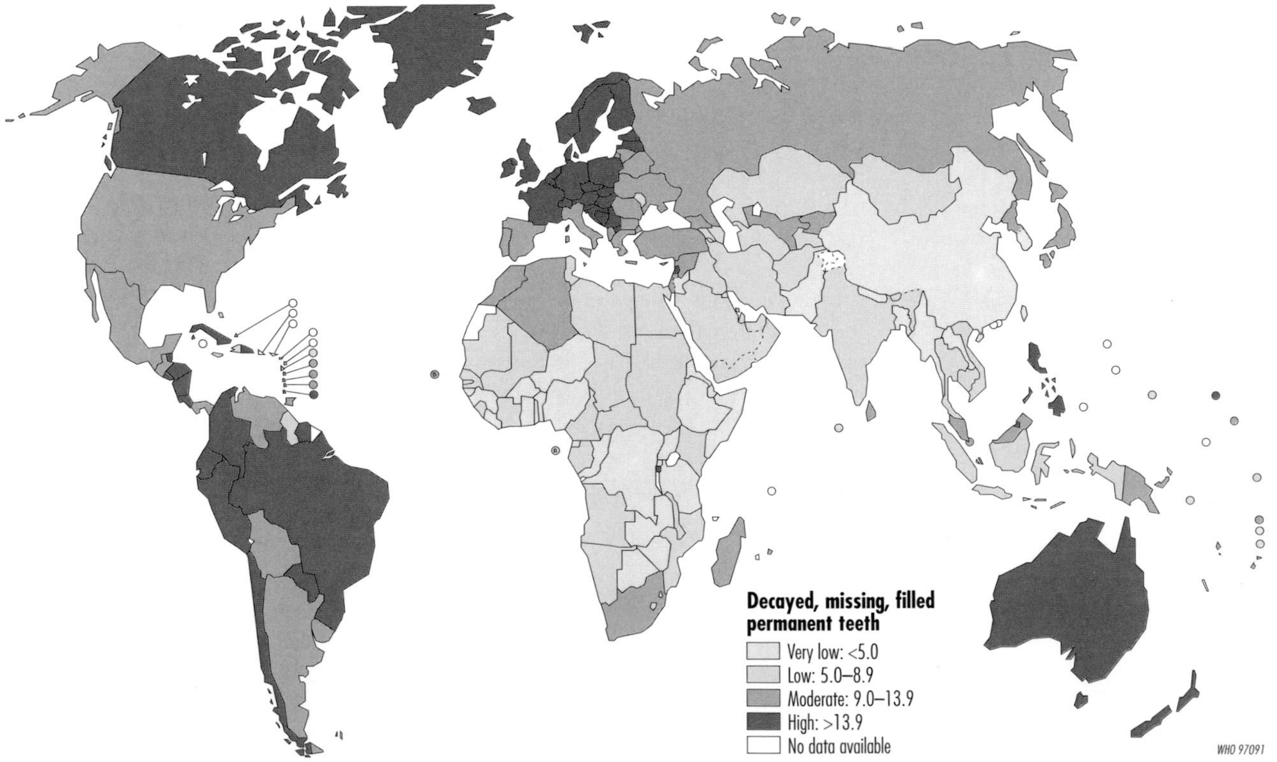

conduct surveys, WHO collates the information so that an accurate global picture is progressively revealed.

The inappropriate use of ototoxic drugs, at all ages, is a considerable cause of hearing impairment in developing countries. Better professional, public and health education is needed to counter this problem, as well as enforcement of drug regulatory measures in some instances to limit access to such drugs. Industrial and other excessive noise is an increasing cause of hearing loss in many settings. Again, public education and hearing conservation programmes and, in some cases, legislation are needed measures.

Chronic otitis media is a major preventable cause of hearing impairment in children; it is a serious problem because it retards language development and educational progress. Chronic otitis media can be managed through primary health care, but it requires proper detection and follow-up of affected children.

Presbycusis is the most common cause of hearing impairment with increasing ageing. It is therefore becoming a major global concern because of the growth of the proportion of elderly persons. The most effective measure in these cases is the fitting of hearing aids, although globally there is still a lack of affordable, good-quality hearing aids in developing countries.

Oral health

Dental diseases are chronic conditions that adversely affect quality of life, especially in the elderly where they may have serious adverse effects on nutrition. Although great progress has been made over the last 20 years in combating them, dental caries and periodontal disease remain the most prevalent dental conditions. Caries, or tooth decay, is the more prevalent of the two.

Dental caries

Dental caries affects almost everyone at some stage of life, and may involve complications such as pain, abscesses, severe infections and teeth extractions. In industrialized countries about 50% of children have dental caries; 15-20% are in the high-risk group of having more than four teeth affected (*Map 3*).

In all industrialized countries up to 40% of people aged over 65 have no teeth at all. The underprivileged – poor, disabled, ethnic minorities, refugees, migrants – all suffer more oral disease than the rest of the population. In countries whose economies are in transition, because of the breakdown in state health care systems and privatization of oral care services, large percentages of the populations cannot get access to or afford preventive, restorative or rehabilitative treatment.

In developing countries, most people get five or six decayed teeth and keep most of their teeth into old age. However, oral diseases are increasing, related to changes in dietary and other habits, and often linked with moves to large cities.

Although bacteria on the teeth are the direct cause of dental caries, many environmental and host factors interact to determine whether the individual will be affected, when, and to what extent. The contribution of sugars to the metabolic activities of the responsible bacteria is well established.

Altered lifestyles and understanding of risk behaviours play a major role in the prevention of a wide range of oral diseases, including dental caries. Current knowledge is sufficient to control caries, if not eliminate it.

In all developing countries the possibility of getting care for oral problems is limited, with perhaps only 5% of decayed teeth treated. For too many people, oral problems are seen as inevitable, painful and costly, and thus are tolerated rather than treated. Appropriate re-

Dental diseases are chronic conditions that adversely affect quality of life, especially in the elderly where they may have serious adverse effects on nutrition.

Research to establish even cheaper and simpler ways of treating early dental caries is needed, as many communities cannot afford even basic instrument sets.

habilitative care – replacement of lost teeth – is often not carried out, which causes further problems such as infections and loss of teeth.

The consumption of fluorides during tooth formation and the application of fluorides to the teeth at any age enhance resistance of the teeth to decay. Fluoridation of community water supplies can reduce tooth decay by at least 50% and the benefits are long-lasting. In the absence of community water supplies, fluoridation of school water can prove effective. The use at home of toothpastes containing fluoride, or their supervised use by children in schools and similar settings are highly desirable as well as avoiding sugar-containing snacks and sticky sweets between meals.

Periodontal disease

There are two main types of periodontal disease: inflammation of the gums (gingivitis) and inflammation of the periodontium (periodontitis). Gingivitis consists of swelling of the gum tissue and destruction of the connective tissue fibres that hold the gum tissue in position. Gingivitis, which occurs most frequently in young adults, may progress to periodontitis if untreated, in which case there is bone damage and loosening and eventual loss of teeth.

Accumulation of the bacterial plaque associated with periodontal diseases is promoted by various conditions including poor oral hygiene, cigarette smoking and diabetes.

Outlook

Traditional dentistry uses expensive equipment dependent on reliable electricity and clean pressurized water, services that are unavailable in most communities in developing countries. A new approach, atraumatic restorative treatment (ART), using basic sets of instruments and simple, easily assembled dental care beds or benches, is both effective and low cost. Essential instruments and materials can be carried in a hand bag, allowing the dental worker to reach isolated communities to provide essential care. This technology is minimally invasive and has successfully been taught to non-dentally-trained personnel, and helps prevent oral diseases in the community.

Research to establish even cheaper and simpler ways of treating early dental caries is needed, as many communities cannot afford even the low costs of ART and basic instrument sets. Thus there is need for developing and using less expensive training equipment so that basic oral care skills can be learned by community health workers.

Chapter 2

WHO's contributions to world health

This chapter gives an overview of WHO's contribution during 1996 to supporting the progress of Member States in improving people's health.

The main focus of this report is on noncommunicable, chronic diseases and disorders, and on such problems as violence, homicides, suicides, accidents and injuries, and their impact on both developing and developed countries. Chapter 1 showed that the burdens of major diseases such as circulatory diseases, cancer and some mental disorders are likely to increase dramatically worldwide, largely because lengthening life spans will make them more common. While infectious diseases pose a relatively minor threat to health in the industrialized world, they will continue collectively to be leading causes of death and illness in many developing countries for the foreseeable future.

This chapter gives an overview of WHO's contribution during 1996 to supporting the progress of Member States in improving people's health. Each of the Organization's programmes consists of an aggregate of activities directed towards the attainment of specific objectives. The totality of the work of these programmes is intended to contribute to global health improvement. While this chapter summarizes the programmes' work in general, it begins by highlighting activities that are particularly relevant to the dominant issues of chronic diseases examined in Chapter 1. As in previous reports, the programme activities are brought together according to their influence on people's health at different stages of life. However, given that the majority of those affected by chronic diseases are elderly or middle-aged adults, and that such diseases in childhood are relatively uncommon, the usual sequence describing activities related to age groups has been reversed.

The Member States of WHO are committed to attaining as a minimum by all people in all countries at least such a level of health that they are capable of working productively and of participating actively in the social life of the community in which they live. This is known as "health for all". The Global Strategy for Health for All by the Year 2000, founded on primary health care and adopted by the World Health Assembly in 1981, provides both the policy framework for the worldwide health action needed to achieve the social target of at least a minimum level of health for all people, and the framework for WHO's programme to support it.

Last year was the first in WHO's ninth General Programme of Work for 1996-2001, which ensures continuity by having the same four interrelated policy orientations that applied in the final two years of the eighth General Programme of Work. The four policy orientations are: (1) integrating health and human development in public policies; (2) ensuring equitable access to health services; (3) promoting and protecting health; (4) preventing and controlling specific health problems. These were established to focus action by the world community, including WHO, on a number of goals and targets as well as to support countries in reaching targets that they might set in the light of their own situations.

The goals and targets in the ninth General Programme of Work are an expression of the commitment of the international health community, including WHO, to support countries in achieving improvements in health status and greater equity in health.

It is not possible for this chapter to reflect the full extent of WHO's work, but examples are given of the different types of action carried out at various levels of the Organization. The evaluation of what WHO has done, and the impact of that work on global health, then provides the framework for Chapter 3 of this report, which outlines the Organization's priority issues and its strategy for tackling them in 1997 and beyond.

Chronic conditions

During 1996 WHO took action on a wide range of chronic conditions. For instance, since chronic diseases have a number of common risk factors, the Organization adopts an integrated approach to their prevention through the INTERHEALTH project. Genetic factors, for example, play an important role in determining individual susceptibility to various types of cancer and to diabetes mellitus, cardiovascular disease and hereditary disorders.

The International Agency for Research on Cancer coordinates and conducts epidemiological and laboratory research and risk evaluations that form the basis of scientific strategies for preventing cancer.

WHO has set up such integrated programmes in all regions of the world, for example, the countrywide integrated noncommunicable diseases intervention (CINDI) programme in Europe, which now comprises 24 countries. In 17 of them, a specially designed survey on experience with policy development in chronic disease prevention has been carried out. The survey showed that successful policy development and the creation of effective partnerships determine the time taken by countries to reorient their health care systems towards prevention and population-based health promotion approaches to chronic diseases. A special action plan to bridge the health gap between the East and the West of the region, based on experience within the CINDI network, has been developed with the aim of building capacity for preventing chronic diseases in eastern Europe. It will be used for planning the activities of the network up to the year 2000. The CINDI action plan on nutrition was also drafted.

In the Americas, the integrated chronic disease intervention project is known as CARMEN. Although the main focus is cardiovascular disease control, other conditions are also included such as diabetes, cervical cancer control and injury prevention. CARMEN is modelled on the North Karelia project in Finland, addressing policy interventions, risk factor reduction, and improvements in the quality of clinical prevention care. The first project, in Valparaiso, Chile, will be followed by similar initiatives in Argentina and other countries. Canada and Spain are providing technical support.

In the Western Pacific, two projects have been carried out in China, which integrate prevention and control of chronic diseases and aim at reducing the main risk factors, with emphasis on tobacco control and hypertension. In Fiji, a series of national workshops trained health workers in methods and skills for reducing risk factors.

Cancer continues to be a threat to health worldwide, as described in Chapter 1. The International Agency for Research on Cancer (IARC) coordinates and conducts epidemiological and laboratory research and risk evaluations that form the basis of scientific strategies for preventing cancer. It assesses the efficacy of various methods of screening and prevention, and disseminates skills and information worldwide through its programme of education, training and publications. Carcinogenic risks posed by a variety of exposures are evaluated and the assessments made are published in the IARC monographs (*Table 4*). The three volumes published in 1996 evaluated the risks posed by printing inks and printing processes; by some pharmaceutical drugs, including tamoxifen; and by retroviruses, including HIV. The Agency launched a programme of genetic epidemiology in 1996 with studies on the role of genetic factors in cancer susceptibility and carcinogenesis, including the search for a third breast cancer susceptibility gene. Publications issued dealt with cancer chemoprevention, cancer mortality in central Europe, fibre carcinogenesis, the role of socioeconomic factors, and cancer incidence and mortality in the European Union.

A cancer profile for the Western Pacific Region has been developed to monitor the epidemiological situation of

Table 4. Carcinogens hazardous to humans, as evaluated in the IARC monographs[a]

Principal target organ/tissue	Carcinogens		Occupational exposures
	Agents/groups of agents	Mixtures	
Blood vessels	Vinyl chloride		
Bone marrow	Benzene; busulfan (1-4-butanediol dimethanesulfonate); chlorambucil; cyclophosphamide; ethylene oxide; melphalan; MOPP (chlormethine, vincristine, procarbazine and prednisone) and other combined therapy including alkylating agents; semustine (1-(2-chlorethyl)-3-(4-methylcyclohexyl)-1-nitrosurea, methyl-CCNU); thiotepa; treosulfan		
Cervix	Diethylstilbestrol; human papilloma-virus type 16; human papilloma-virus type 18		
Digestive tract, upper		Alcoholic beverages, betel quid containing tobacco; tobacco smoke	
Kidney		Analgesic mixtures containing phenacetin; tobacco smoke	
Liver	Aflatoxins, naturally occurring; hepatitis B virus (chronic infection with); hepatitis C virus (chronic infection with); oral contraceptives, combined[b]	Alcoholic beverages	
Bile ducts/liver	*Opisthorchis viverrini* (infection with)		
Lung	Arsenic and arsenic compounds[c]; asbestos; beryllium and beryllium compounds[c]; bis (chloromethyl) ether and chloromethyl methyl ether (technical-grade); cadmium and cadmium compounds[c]; nickel compounds[c]; radon and its decay products; talc containing asbestiform fibres	Tobacco smoke	Aluminium production; coal gasification; coke production; haematite mining (underground) with exposure to radon; iron and steel founding; painter (occupational exposure as); silica, crystalline (in the form of quartz and cristobolte from occupational sources)
Lymphatic tissues	Azathioprine; ciclosporin; ethylene oxide; human immunodeficiency virus type 1 (infection with); human T-cell lymphotrophic virus type 1 (infection with)		
Nasal cavity		Wood dust	Boot and shoe manufacture and repair; furniture- and cabinet-making
Nasopharynx		Salted fish (Chinese-style)	
Oral cavity		Alcoholic beverages; betel quid containing tobacco; tobacco products, smokeless; tobacco smoke	
Paranasal sinuses		Wood dust	2-Propanol (isopropanol) manufacture (strong-acid process)
Pleura	Asbestos; erionite		
Respiratory tract, upper	Mustard gas (sulfur mustard); nickel compounds[c]		Strong-inorganic-acid mists containing sulfuric acid (occupational exposure to)
Skin	Arsenic and arsenic compounds[c]; methoxsalen (8-methoxypsoralen) + ultraviolet A radiation; solar radiation	Coal-tar pitches; coal-tars; mineral oils, untreated and mildly treated; shale-oils; soots	Coal gasification
Stomach	*Helicobacter pylori* (infection with)		
Urinary bladder	4-Aminobiphenyl; benzidine; chlornaphazine (*N,N*-bis(2-chlorethyl)-2-naphthylamine); 2- cyclophosphamide; 2-naphthylamine; *Schistosoma haematobium* (infection with)	Tobacco smoke	Auramine, manufacture of; coal gasification; magenta, manufature of; rubber industry
Uterus	Estrogens, steroidal and nonsteroidal; oral contraceptives, sequential; tamoxifen[d]		
Vagina	Diethylstilbestrol		

[a] The full list with references can be found on Internet at http://www.iarc.fr.
[b] There is also conclusive evidence that these agents have a protective effect against cancers of the ovary and endometrium.
[c] Evaluated as a group.
[d] There is also conclusive evidence that this agent reduces the risk of contralateral breast cancer.

A multinational WHO study in China, Japan, Philippines, Republic of Korea and Viet Nam investigated health workers' knowledge of cancer pain relief, with a view to developing an appropriate approach for training.

the most common cancers, summarizing the age-adjusted incidence of cancer in different parts of the body in 29 countries and areas. A WHO working group on cancer prevention and control convened in the Philippines in 1996 and funded by Australia reviewed the situation and made recommendations for the planning and implementation of cancer control programmes. IARC is conducting a randomized controlled trial of breast cancer screening by physical examination in 340 000 women in the Philippines. Cancer registries are in use in most countries, although with varying degrees of effectiveness and coverage of population.

A multinational WHO study in China, Japan, Philippines, Republic of Korea and Viet Nam investigated health workers' knowledge of, and attitudes to, cancer pain relief, with a view to developing an appropriate approach for training. Cancer pain relief methods were introduced in Fiji, Mongolia and Samoa.

In order to prevent liver cancer, the Gambia and Zimbabwe are undertaking systematic immunization against hepatitis B (*Box 9, page 32*). Cancer of the urinary bladder, which is associated with *Schistosoma haematobium* infection, will gradually come under control as some countries have started mass chemotherapy with praziquantel and improvement of water and sanitation of communities at risk.

The 10-year-old, 26-country MONICA project continues to monitor trends and determinants of ***circulatory diseases*** and measures the effectiveness of interventions. In 1996, WHO disseminated the first 5-year trend data on risk factors and incidence of heart attacks and strokes. The Organization made available a set of protocols and a training manual for monitoring cardiovascular disease risk factors in developing countries, as well as guidelines for promoting physical activity as part of a prevention strategy.

In China, community-based population strategies for prevention and control of circulatory diseases were initiated with the development of national guidelines for intervention on risk factors. WHO collaborated with the Republic of Korea in a national workshop aimed at strengthening community-based hypertension prevention and case management. Information on promotion of healthy lifestyles and prevention of cardiovascular diseases was disseminated through mass media in Mongolia. In view of the importance of nutrition in the prevention of cardiovascular diseases, WHO collaborated with Malaysia in re-examining the role of unhealthy nutrition as a risk factor for these diseases and developing nutrition intervention strategies for preventing them.

WHO published a regional plan for control of cardiovascular diseases and specific guidelines for countries in the Eastern Mediterranean (EMRO Technical Publication No. 22, *Prevention and control of cardiovascular diseases*). Following a pan-European consensus conference on stroke management held in cooperation with the European Stroke Council, at which a series of quality indicators were identified and the establishment of databases for stroke discussed, long-term cooperation for improving the quality of such care in Member States began. This initiative was further pursued in the joint third world and fifth European stroke conference in 1996.

During 1996, WHO conducted a study to determine the worldwide prevalence of ***diabetes mellitus***. It concluded that the population affected will more than double in the next 25 years. World Diabetes Day on 14 November was an important vehicle for maintaining awareness and increasing understanding of what can be done to prevent and control diabetes. The 1996 theme "Insulin for life" highlighted the continuing unavailability or unaffordability of this essential medication in many of the world's poorest countries.

Diabetes liaison offices are in place in all European Member States, 46% of countries have a national diabetes programme, 80% have a national diabetes task force and 85% have a diabetes patient organization. WHO has set up a computerized information system (DIABCARE), which aggregates and evaluates data provided by countries. Diabetes is the subject of a priority chronic disease programme in the Americas. In 1996, the Declaration of the Americas on Diabetes, developed with the International Diabetes Federation (IDF) and regional partners, was endorsed by the ministries of health of the region as a guide for national programme development. A national programme on prevention and control of diabetes was formulated at a WHO-supported national symposium in China. Education for diabetic patients, training of health workers to update skills and knowledge on diabetes, and diabetes management programmes have been carried out in China, Fiji and the Republic of Korea. WHO is collaborating in a national diabetes survey in the Philippines to assess the burden of the disease and to identify the most common risk factors for diabetes and cardiovascular disease. The regional task force on diabetes established in the Eastern Mediterranean developed a regional plan for diabetes control. WHO has also produced a protocol for a diabetes prevalence survey for use in countries and a document, *Diabetes prevention and control: a call for action*, which includes technical guidelines and a regional plan for diabetes prevention and control. IDF and WHO issued a consensus document for the whole of Africa, with guidelines for the management of non-insulin-dependent diabetes mellitus.

WHO continues to support studies on and the application of primary prevention approaches for a variety of ***hereditary disorders*** including familial hypercholesterolaemia, haemophilia and cystic fibrosis. A landmark technical report, *Control of hereditary diseases*, was published in 1996 (see *Box 13*, page 53).

WHO is also concerned with ***other chronic conditions*** such as asthma and arthritis. WHO and the National Heart, Lung and Blood Institutes (United States) have jointly instigated a global initiative on asthma (GINA) to assist health care professionals and public health officials in appreciating the magnitude of the problem and in designing and delivering effective asthma management and prevention programmes in their countries. Following the preparation of a strategy and plan of action for GINA by 24 international experts, 27 national and international organizations have agreed to implement this strategy in all WHO regions. A joint WHO/International League of Associations of Rheumatology meeting was convened to address treatment decisions, relations of physicians with the pharmaceutical industry and coordination of drug regulation, and WHO has issued the resulting guidelines. The WHO low back pain initiative began comparative studies of a variety of common treatments (medical, chiropractic, alternative medical, etc.) to find the most appropriate approach for management of this prevalent debilitating disorder.

WHO's work in 1996 on the epidemiology of ***mental and neurological disorders*** included a study of the prevalence, severity and cost of neurological disorders such as dementia, stroke, epilepsy and headache. An internationally accepted nomenclature and diagnostic categories are essential for carrying out epidemiological research. This common nomenclature is provided by the ICD-10, Chapter V, which has been expanded to include diagnostic guidelines and has now been translated into more than 25 languages.

A WHO collaborative project, involving 14 countries and completed in 1996, assessed psychological problems in general health care and indicated that one in four adults visiting a general doctor had a current and diagnosable mental disorder. The results of the research further suggested that only half of the patients suffering from well-known mental disorders such as depression, anxiety or alcohol abuse consulted a doctor. Of those, only half are diagnosed and only half of those diagnosed are treated. While a third of those using general health services need careful attention for psychological problems, no more than "the tip of the iceberg" is dealt with by the health services; and only 1% of people with mental disorders receive specialized care although

A landmark technical report, Control of hereditary diseases, *was published by WHO in 1996.*

even severe mental illnesses can be managed outside the hospital.

Countries in all regions have prepared national mental health programmes. In Africa, 45% of countries have prepared a national programme on mental health, and 32% on prevention and control of substance abuse; 17% have set up a national coordination mechanism for implementation of mental health activities; 32% have integrated mental health into primary health care services; and 25% have a community-oriented programme. In the Eastern Mediterranean, national programmes have been set up in 20 out of 23 countries, and are evaluated regularly. In the Western Pacific, a regional mental health database has been established to facilitate problem identification and prioritization, and for planning, implementing, monitoring and evaluating mental health programmes and services.

WHO has prepared simple and user-friendly primary care versions of diagnostic and treatment guidelines for the common mental disorders.

Much psychiatric and psychological distress can be managed in general health care settings. Education on mental health interventions for those working in primary care is a priority, especially in war-torn countries. WHO has prepared simple and user-friendly primary care versions of diagnostic and treatment guidelines for the common mental disorders, based on the ICD-10, and educational kits. Two versions of the guidelines for the primary prevention of mental, neurological and psychosocial disorders were produced: one for professionals with a post-college degree and the other for mid-level health workers. A document on essential psychosocial interventions was prepared as part of the WHO series *Essential treatments in psychiatry*.

In 1996 WHO published *Ten basic principles of mental health care law*. These were based on a comparative analysis of mental health laws in 60 jurisdictions at provincial, state and federal levels in 45 countries. Another WHO document issued in 1996 gives guidelines for promoting the human rights of people with mental disorders.

In order to increase public and professional awareness of epilepsy as a treatable brain disorder, WHO and the International League against Epilepsy announced a worldwide campaign against epilepsy in 1996.

Nicotine dependence affects around one-third of the global population above 15 years of age. Patterns and trends of tobacco, alcohol and illicit substance use were studied and their health and social consequences analysed. A status report on the global tobacco or health situation was finalized. Action to fight smoking is a central priority for the CINDI programme in Europe, and a multinational collaborative smoking cessation campaign, "Wait and win", was organized in 1996 by the Finnish CINDI centre. Altogether 24 countries participated and some 70 000 smokers registered. Nicotine dependence is becoming a public health problem in Africa, and countries have expressed their desire to diversify their crops and eventually to replace tobacco cultivation by other commercial crops if they have a guarantee that this will not result in economic hardship. All Member States have now appointed a national focal point to manage their control programme, developed an education programme to sensitize the public on the health risks associated with tobacco use, and introduced teaching modules into their school curricula. They will need the support of the United Nations specialized agencies, especially WHO, FAO and the World Bank, if these efforts are to succeed.

A conference on the very sensitive subject of ***alcohol dependence*** brought together participants from 46 Member States, mainly in the European Region, who unanimously adopted a European Charter setting out five basic ethical principles and 10 action strategies for use at country level. WHO has undertaken comprehensive policy missions on alcohol, drugs and tobacco in eastern European countries to support the development and implementation of policy and action programmes to help prevent and reduce the severe problems they face.

In the area of ***psychoactive drug dependence***, WHO's activities include epidemiological surveillance and risk assessment, dissemination of information, development of primary prevention programmes, identification and development of treatment, and rehabilitation. WHO has a global epidemiological surveillance system to assess and describe patterns and trends of substance abuse, together with the health consequences and national policy responses, and is working on a multisite opioid drug substitution pharmacotherapy trial involving countries in the Western Pacific and South-East Asia. A project to assist with the development of culturally appropriate programmes has been designed to reduce the harm associated with the use of psychoactive substances among indigenous populations.

Most of WHO's activities related to ***blindness and deafness*** are directed specifically to the elderly and to children. A new global initiative for the elimination of trachoma was launched in collaboration with the Edna McConnell Clark Foundation and a group of nongovernmental organizations, following a global scientific meeting convened in 1996. Work will focus on planning and coordination of interventions in selected countries.

In the Eastern Mediterranean, a collaborative agreement between WHO and IMPACT (the International Initiative against Avoidable Disablement) has resulted in a combined approach to improved eye health in Yemen, with IMPACT providing assistance to reduce the backlog in cataract surgery and WHO providing funds and technical assistance for the establishment of a diploma course in ophthalmology. In Africa, a review of human resource development for prevention of blindness was completed in 1996. More nurses or medical assistants are to be trained as cataract surgeons and plans are at an advanced stage to open another training centre for Central African countries.

WHO has devised a new evaluative approach to enable Member States to improve ***oral health*** and care, making use of information on epidemiology, the fourth edition of *Oral health surveys: basic methods* (1996) and the country programme profile. Field tests in developing countries have shown that a new method for caries control – atraumatic restorative treatment – is scientifically valid and affordable for immediate use in all countries. The acceptability and effectiveness of a new type of fluoridated toothpaste has been demonstrated in Indonesia. Milk fortified with fluoride, in addition to its high nutritional value, now benefits children in Bulgaria, Chile, China, the Russian Federation and the United Kingdom. WHO guidelines on this subject are available. Of the six global goals for oral health by the year 2000 adopted by WHO and the World Dental Federation, the one concerning the establishment of databases to monitor and evaluate changes in oral health is now seen as a priority, especially for the countries in eastern Europe. Software to be used by health care providers and administrators at community and national levels has been developed by WHO and is currently being tested in five Member States.

As regards safety promotion and ***injury control***, WHO, in cooperation with the Government of Australia and with the active involvement of WHO collaborating centres on injury prevention, cosponsored the third international conference on injury prevention and control in 1996. The effectiveness of prevention in this area has been demonstrated in the Americas (*Box 16*). WHO convened a global consultation on violence and health to assist in the formulation of a plan of action.

Over the past two decades, WHO has been promoting community-based ***rehabilitation*** as a component of primary health care, and continues to do so as an effective strategy to increase access to rehabilitation for persons with physical disabilities and mental retardation, and to promote opportunities for their full integration into community and society. Close collaboration is maintained with ILO and UNESCO, with disability organizations and international nongovernmental organizations, and over 80 countries have now initiated programmes. An important trend in such programmes is to broaden the focus to "persons with social disadvan-

WHO has a global epidemiological surveillance system to assess and describe patterns and trends of substance abuse, together with the health consequences and national policy responses.

Box 16. Injury prevention in the Americas

In Latin America and the Caribbean, injuries account for 10% of mortality and 18% of years lost to disability. Injury is the first ranked cause of death in the age group 5-45 years. Leading causes of unintentional injuries are motor-vehicle collisions, falls, burns and drowning. Although deaths due to unintentional causes exceed those due to violence by a ratio of 2:1, violence recently superseded motor-vehicle collisions as the leading contributor to deaths from external causes in Latin America. During the 1980s, several countries suffered an increase in violence during times of internal conflict. Although such conflict has generally subsided, the trend in violence (e.g. homicide, suicide) as a cause of death continues upwards in several countries, while the trend in death from motor-vehicle collisions is more generally downwards.

Many countries have taken effective action against unintentional injuries. For example, both Chile and Saint Lucia have formed interministerial commissions to address road traffic injuries; in Bogota (Colombia), a surveillance project is under way, utilizing emergency department records, and a similar approach is being piloted in the eastern Caribbean by the WHO Caribbean Epidemiology Centre with financial support from the International Development Research Centre (Canada). Such surveillance is potentially valuable for the recognition of risk factors and for the design of specific interventions. Suriname, among other countries, recently introduced legislation requiring the use of helmets by riders of motorcycles. Despite limited resources, many countries have been able to reduce the impact of road traffic accidents by introducing highly cost-effective interventions such as improved traffic engineering (one-way roads, signs, speed bumps), as well as seat-belt legislation and safety promotion. Nonetheless, all countries could still achieve significant reductions in the impact of unintentional injuries through a more assertive approach to this area of public health.

Violence is becoming a serious issue in many countries, and takes many forms. The patterns differ significantly among countries; in most, domestic violence is a serious concern (e.g. spouse abuse, child abuse, elder abuse). In most countries, violence is increasing in virtually all age groups. Violence may be addressed effectively by adopting a public health approach consisting of surveillance, risk factor identification, intervention evaluation, and implementation. The following questions need to be asked: "What is the problem?" "What is the cause?" "What works?" "How do you do it?". The causes of violence are, in principle, as amenable to intervention as the causes of unintentional injury, although there is a great need for studies that will answer the questions just posed in specific cultural contexts. Nonetheless, some factors are sufficiently well understood to be generally applicable across cultures, such as the role of drugs and alcohol, and ease of access to deadly force (e.g. firearms).

National leadership is essential in the prevention of injury, whether due to unintentional causes or to violence. This has become a major public health challenge for the 21st century.

tages" or "persons more in need" and to include vulnerable and special population groups, such as displaced persons and war victims. WHO's activities in 1996 included training senior personnel from 26 countries in managing community-based rehabilitation, the introduction of the strategy in Brazil and Kenya, and the preparation of documents (including *The multisectoral approach to community-based rehabilitation*, in collaboration with ILO and UNESCO) and training materials for work with children (on spina bifida, hydrocephalus and communication) and on spinal cord injuries.

WHO is currently undertaking a major revision of the International Classification of Impairments, Disabilities and Handicaps (ICIDH), which covers all disabilities. A measure of subjective quality of life is being developed, covering areas such as physical and psychological functioning, level of independence and social relations. Field trials of a questionnaire with 100 items were completed in 15 countries in 1996, while a short version with 26 items is currently being field-tested.

Activities directed to specific age groups

Health of the elderly

While elderly people have much to offer the world in terms of skills and talents developed over a lifetime, they can also become a burden on their families and society. Ill-health is increasingly frequent, and often chronic. Ageing is often accompanied by persistent poverty and isolation, and the biggest impact is on women.

WHO emphasizes the concept of healthy ageing and stresses the need to avoid compartmentalizing older persons in "the elderly" category. For example, in collaboration with the Institute of Gerontology of the University of Heidelberg, Germany, WHO published the first of a series of guidelines on healthy ageing. Endorsed by the scientific community, these guidelines are now being translated into several languages, adapted to different cultural settings and triggering multiple activities – such as "walk events" to mark worldwide the celebration of 1 October, the International Day of Older Persons. The focus is on active ageing for healthy ageing. The model used for producing these guidelines has now been adopted for preparing guidelines on a range of topics such as back pain, incontinence, healthy eating for healthy ageing and oral health.

In 1996 WHO developed a conceptual framework for establishing the priority areas for research on ageing and health worldwide. A joint conference with the United Nations took place in New York, attended by 40 experts representing 28 countries from North and South. Its final report focuses on three main areas: priority research topics on healthy ageing; policy development; and ageing-related conditions (which include most of the chronic diseases referred to in Chapter 1). In order to look more closely at the different policy implications of population ageing, WHO collaborated in an international conference in 1996 which culminated in the Brasilia Declaration on Ageing.

Untreated ***cataract*** greatly adds to the dependence of old people and can aggravate the confusion associated with both normal age-related memory loss and the more serious dementias. WHO has developed a simplified grading system for cataract which will help in implementing preventive strategies. Up to 20% of cataract operations could be prevented or delayed by informing people about the influence of ultraviolet light on cataract formation and through simple techniques such as wearing sunglasses to protect against excessive exposure. WHO has developed guidelines for training in community ophthalmology, in collaboration with the Task Force of the partnership committee on collaborating nongovernmental organizations, and the International Centre for Eye Health (United Kingdom). Visual loss from chronic diseases often leads to poor vision (severe visual disability), but leaves residual vision which can be enhanced through training and the use of optical devices. A workshop on low vision care for the elderly was hosted by *Organización Nacional de Ciegos de España* in Madrid, together with the above-mentioned Task Force, and led to the development of a global estimate of low vision and guidance for the basic content of a low-vision care model.

Dementia afflicts people over the age of 60 in rich and poor countries alike. Early diagnosis helps delay the onset of the disease and depends on understanding the clinical manifestations and on training health personnel to recognize the signs of change. In that regard, WHO cosponsored a meeting of the International Psychogeriatric Association on clinical and other methods in use and being developed, to make as early a diagnosis as possible in Alzheimer disease.

Health of adults

In the area of ***reproductive health***, WHO emphasizes the importance of enabling people to achieve their reproductive intentions – the desired number and timing of children within the context of the reproductive health of each individual. In Europe, several Member States have developed national policy documents on reproductive health, the main aim being to move from the use of abortion as the main method of fertility control to modern contraceptive methods. A scientific working group on training in reproductive health was established for the countries of central and eastern Europe and the newly independent States, involving all the major European schools and institutions of public health as well as nongovernmental organizations. In Africa, WHO cosponsored the first forum on teaching reproductive health in medical schools and other basic training institutions in 16 countries, where a version of the reproductive health training curriculum was also launched.

In collaboration with a large number of national and international groups, WHO has made recommendations on the medical criteria for prescribing various contraceptives, which will help national family planning programmes to simplify current contraceptive screening procedures and improve access to the services concerned. WHO regularly provides technical support to UNFPA on

In Africa, WHO cosponsored the first forum on teaching reproductive health in medical schools and other basic training institutions in 16 countries.

Box 17. Ergonomics and health

Two-thirds of the world's population spend one-third of their lives in earning a living for themselves and their families. These occupational activities generate revenue estimated at \$21.6 trillion to sustain the world's economies and social programmes. But these essential occupations present hazards to workers' health. WHO and ILO estimate that they result in 160 million cases of occupational diseases and more than 120 million occupational accidents and injuries per year (including at least 200 000 fatalities). A significant number develop into chronic debilitating disorders and diseases which, since they are preventable, are needlessly afflicting human health.

Many occupational diseases are musculoskeletal in nature, e.g. low back pain and repetitive strain injury. Musculoskeletal injuries have known causes such as excessive force, awkward postures, repetitive tasks – all resulting in overexertion.

The quality of life of workers can be improved markedly by designing or modifying the work processes, products and environment, in accordance with ergonomic considerations and adapted to different cultures and practices in manufacturing and service industries. With this in mind, the International Ergonomics Association (IEA) has designed ergonomic packages and strategies adjusted for gender and age that are relevant, efficient and acceptable for the emerging industrial countries of the developing world.

Rehabilitation for musculoskeletal disorders is needed most urgently, and highest priority is being given to research into these disorders, which should result in the formulation of appropriate standards for the prevention of injuries, chronic diseases and disability. To this end, IEA has taken the lead in advocating and supporting the development of rehabilitation ergonomics. The IEA organized an international symposium on the subject in Toronto, Canada, in 1994. Another is to be held in Tampere, Finland, in 1997.

IEA, which is a nongovernmental organization in official relations with WHO, recommends that to minimize human suffering due to occupational injuries, priority should be given to: reducing or eliminating ergonomic hazards in the workplace; setting up "return-to-work" programmes with special emphasis on the disabled and ageing population; designing control strategies for the increasingly sedentary occupations associated with the microcomputer revolution; and promoting the adoption of legislative measures to protect workers' health.

At the international level, IEA advocates the establishment of regional networks of ergonomics research centres to address and develop standards to remedy locally relevant problems, and of a global ergonomic information system and databases.

Based on a personal communication from the International Ergonomics Association.

reproductive health programmes. Existing family planning services have been assessed in eight countries with varied contraceptive prevalence, method mix, geographical position, and political and social systems, including Brazil, Viet Nam and Zambia. The assessments revealed that improved utilization of existing methods is of a higher priority than the introduction of new ones, and that, in general, service delivery management capability is not strong enough to introduce new methods widely with adequate quality of care without significant change and adaptation. One of the specific outcomes in Zambia was the development of a national document entitled *Family planning in reproductive health: policy framework and guidelines*. This is the first component of a national reproductive health policy and plan of action being developed to incorporate reproductive health in the health reform and district health planning processes.

Men still have relatively few contraceptive options, and WHO has supported the development of research on the contraceptive efficacy of suppressing sperm production by using exogenous steroids. The Organization has developed an improved formulation of a non-hormonal contraceptive based on immunological methods, which may provide protection for between 6 and 12 months.

Women and men of all ages at work are exposed to many potential hazards to health and to life (*Box 17*). WHO supports technical cooperation, information exchange, research and training through its global network of collaborating centres in ***occupational health***.

Health of women

In the domain of maternal and neonatal well-being and the reduction of maternal and newborn deaths, straightforward and effective strategies and action can have an immediate as well as long-term impact on women, their families and their communities. Women suffer a disproportionate burden of ill-health, which cannot be explained by biological differences alone. Their social, economic and political disadvantages have a detrimental effect on their health (*Box 18*).

WHO assists countries in the implementation of national plans for safe motherhood by providing technical input on research or programming issues. The WHO data banks on maternal mortality, coverage of maternity care, anaemia, unsafe abortion, infertility, perinatal mortality, low birth weight and preterm birth are a source of up-to-date information, and invaluable advocacy tools that contribute to the development and maintenance of standards and normative guidelines. The *Safe motherhood* newsletter regularly makes recent developments known to a wide audience of health care providers and decision-makers. WHO's midwifery education modules, designed to equip health care workers to manage the major obstetric complications which threaten women's lives, have been field-tested and are already being used in a number of countries. WHO's technical support for research projects such as those on neonatal resuscitation, oxytocin administration and the measurement of haemoglobin focused on the development of simple technologies for vital interventions that will also help to reduce the morbidity and mortality associated with childbirth.

Work began on a literature review paper on *Achievements and pitfalls of supplementary feeding programmes for women and children* with the aim of drawing lessons for the future. Later, guidelines will be developed to ensure that such programmes not only result in short-term nutritional benefits, but contribute to sustainable improvements in maternal and child health.

In 1996 WHO issued the report of an informal consultation on hookworm infection and anaemia in girls and women as well as a document defining indicators and measurement methods for assessing iron deficiency, which complemented earlier publications on iodine and vitamin A deficiencies. The Organization participated in multicountry studies of the effectiveness of weekly iron supplements (instead of daily supplementation) for pregnant women, adolescent girls and young children and the results so far are promising. In 1996, WHO issued a report on the menopause in the 1990s (*Box 19*).

A group of experts on ***osteoporosis***, including officers from national drug regulatory authorities and scientists, are preparing draft guidelines on the preclinical evaluation of and clinical trials on drugs which are being considered for use in osteoporosis. WHO will consult with the pharmaceutical industry and others concerning the draft guidelines. The objectives are to offer advice to the medical profession on which type of clinical study provides evidence of efficacy and safety, and to offer guidelines to the pharmaceutical industry to enable it to apply appropriate techniques and methodologies in the development of cost-effective interventions in osteoporosis. These final guidelines will be issued by WHO in 1997. This document, which will provide a scientific basis for the development of suitable drugs, will be of use not only to regulators and the pharmaceutical industry but also to academics and practising physicians. A shorter précis of the document

Box 18. Gender as a determinant of health

The gender concept was first used in the 1970s to describe those characteristics of men and women which are socially constructed, in contrast to those which are biologically determined. Essentially, the distinction between sex and gender aims to emphasize that everything women and men do, and everything expected of them, with the exception of their distinct biological functions (for women, pregnancy, childbirth and breast-feeding) can and does change over time, and according to changing and varied social and cultural factors. But in practically all cultures the role of women is subordinate to that of men. People are born female or male, but learn to be girls and boys who grow into women and men. They are taught what the appropriate behaviour and attitudes, roles and activities are for them, and how they should relate to other people. This learned behaviour is what makes up gender identity and determines gender roles.

A gender approach to health moves beyond describing women and women's health in isolation, but rather brings into the analysis how the different social roles, decision-making power and access to resources between women and men affect their health status and their access to health care. It examines how these differences determine, for example, differential exposure to risk, access to the benefits of technology, information and services, and the ability to protect oneself from disease and ill-health.

In order to meet the special needs of women and remove inequities, WHO's activities to improve women's health include setting norms and standards, developing guidelines and policy, the provision of technical support, and research. Increased efforts will be directed towards:

- advocacy for women's health and gender-sensitive approaches to health care delivery and development of practical tools to achieve this;
- promotion of women's health and prevention of ill-health;
- making health systems more responsive to women's needs;
- policies for improving gender equality; and
- ensuring the participation of women in the design, implementation and monitoring of health policies and programmes, in WHO and in countries.

Box 19. After the menopause: implications for women's health

In 1990, it was estimated that there were 467 million postmenopausal women worldwide, 60% of whom were living in developing countries. This number is expected to rise to 1200 million by the year 2030, with the proportion living in developing countries reaching 76%. Until now, however, almost all of the research into the health implications of the menopause has been conducted in industrialized countries, leaving a huge gap in understanding the health needs of the great majority of postmenopausal women in the world.

To redress this imbalance, a WHO scientific group has reviewed current research, including studies on the symptoms of the menopause and their treatment, and the effects of this crossroads in women's life on their cardiovascular and skeletal systems. In its report, published in 1996, the group has identified and described the areas where research needs are greatest, and emphasized the need to gather information on women in the developing world.

The menopause occurs between the ages of 45 and 55, when reproductive capacity ceases. The ovaries stop functioning and their production of hormones falls. A variety of physiological changes occur, and many women experience symptoms which are unpleasant and sometimes disabling. More important than the immediate symptoms are the effects of hormonal changes on many organs of the body.

Both the cardiovascular and the skeletal systems are adversely affected, as they also are by the ageing process. Numerous studies show that compared to premenopausal women of the same age, postmenopausal women have more risk factors for coronary heart disease, including higher blood cholesterol levels. A serious hazard for postmenopausal women is osteoporosis, sometimes called "brittle bone disease", which makes bones more liable to fracture, especially the long bones such as the femur, and vertebrae. Fractures of the vertebrae are painful and cause spinal deformity. Long bone fractures, especially of the neck of the femur, cause the greatest disability and death. Osteoporosis and associated fractures are a major cause of death, disability and medical expense worldwide.

The condition affects an estimated 75 million women in Europe, Japan and the United States combined, including one in three postmenopausal women and most elderly people. About 1.3 million osteoporotic fractures occur annually in the United States alone, with an annual cost approaching $10 billion a year. As the world population ages, the condition will become an ever greater public health problem. Thus early detection, prevention and treatment will be of greater importance. Prevention of osteoporosis can be aided by supplements of calcium and vitamin D, by physical exercise, by hormone therapy and by avoidance of smoking and heavy consumption of alcohol, but prevention should begin much earlier in life, with young women being encouraged to take appropriate steps to safeguard their own health.

To ameliorate the immediate and long-term consequences of the menopause, hormonal therapies are being used extensively in some societies. The therapies themselves have created new concerns about the increased risk of cancer of the endometrium and possibly the breast, and raise complex issues regarding the health benefits achieved relative to their cost in both health and monetary terms.

Research on the menopause in the 1990s: report of a WHO scientific group. Geneva, WHO, 1996 (Technical report series, No. 866.)

in lay language will be developed in parallel which may in turn be used by consumer groups as an educational tool.

Violence against women is a major public health issue. Studies show the impact of violence on women's mental and physical health, and its far-reaching effects for the woman and her children. In 1996 WHO held a consultation on violence against women, and the WHO Global Commission on Women's Health addressed the issue at its 1996 meeting. Both meetings focused on the topic of violence against women, but their findings and recommendations are relevant to all other situations where violence unfortunately may occur. WHO is carrying out a multicountry study on the prevalence, health consequences and risk factors of violence against women, especially violence in the family, and has identified information gaps and made recommendations for appropriate research methodologies, for ways to improve access to information, for advocacy and for interventions to prevent and address the consequences of violence.

Health of school-age children and adolescents

During adolescence, young people acquire new capacities and are faced with many new situations, presenting both opportunities for progress and risks to health and well-being. The patterns of behaviour which are initiated or consolidated during the second decade of life have long-term consequences, especially for chronic diseases.

Programmes for adolescents provide them with support and opportunities to acquire accurate information, to have access to health services and counselling, and to contribute to the well-being of their family and community. WHO's life skills education project assists education authorities to introduce problem-solving, communication and interaction skills into school curricula. In addition to helping young people to handle emotions and tension, it promotes a more positive view of health and the self, which will favourably affect their future physical and mental health status.

Education and health complement and enhance each other. In order to mobilize broad support for health promotion through schools, WHO launched the global school health initiative. In 1996, for example, teachers' unions in 18 Latin American countries benefited from training of trainers programmes based on the WHO/UNESCO resource package *School health education to prevent AIDS and STDs*. The long-term outcome is that spin-off programmes are launched to train others. Guidelines on strengthening interventions to prevent helminth infection through schools were issued, and financial and technical support was provided to China to use this document as an entry point for the development of health-promoting schools. In Europe, demonstration projects on school-based oral health promotion are being carried out in five countries.

Jointly with UNFPA and UNICEF, WHO has developed a human resources roster for adolescent health, aimed at helping countries to identify and deploy people with expertise in all aspects of programme development and delivery. WHO provides technical input to countries, partners in the United Nations system and key nongovernmental organizations and professional associations.

Rheumatic fever/rheumatic heart disease often result in significant chronic morbidity for schoolchildren and young adults. With a view to cooperating with countries in establishing a joint prevention and health promotion project with the support of the educational system, WHO signed a joint memorandum of understanding with UNESCO and the International Society and Federation of Cardiology in 1996.

WHO and the Arab Gulf Programme for United Nations Development Organizations (AGFUND) support an intensified programme on prevention and control of rheumatic fever and rheumatic heart disease in China, the Philippines, Tonga and Viet Nam. Studies on primary prevention among schoolchildren were carried out in China and the Philippines; the results showed that application of penicillin to streptococcal infection of the throat in schoolchildren and young people is an effective measure for primary prevention. National and regional registry centres for rheumatic fever and rheumatic heart disease were established, connecting to the computerized disease monitoring network in the Philippines.

A health and ***nutrition*** school feeding manual was completed, providing guidance to countries and the World Food Programme on the design and implementation of school feeding programmes. It sets out nutritional principles for establishing food requirements with emphasis on micronutrients as well as school-based health-related activities in areas such as food safety, safe water supply, sanitation and solid waste disposal, and intestinal parasite control.

WHO has established a project on ***substance abuse*** to address the needs of street children and other young people in especially difficult circumstances, recognizing their unique risk of substance-related harm. The project includes initiatives to train street educators working with young people.

WHO has developed a protocol for health services research on providing easier access for young people to reproductive health services. A guide on analysing sexual and ***reproductive health*** in adolescents was field-tested, and with UNICEF and the Commonwealth Medical Foundation a series of short training modules are being developed to strengthen knowledge, interpersonal communication skills and the sensitivity of health and other sectors to adolescent health and development issues. In Ghana, WHO participated in organizing the first African youth conference on sexual health, which was attended by more than 200 adolescents and young people, and which reviewed various activities relating to education on sexuality and sexual health in that age group in the participating countries.

WHO participated in organizing the first African youth conference on sexual health.

Child health

Recent data indicate that more than half of child deaths in developing countries are attributable to ***malnutrition***. Undernutrition retards the development of the infant's immune system, resulting in an inadequate response to immunization and resistance to infection, and stunted physical and intellectual growth. To date, over 140 countries have drafted, finalized or adopted national plans of action for nutrition. Most successful programmes involve communities in identifying the problems and mobilizing action and resources to solve them. WHO support was channelled particularly to the least developed countries, in collaboration with national institutions, FAO and UNICEF. In Europe, the first nationally-representative food consumption survey in the countries of central and eastern Europe and the newly independent States was carried out in Kazakstan in collaboration with UNDP.

In order to help monitor and prevent protein-energy malnutrition, WHO has published an expert committee report on *Physical status: the use and interpretation of anthropometry*. This and the WHO global database on child growth and malnutrition (now also accessible on the Internet) have become standard reference works for those active in this field. As existing international reference values for the growth of children have been found to be inappropriate, WHO has started work to develop and establish new standards. *Trace elements in human nutrition and health*, also published in 1996, gives reliable criteria and new knowledge on the global status and assessment of deficiency and excess of 19 trace elements.

By the end of 1996, more than 7700 hospitals in 171 countries had been designated as "baby-friendly". A new training course for administrators and policy-makers on promoting breastfeeding in health facilities is now available, and WHO has finalized the *Common review and evaluation framework* for use by countries in reviewing action to give effect to the International Code of Marketing of Breast-Milk Substitutes. The WHO global data bank on breastfeeding has been updated with new definitions and indicators, which will facilitate comparisons and monitoring of trends. With the collaboration of UNICEF, the University of Davis, California (United States), and the Nutrition Department of the *Office de la recherche scientifique et technique*, Montpellier (France), and other WHO collaborating centres, WHO has prepared a paper examining complementary feeding practices of infants and young children worldwide as well as guidelines for future research and survey procedures.

Sustainable elimination of new iodine deficiency disorders appears feasible by the target year 2000, provided that national and international commitment are maintained.

Infant and child health are affected by the mother's nutritional status during pregnancy. ***Iodine deficiency*** in the mother, for example, can lead to iodine deficiency and mental retardation in the child, with devastating consequences lasting into old age. Universal iodization of salt for human and animal consumption is the optimal way of correcting iodine deficiency and should continue to be the primary focus for preventing and controlling iodine deficiency disorders. Through the efforts of national governments, WHO, UNICEF, the International Council of Iodine Deficiency Disorders and the salt industry, and with the support of bilateral development agencies, financial resources required to achieve universal salt iodization have been mobilized. An estimated $30 million worth of investment in salt iodization has been made available to countries since 1990 from external sources, over and above national investments. Salt iodization programmes now exist in 110 countries. By 1996, 57% of all salt consumed in 83 countries was adequately iodized. WHO has confirmed that it is safe to administer periodic large doses of iodized oil at any time during pregnancy, pending successful establishment of salt iodization in areas of moderate and severe iodine deficiency. Sustainable elimination of new iodine deficiency disorders appears feasible by the target year 2000, provided that national and international commitment are maintained.

The WHO/UNICEF ***Integrated management of childhood illness*** strategy provides a systematic process for diagnosing and treating five conditions: diarrhoea, acute respiratory infections, malnutrition (including problems with breast-feeding), measles and malaria, which together are responsible for approximately 70% of all child deaths. WHO provides technical support to national programmes and contributes to worldwide research aimed at the prevention and control of these problems. Six African countries are already implementing the programme.

WHO makes regular contributions to the newsletter *Child health news* which disseminates information on prevention and case management of childhood illness, aimed at programme managers and health workers taking care of children. It is published in English by the Appropriate Health Resources and Technologies Action Group in the United Kingdom, with regional or country-specific editions in a range of languages including Gujarati, Portuguese and Vietnamese.

Similar materials on diarrhoeal and respiratory diseases are being tested now for use in nursing and paramedical schools. The first country experience in using a self-instructional course on clinical skills in the control of diarrhoeal diseases was carried out in 1996.

In a trial in Kenya, WHO has shown that impregnated bednets not only prevent deaths from ***malaria***, but also significantly reduce hospital admissions for severe malaria, which can thereby significantly reduce the burden on health services. Operational research is now focusing on such problems as how to promote wider use of insecticide-treated bednets and how to lengthen the time between retreatment of nets.

As a result of WHO's activities, 500 million ***immunization*** contacts a year are made with children. Immunizing children also opens the door to other elements of care – for the children concerned, their siblings and the adults who take them to be vaccinated. Unfortunately, the relative success of global immunization is breeding complacency among donors. Resources for basic programmes are shrinking and interest is shifting to newer but much more expensive products.

One of WHO's goals is to enable the provision of sufficient quantities of high-quality affordable vaccines to be sustained. A network was established to train the staff of national control authorities so that a uniform high standard for all vaccines used within each country can be ensured. A new evaluation tool is enabling countries to rapidly assess their production facilities and also to determine the investments needed to meet quality standards and ensure the long-term financial viability of immunization programmes.

A new vaccine against rotavirus is now ready for clinical testing. Vaccines against both strains of cholera have been produced and are being used in refugee camps. Standardization has been completed of animal models for testing and assessment of four newly developed tuberculosis vaccines, including a DNA vaccine. Examples of novel vaccination approaches include preclinical studies of a single-dose tetanus vaccine using a controlled release system, clinical trials for a nasal meningococcal vaccine, and research to develop optimal mucosal delivery systems for DNA vaccines. WHO has coordinated field trials of new vaccines against meningococcal meningitis in Niger, clinical trials of a locally produced cholera vaccine in Viet Nam, and of an oral cholera vaccine in Mali.

Vaccines against meningitis and pneumonia caused by *Haemophilus influenzae* type b have recently been shown in studies supported by WHO, the Children's Vaccine Initiative, USAID and other funders to be capable of preventing at least 250 000 child deaths per year worldwide. The Children's Vaccine Initiative has therefore entered into broad collaboration with WHO, UNICEF and vaccine producers to promote the wider use of this and other vaccines against acute respiratory disease.

Hearing impairment is a serious problem in young children because it retards language development and

Immunizing children also opens the door to other elements of care – for the children concerned, their siblings and the adults who take them to be vaccinated.

school progress – both of which have a significant impact in later life. Some children have inherited severe inner-ear deafness, but most children who develop hearing impairment have had chronic otitis media which has not been recognized and not treated. In 1996 WHO and the CIBA Foundation developed guidelines on detection and proper management, especially at the primary care level.

Infectious diseases

Whatever their mode of transmission, most infectious diseases are chronic problems for all age groups. Chronic because of the persistence of the pathogens themselves and of the conditions they need for survival and transmission, and because in addition to the immediate impact that diseases such as leprosy, malaria or onchocerciasis have on individuals and communities, they have devastating consequences that can last a lifetime.

WHO issued guidelines for malaria control among refugees and displaced populations in 1996.

By end-1996, a cumulative total of 29.4 million children and adults had been infected with ***HIV*** and a cumulative 8.4 million ***AIDS*** cases had been documented worldwide. The Joint United Nations Programme on HIV/AIDS (UNAIDS) became operational on 1 January 1996. WHO, one of its six cosponsors, provides epidemiological and technical support by maintaining the epidemiological surveillance and tracking of HIV/AIDS and STDs. Publications include *A source book on HIV/AIDS counselling* and the results of a study on AIDS orphans carried out with UNICEF entitled *Action for children affected by AIDS: programme profiles and lessons learned*. WHO began publication of a quarterly newsletter in 1996, and information is accessible electronically on WHO's Internet site. A policy and advocacy document was issued in collaboration with UNAIDS entitled *A deadly partnership: TB in the era of HIV*. The WHO publication *TB/HIV: a clinical manual* will help clinicians cope with the growing problem of TB/HIV co-infection. WHO, UNICEF and UNDP collaborated to produce a policy guide on HIV and infant feeding.

In the fight against ***tuberculosis***, WHO promotes the adoption and implementation of the directly observed treatment, short course (DOTS), which entails the use of standardized regimens of effective drug combinations, direct supervision of treatment for at least the first two months, and evaluation of treatment for each patient. Over 80 Member States have adopted, or are starting to use, the DOTS strategy, with an increase in cure rates to 90% in some countries. WHO continues to identify ways to facilitate DOTS adoption in different environments. An operational research project in Malawi improved the efficiency of diagnosis and treatment. Studies are under way to show the potential economic benefits of DOTS in India and how good-quality care might be delivered through a network of private providers. Advocacy workshops help translate programme review findings into action, and WHO's new training modules, *Managing tuberculosis at national level*, and guidelines aim to reinforce national technical expertise (e.g. tuberculosis control among refugees, and the management of drug-resistant tuberculosis). A new WHO newsletter, the *TB treatment observer*, highlights the success of DOTS in many countries.

WHO works with ministries and donors in developed countries to ensure continued financial support from them to countries where ***malaria*** is endemic. WHO organized training in epidemic preparedness and control with support from donors in 17 African and 3 Asian countries, trained 35 entomologists from national programmes in Asia and Africa in selective vector control in intercountry workshops, and provided technical assistance for malaria prevention and control in refugee camps in Azerbaijan and in 10 other countries affected by epidemics. The Organization issued guidelines for malaria control among refugees and displaced populations in 1996. WHO collaborated with UNDP in Myanmar; with the World Bank in Bangladesh, Lao People's Democratic Republic, Madagascar and Viet Nam; and with the European

Union in Cambodia, Lao People's Democratic Republic and Viet Nam. Community-based malaria control activities have been established in parts of Eritrea and Ethiopia, with support from Italy and the Netherlands, and in Uganda with the German Agency for Technical Cooperation (GTZ).

Onchocerciasis is prevalent in tropical Africa, Yemen and parts of Latin America. The two principal intervention methods for its control are vector control through larviciding and chemotherapy by ivermectin. In January 1996, a new African Programme for Onchocerciasis Control was started, covering 19 African countries where onchocerciasis affects about 15 million people.

Leprosy is declining in most endemic countries and variations in case detection observed in some countries are often related to intensified case-finding activities and the expansion of geographical coverage, rather than to an increase in the incidence of the disease. Different WHO regions and countries are expected to reach elimination levels at different dates. Each endemic country is expected to identify districts where leprosy is still endemic and give priority to them. WHO, by collecting information at the global level, assists in defining high-priority zones and in mobilizing adequate resources (*Map 4*). The leprosy elimination campaign is an initiative implemented by national staff with technical cooperation from WHO and other agencies, which aims at providing national programmes with additional external inputs to intensify elimination activities. The involvement of community volunteers and general health workers reduces the delay in managing cases and ensures that the existing health services are able to treat them.

1996 was the 200th anniversary of Jenner's ***smallpox*** vaccine. The World Health Assembly recommended that the world's remaining stocks of variola virus should be destroyed on 30 June 1999. The smallpox vaccine seed virus will be maintained in the WHO collaborating centre on smallpox vaccine at the National Institute of Public Health and Environmental Protection, Bilthoven, Netherlands.

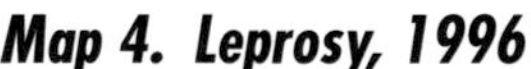

Map 4. Leprosy, 1996

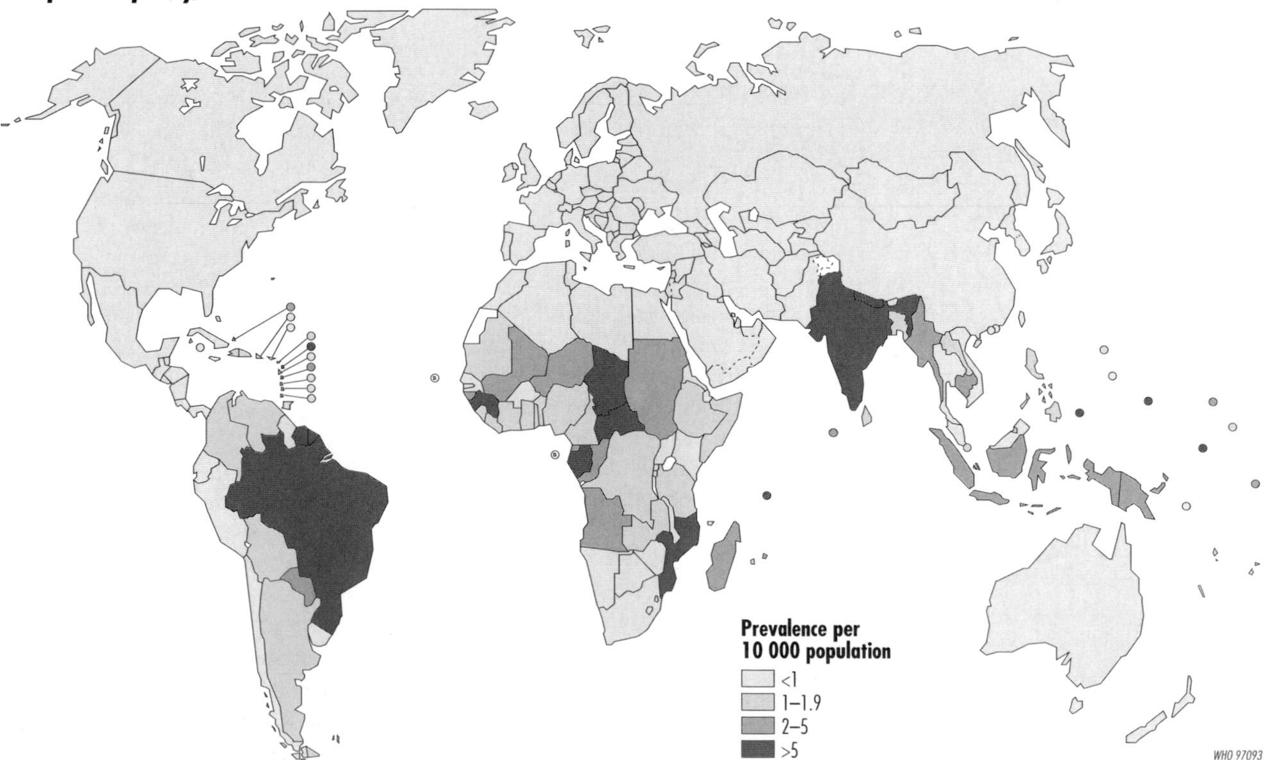

WHO remains active in ***tropical disease research***. Preclinical trials of UMF 078, a drug which is proving to be effective against adult worms of *Onchocerca*, *Wuchereria* and *Brugia* (which cause river blindness and lymphatic filariasis) have been successfully completed. The drug has now been shown to be effective against adult worms after a single injection.

Promotion and protection of health

WHO and FAO have jointly published recommendations concerning the use of fermentation as a household technology for improving food safety.

Promotion and protection of health cover a wide range of actions: from promotion of individual healthy lifestyles and human behavioural changes to management of risk to human health by governments, communities and the private sector.

WHO encourages the adoption of ***healthy lifestyles*** by focusing on advocacy for health, empowerment of communities and design of media strategies for health. In order to achieve this, a *Five-year action plan, leading health promotion into the 21st century* has been launched. Feasibility discussions on infrastructures for health promotion and education to mobilize support and action were held in the Centers for Disease Control and Prevention (CDC), Atlanta, United States, with representation from China, India, Indonesia, Japan, the Russian Federation and the United States – the mega country initiative; and with networks of countries which are geographically close – such as the Mediterranean country network for health promotion. Two new collaborating centres were established in Sydney (Australia) and Toronto (Canada) and two more are being designated in CDC and the African Medical and Research Foundation (AMREF), Kenya, bringing the total to 18. WHO also carried out targeted activities at country level, such as a workshop in Gabon on health education programme planning and evaluation techniques for health personnel.

Safe food and good nutrition are cornerstones of socioeconomic development and basic human rights. In 1996, enterohaemorrhagic *Escherichia coli* (EHEC), a newly emerging foodborne pathogen, struck in Japan and in the United Kingdom. WHO kept the international public health community informed by issuing articles in the *Weekly epidemiological record* and fact sheets on *E. coli* O157:H7 and emerging foodborne diseases. WHO is organizing a consultation in 1997 to propose measures for the prevention of epidemics caused by EHEC, and to outline steps which should be taken when an epidemic strikes, in order to control its spread. To draw the attention of public health authorities to the role of food technologies in health protection, WHO has prepared a document on *Food technologies and public health*, as well as guidelines for developing or strengthening a national food safety programme. As contaminated food plays an important role in the spread of infant diarrhoea and as many families in developing countries have only limited, if any, access to facilities to control contamination (e.g. refrigeration), WHO and FAO have jointly published recommendations concerning the use of fermentation as a household technology for improving food safety.

In recent years, official food control as well as the food industry's safety activities have increasingly been based on a relatively new food safety assurance system: the hazard analysis and critical control point system (HACCP). In order to promote the application of this system, WHO convened a workshop on the basis of which training materials for different target groups (decision-makers, food and public health inspectors, managers in the food industry) were developed in collaboration with the Industry Council for Development. A regional training course was convened in Harare to field-test this material. In 1996, WHO published *Preparation and use of food-based dietary guidelines*, which demonstrates how national authorities can emphasize locally available foods in their dietary advice, and integrate the messages in the guidelines into other health-related policies such as those on smoking, physical activity and alcohol consumption.

In 1996, WHO published the report of the joint FAO/WHO Expert Consultation on Biotechnology and Food Safety which addresses the evaluation of the safety of foods and food products produced using biotechnology.

Human health continues to be adversely affected by a wide array of ***environmental factors***, ranging from climate change to water supply. In 1996, WHO provided information to the Intergovernmental Panel on Climate Change which was instrumental in securing new international commitments to deal with the root causes of global climate change. A related issue is increased exposure to ultraviolet radiation due to ozone layer depletion. During 1996, WHO produced information on health hazards and protection measures, including guidelines on a simple ultraviolet index to be used in risk communication in collaboration with UNEP, WMO and the International Commission on Non-Ionizing Radiation Protection.

As part of the GEMS/AIR programme, a system for making information on air quality more accessible was set up. Preliminary estimates show that many more "excess deaths" are caused by air pollution in the developing countries than in the developed countries, and that indoor air pollution in rural dwellings may present the greatest threat to health.

WHO emphasizes the low-cost and community-based aspects of water and sanitation programmes, serving populations at greatest risk from sanitation-related diseases. Practical training and guidance manuals produced by WHO are used throughout the world. Two of the most popular titles are *Operation and maintenance of urban water supply and sanitation systems* and *Management of operation and maintenance in rural drinking-water supply and sanitation.*

At the HABITAT II Conference in Istanbul in June 1996, WHO organized a panel discussion of international personalities on the theme "Creating healthy cities in the 21st century", which stressed the participatory approach and the important role of local authorities in addressing health and environment issues in urban areas. World Health Day 1996, on the theme "Healthy cities for better life", involved over 1000 participating cities around the world. The concept is now being extended to municipalities, villages and islands.

WHO is the executing agency of the International Programme on Chemical Safety (IPCS), operated jointly with ILO and UNEP, and the administering agency of the Intergovernmental Forum on Chemical Safety and the Inter-organizational Programme for the Sound Management of Chemicals. In the field of assessment of risks to human health and the environment from exposure to chemicals, validated information was produced in the form of international chemical safety cards, data sheets on pesticides and the classification of pesticides by hazard. A new project was launched to accelerate international assessment of priority chemicals by producing concise international chemical assessment documents based on national and regional assessments. The first seven documents were reviewed in 1996. More than 30 poison information monographs and 14 treatment guides were reviewed and finalized. Several working groups met in the framework of the IPCS INTOX project which dealt with various aspects such as analytical toxicology and aquatic biotoxins, as well as an international seminar and workshop on poison control in eastern Europe. At a consultation on methodology for collection of pesticide poisoning data, a pilot study to be conducted in four countries was launched. A project to provide national training for developing countries on toxic chemicals, environment and health, was launched in 15 countries in Africa, Asia and Latin America, addressing decision-makers and risk managers at different levels and in different sectors dealing with chemicals.

IPCS has produced the first edition of a CD-ROM (IPCS-INCHEM) containing all IPCS publications which will be updated periodically. The INTOX CD-ROM IPCS publication relevant to the management of poisonings was updated, and the second issue finalized and distributed in 1996. IPCS now also has a home page on the World Wide Web.

A project to provide national training for developing countries on toxic chemicals, environment and health, was launched in 15 countries in Africa, Asia and Latin America.

Box 20. Essential Health Interventions Program

With many governments and international aid agencies forced to tighten spending in recent years, funding for essential health services is in short supply. The challenge now is to find ways of improving health delivery systems so as to ensure sustainable delivery of limited health resources.

The Essential Health Interventions Program (EHIP) is a response to this challenge. An initiative of Canada's International Development Research Centre (IDRC) with support and input from the Canadian International Development Agency (CIDA), EHIP is a four-year health research and development initiative designed to generate new knowledge in support of the planning and delivery of essential public and clinical health services. It will assist, at the district level, with the selection of essential clinical and public health interventions, taking into consideration community perceptions and preferences for health services. It will also study the usefulness of burden of disease and cost-effectiveness measurements for setting priorities and allocating health resources.

The initiative is already under way in the United Republic of Tanzania, where it is known as TEHIP (Tanzania Essential Health Interventions Project). Over time, and with additional funding, it is hoped that EHIP may expand to other countries with different environments and challenges, thereby adding to the knowledge base surrounding the universal applicability of this approach to health planning.

Over the past few years the Government of Tanzania has been working to strengthen health planning and service delivery capacity at district level through its health sector reform. TEHIP provides an excellent opportunity both to build on the existing health system and to test selected aspects of initiatives for health sector reform. The project is an excellent example of collaboration between all partners concerned: the Government of Tanzania, WHO, the World Bank, UNICEF, CIDA and the Edna McConnell Clark Foundation.

TEHIP will focus primarily on two strategies for improving health:

- financing and delivering essential clinical and public health interventions; and
- improving the planning and management of health services at the district level.

Tanzanian researchers will endeavour to answer the following three key questions:

- In the context of decentralization, how and to what extent, can district health management teams establish priorities and plan the allocation of resources according to local estimates of burden of disease and knowledge of the cost-effectiveness of relevant interventions?
- How, and to what extent, are the district health plans translated into the delivery and use of essential health interventions?
- How, to what extent, and at what cost, does this have an impact on burden of disease?

If the principles of health care planning being tested through EHIP prove workable, this Canadian initiative will have implications for improving health resource allocation in low-income countries around the world, and the use of limited health resources could be considerably improved.

Health services and health policy

Improving health services

In the decade ahead many countries will make decisions on their ***health systems*** development strategy which may prove irreversible. They will also have to strike a balance among health policy objectives such as service quality, cost effectiveness and acceptability (*Box 20*). These decisions should be made in the light of the best available evidence and in the most accountable and consultative manner possible. In 1996, a WHO conference on health care reform, which united participants from 45 countries and representatives of the World Bank, the Council of Europe and nongovernmental organizations, adopted the Ljubljana Charter, which places strong emphasis on developing health care systems governed by the principles of human dignity, equity, solidarity and professional ethics.

Many countries and agencies look to WHO for leadership on health systems issues. More specifically, strategic support is provided to countries in greatest need through public information programmes such as in the Republic of Moldova; a telecommunication programme in Bhutan; the development of rural medical cooperatives in China; the production of latrines in Guatemala; political mapping for health reform in Zambia; and the integration of health activities in agricultural projects in Mali and Uganda. WHO creates opportunities for countries to learn from each other's experience in health systems development, carrying out comparative studies and distilling key lessons in order to understand how individual country contexts affect policy. To this end, a series of discussion papers are produced, covering topics such as "Applying planned market logic to developing countries' health systems". Technical support is given to the poorest population groups with their own participation (e.g. in Bolivia, Guinea-Bissau and Viet Nam), emphasizing local processes and basic health services.

Reform strategies in ***health financing***, organizational change and innovations in service delivery often involve trade-offs between different objectives of health policy. There is frequently a conflict between the demands of equity and the need to mobilize more private financing. While there is a growing awareness of the size and potential of private finance, few countries have reassessed the role of government in relation to the private health care sector. However, a clear message from reform experiences is that greater reliance on market mechanisms requires more regulation, not less. WHO guidelines, for example on social health insurance, have been widely used and cited.

Quality of care

Ensuring access to and availability of ***essential drugs and vaccines*** at low cost, their rational use, and their quality and safety are a major goal for WHO. The WHO *Model list of essential drugs*, which contains drugs that satisfy the health care needs of the majority of the population, was updated having regard to the increasing problem of resistance to antimicrobials. A new category of drugs with restricted indications was introduced. WHO provided support to over 50 countries, covering all elements of national drug policies. More than 110 countries now have an essential drugs list. Some 60, including countries as diverse as Australia, Kazakstan and Viet Nam, have formulated, and are implementing, a national drug policy. To this end, the *Guidelines for developing national drug policies* are being updated. Innovative materials for training such as the *Model guide to good prescribing* and *Guidelines to the economic aspects of drug supply*, have been widely disseminated and used. *Indicators for monitoring national drug policies* were applied in research on comparative analysis of national drug policies which took place in 12 countries. Information was provided during 1996 on the essential drugs concept, national drug policies and rational use of drugs through a wide range of publications including technical documents and reports and the *Essential drugs monitor*, published in English, French, Spanish and Russian.

In the field of ***drug quality and efficacy***, WHO supports the rational prescribing and use of essential drugs by regularly producing the series *Model prescribing information*. Other publications include *WHO guidelines for good clinical practice for trials on pharmaceutical products* (to set globally applicable standards for the conduct of biomedical research on human subjects); *Drugs used in parasitic diseases*; *Drugs used in sexually transmitted diseases and HIV infection*; and *Drugs used in skin diseases*.

Biotechnology will contribute significantly to the introduction and development of new therapies for chronic and debilitating diseases such as diabetes, dementia and cancer. To meet the vital need for respected worldwide standards of quality, efficacy and safety for biotechnology products, WHO regularly formulates guidelines and requirements on relevant biotechnology-derived biologicals that form a basis for globally harmonized norms and standards.

In spite of the increase in international trade in herbal medicines and other types of alternative medicine worldwide, the potential of ***traditional medicine*** is far from being fully utilized in most national health systems (*Box 21*).

WHO prepared a number of documents concerning national policy and regulation of traditional medicine and technical guidelines during 1996 (e.g. *Guidelines on basic training in acupuncture* and *Guidelines for safe acupuncture treatment*). With the aim of facilitating research and development of traditional medicine and scientific information exchange at the country level, the Organization issued a report summarizing the latest research achievements and activities in 17 WHO collaborating centres for traditional medicine during the last five years.

Technology assessment

Technology assessment is fundamental to quality of care as it provides the basis for rational decisions on selection of

In spite of the increase in international trade in herbal medicines and other types of alternative medicine worldwide, the potential of traditional medicine is far from being fully utilized.

Box 21. Traditional medicine

Many elements of traditional medicine are beneficial, but others are not. WHO encourages and supports countries in their efforts to find safe and effective remedies and practices for use in health services while not endorsing all forms of traditional medicine. Traditional medicine is examined critically, with an open mind.

Most of the population in developing countries still rely mainly on traditional practitioners and local medicinal plants for primary health care, and interest in traditional and alternative systems of medicine has grown in industrialized countries during the last decade. In the United States it is estimated that one-third of the population uses at least some form of alternative treatment such as herbal medicines, acupuncture, chiropractic and homeopathy. Surveys in European countries have shown similar interest: 60% of the Dutch and Belgian public have expressed their willingness to pay extra health insurance for alternative medicine, and 74% of the British public favour complementary medicine being available on the national health service.

Despite the existence of *herbal medicines* for many centuries, only a relatively small number of plant species – about 5000 – have been studied for their possible medical applications. Safety and efficacy data exist only in respect of a much smaller number of plants, their extracts and their active ingredients. The establishment and use of regulation procedures and quality control have become major concerns in both developing and industrialized countries.

Acupuncture is used worldwide because of the simplicity of its application, its minimal side- effects and its low cost. It has been in constant use in China for thousands of years, and spread to other oriental countries long ago. By 1990, the total number of acupuncturists in Europe had reached 88 000, of whom 62 000 were medical doctors, while acupuncture users totalled 20 million . Consumer surveys consistently show positive public attitudes to complementary medicine – 90% of the pain clinics in the United Kingdom and 77% in Germany use acupuncture. Important advances have been made in our understanding of the mechanisms of acupuncture. In particular, great progress has been made in clinical research on acupuncture analgesia which has been used during surgery and for the treatment of acute and chronic pain.

There are 19 WHO collaborating centres for traditional medicine, eight of which are involved in training and research on acupuncture, while the others are conducting research on herbal medicines. These centres have made a major contribution to the international standardization of herbal medicines and acupuncture, and the exchange of information.

In China, where traditional medicine is widely practised, each province has a college and a research institute for Chinese traditional medicine. In India, the government provides financial support for the research and development of the Ayurvedic and Unani systems and their increasing involvement in the delivery of health services. Such systems are seen as allies in the delivery of primary health care. Research institutes and foundations have also been established in industrialized countries, such as the Office of Alternative Medicine in the United States. A group set up by the European Commission is investigating the therapeutic significance of unconventional medicine, its cost-benefit ratio and its sociocultural importance as a basis for the evaluation of its possible use in public health.

WHO strongly supports the further promotion and development of the rational use of traditional medicine throughout the world.

technologies and procedures. Jointly with the WHO collaborating centre for essential technologies in Tygerberg (South Africa), work started on preparation of guidelines on determination of needs for technologies at the district level. The first meeting of a regional group of experts on essential health technologies in Africa was held in 1996, launching a survey of existing and potential resources for training and technology assessment in that region. In the area of clinical technology, teaching video tapes based on WHO publications on surgery and anaesthesia at the district hospital were produced. Guidelines on day surgery, simple external fixation of fractures and management of bone and joint infection were drafted in collaboration with the United States Food and Drug Administration.

In the area of ***blood safety***, WHO works regularly with UNAIDS in testing strategies, bulk procurement of testing assays and blood donor counselling. WHO's simple reusable haemoglobin (Hb) colour scale has been extensively evaluated in laboratory settings and some controlled field studies, showing that it is sensitive and specific and meets the requirements for screening for anaemia at a cost estimated at less than 1 US cent per test overall. It is anticipated that the device will be ready for production in the second half of 1997.

In collaboration with UNDP and with specialists in Nigeria and Switzerland, WHO has developed a device that will salvage patients' blood that has been lost in trauma as a result of childbirth and other conditions, thus avoiding the risk of receiving infected blood, at less than the cost of blood donation. The Organization has also developed a blood cold chain to ensure the safety of blood and blood products from donor to recipient, with financial support from the Government of Luxembourg. As a result, cold boxes, refrigerators and freezers specifically designed for blood and blood products have been improved in four developing countries. Three regional workshops utilizing the WHO *distance learning material on safe blood and blood products* to train trainers were held in the Americas, Europe and the Western Pacific. With funding from the Japanese Ministry of Health and Welfare, the material has been translated from English into Chinese, French, Portuguese, Russian and Spanish.

WHO continuously monitors the establishment of national external quality assessment schemes as an indicator of the implementation of agreed principles to ensure ***good laboratory practice***. To date, more than 60 countries have established national and/or regional schemes in at least one of the main laboratory disciplines. The Organization gave a training course on good diagnostic practice in collaboration with AMREF, to discuss and overcome major problems in communication between health laboratories and their users. A laboratory procedure for screening and monitoring diabetes mellitus in children was developed, and studies in central and eastern Europe proved the efficiency of the method in the long-term monitoring of patients, and in achieving comparability of epidemiological data. WHO issued a document entitled *Safety in health laboratories*.

In the area of ***radiation medicine***, the technical specification for the WHO basic radiological system published in 1985 was updated and printed for worldwide distribution as the *Technical specifications for the world health imaging system for radiography*. Operation of the IAEA/WHO network of secondary standard dosimetry laboratories covering 73 laboratories in 56 countries (43 in developing ones), and the IAEA/WHO postal dose intercomparison programme, continued in all regions.

Health personnel

Since the health workforce accounts for some 70% of the recurrent health budget in many countries, it becomes a natural focus for improving cost-effectiveness in health services (*Box 22, Fig. 8*). Changes taking place in some Member States provide excellent lessons on how financial and economic forces modify the way care is provided and who provides it. International comparison in human resources for health is complicated by the lack of uniform nomenclature and standards. In addition, the data available are generally from the public sector only.

In order to strengthen ***health workforce planning*** and management in countries, WHO has developed a range of methods and instruments including computerized models of supply and requirement projections, among them a method for calculating staffing norms and a guide on the selection of planning methods to match specific situations. Trainers from some 40 countries have taken part in workshops on the use of these health workforce planning tools. Three countries in the South-East Asia Region have developed master plans for human resources for health, and two others have reviewed existing plans; all countries in the Region now recognize the need to continually review existing plans. The Kellogg Foundation and Japan provided funds for health workforce planning and policy analysis. Successful collaboration with nongovernmental organizations, foundations and individual institutions in the field of education of health professionals enabled WHO to maintain a wider spectrum of activities than would otherwise have been possible.

The *World directory of schools of public health* has been made available on microcomputer diskettes from an electronic database now being maintained in Geneva. The sixth edition of the *World directory of medical schools* was reprinted in 1996, with supplementary information. Future editions of this directory will be in electronic format only.

The importance of the role of ***nursing and midwifery*** is now widely acknowledged. A nursing management information system has been successfully tested and set up as part of an effort to establish national human resources information systems. In Africa, WHO is working towards legislative recognition of the role of nurses and midwives. In the Western Pacific, WHO is working with China to upgrade nursing education for the more than 1 million nurses

Changes taking place in some Member States provide excellent lessons on how financial and economic forces modify the way care is provided and who provides it.

Box 22. Health personnel

Ministries of health are faced with chronic problems of imbalance of three types in the health workforce: (i) numerical – the difference between the numbers of health care providers of various categories and the numbers a country or community needs and can afford; (ii) qualitative – the mismatch between the type and level of training and the job that needs to be done; and (iii) distributional – mismatch between the geographical, occupational, institutional and specialty mix, or between the public and private sector. These types of imbalance result in an inappropriate mix of skills, poor distribution of personnel and skewed allocation of resources to certain categories of health personnel.

Identifying the appropriate mix of health personnel is one of the major challenges that countries face. The number of each category of health worker is influenced by traditional ways of delivering services and by the available financial resources for salaries and equipment. Countries are attempting to find the most cost-effective combination to provide high-quality health care. In this context, countries must first make an assessment of the prevailing situation, based on the best available information.

WHO has taken the initiative to make a global comparison of health workforce ratios between countries. These can be misleading as they depend on methods of organization, financing and the public-private mix. Comparisons can, however, indicate genuine differences worldwide. Difficulties in comparisons between countries and regions occur because of variations in the level of education and number of years required for admission to practise in the respective disciplines, different terminology* and differences in the scope of responsibilities. The average ratio of physicians, nurses and midwives, and dentists per 100 000 population, by region, is given in *Fig. 8*. Ratios by country and rates by level of development are given in *Annex 2*.

The number of ***physicians*** per population varies significantly between and within countries. Globally, the developed market economies have a ratio of over 250 physicians per 100 000 population, compared to 14 per 100 000 in the least developed countries (LDCs), or almost 20 times as many. Developing countries (other than LDCs) have 85 physicians per 100 000. These differences reflect that access to services provided by physicians varies significantly between these three categories of countries. The economies in transition have a ratio of 360 physicians per 100 000 population, reflecting past policies in this group of countries to produce and employ large numbers of physicians in government service.

LDCs often do not have the capacity to train appropriate numbers of physicians and are unable to retain physicians trained in their country (when national medical schools exist) or abroad. Poor salaries and working conditions are often cited as factors contributing to poor retention rates. Shrinking public sector budgets have restricted the employment of health providers.

One of the most significant changes in the deployment of medical personnel during the past decade is the extended use of the general practitioner and the development of the "specialist" family physician. These practitioners are medical primary care providers, who are intended to interact more closely with the community than their more specialized colleagues. Their work encompasses health promotion, disease prevention and curative care for both individuals and the community.

The work of ***nurses and midwives*** ranges from carrying out high-technology investigations in the most industrialized countries to providing the whole range of primary health care services in remote regions in developing countries. Nursing and midwifery personnel are the largest group of health care professionals accounting for the largest share of the budget for human resources in most countries.

A survey of 94 countries in 1994 found that the demand for nursing and midwifery services is increasing. Factors affecting this demand include changing disease patterns and demographic profiles, resulting in higher demands for chronic care and home-based care. There are shortages of nurses and midwives, which are often compounded by inappropriate deployment, underuse or inappropriate use. The effective use of nurses and midwives within health care systems is affected by a number of interrelated issues such as a lack of clear definition of roles and responsibilities of this category of personnel in relation to others; traditional relationships between nurses and midwives, and physicians; the status of women in general and of nursing and midwifery as a career (in some countries) in particular; and poor working conditions (e.g. remuneration and physical safety).

Issues of substitution, delegation and complementarity of providers and their skills are being tackled as health care delivery systems and their managers struggle with questions of economic efficiency and effectiveness. Studies have indicated that some sets of activities and

Box 22. Health personnel (continued)

individual tasks traditionally performed by one category of health care worker can be performed by a worker who has been educated differently.

A comparison for recent years of the availability of nursing and midwifery services in countries at different levels of economic development shows that economies in transition report an estimate of 800 nurses and midwives per 100 000 population and developed market economies report around 750, whereas LDCs have around 20 per 100 000.

There are great differences between regions in terms of access to dental services provided by ***dentists***. Other oral care personnel include operating therapists, who work in more than 40 countries and provide a high proportion of oral treatment in many developing countries, and dental hygienists, employed in at least 57 countries, who also play a major role in the prevention of oral diseases at individual and community levels. Chairside assistants are employed in most countries and greatly increase the safety and efficacy of oral care, as well as, in some countries, transmitting health education messages to patients. Dental technicians are also involved in providing oral prosthetic services.

Pharmacists, who are key members of the health care team, work in hospitals, clinics and government and private pharmacies. When they dispense medicines they complement information given by the medical prescriber to ensure that the patient stores and uses the drugs correctly. Pressures of health care reform in countries are resulting in a growth in private sector pharmacies and privately employed pharmacists. The role of the pharmacist as a community health care provider is being supported in both developed and developing countries.

The differences observed between and within countries are the result of very complex factors, such as the availability of finances and human capacity to train, employ and adequately remunerate health personnel. Other factors include: opportunities to practise in other jurisdictions; the expectations of consumers or perceptions about what constitutes good care; and the relative power exercised by interest groups (e.g. medical associations, nursing groups).

Countries continue to emphasize education, training and skill development in the building of capacity, and are concerned with ensuring that their public health systems address current and emerging complex health issues. Accordingly, the interdependence of all health care workers and the need to strengthen linkages between medical and public health institutions are increasingly being recognized as desirable policy objectives. Some countries are engaged in designing policies for clearly formulated human resources for health within the national health policy, as a sound basis for continued progress in this area.

** For definitions of the categories, please refer to Annex 2.*

Fig. 8. Human resources, regional estimates, around 1993

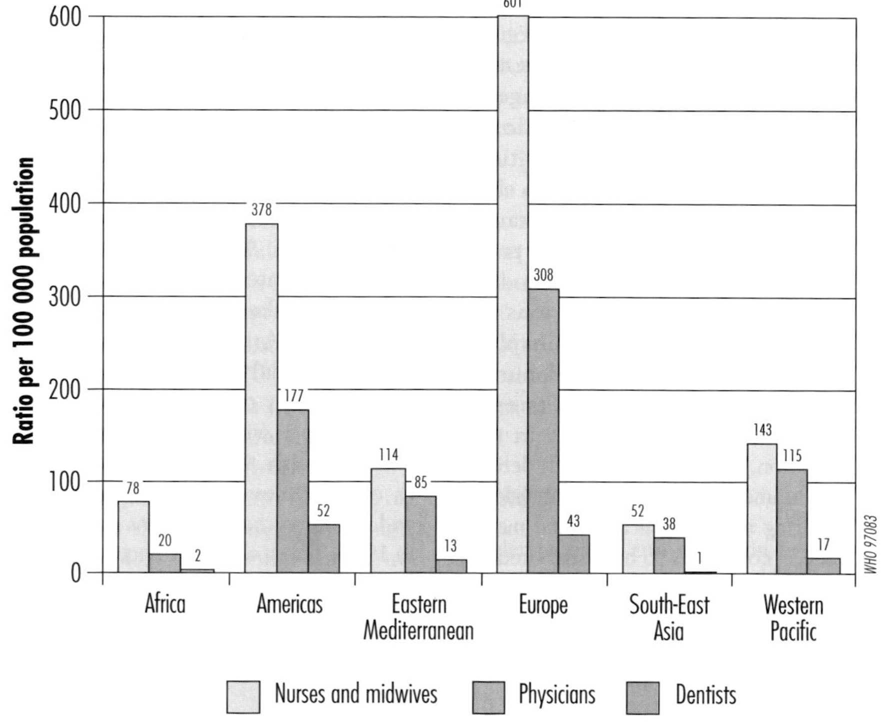

Box 23. Investing in health research and development

One of WHO's constitutional functions is to promote and initiate health research development at national and international levels. Its Advisory Committee on Health Research (ACHR), and its regional counterparts established in the 1980s, have guided WHO's work in this field. Since then the ACHR has increasingly become a catalyst for scientific research and cooperation, encouraging and welcoming contributions from all sources, including governments, research institutes, and universities.

In that context, it reviewed an important contribution in 1996, a report of the Ad Hoc Committee on Health Research Relating to Future Intervention Options entitled *Investing in health research and development.* The report analyses current and projected disease burdens and investment patterns in research and development (R&D) in health, and offers both national and international investors ways to make informed decisions about resource allocation in a climate of scarce resources.

Among its main conclusions, the report finds that childhood infections and poor maternal health continue to dominate the health needs of low-income countries. Research is needed to determine the most effective application of existing packages of essential services and to improve the content of the packages – for example, vaccines for major childhood diseases. The report identifies particularly attractive R&D investment opportunities with a high potential for reducing disease burden.

The focus for R&D against the threats of tuberculosis, pneumococcal infection, HIV, STDs and malaria should be primarily biomedical, and aimed at developing new tools for their prevention, treatment and control. A list of "best buys" is identified and mechanisms to foster cooperation between the pharmaceutical industry and public sector are proposed as a means to focus all efforts at cooperation on key products for low-income and middle-income countries.

The report shows that demographically developing regions face a rapidly growing epidemic of noncommunicable diseases and injuries. Many of the interventions developed in industrialized countries are not cost-effective and will not offer solutions for poor countries. To address these challenges, two new initiatives are proposed.

Health services in many countries remain inefficient and poor in quality, and costs are spiralling. An initiative to strengthen national health policy development is outlined which would include indicators of performance, tools that assist the translation of policy into practice, and sharing of information, data and experience of health systems.

The creation of an informal forum for investors in international health R&D is also proposed to stimulate action for investment globally and nationally.

of resources for health, WHO has developed strategic alliances with the international scientific community, intergovernmental organizations within and outside the United Nations system, and nongovernmental organizations and other bodies.

WHO's ***Advisory Committee on Health Research***, which deals with all issues related to research, including ethical concerns, provides a privileged link with partners in the scientific community. Following the Committee's recommendations, WHO established a task force on organ transplantation in 1996, to identify and clarify the medical, social, economic, ethical and related issues implicated in the potential advance in health care that cadaveric organ recovery and transplantation represent. Critical research issues of major significance to global health include multisectoral determinants and borders health. In the wake of the DALY debate, a subcommittee on health measurement was set up. In 1996, ACHR reviewed the report of an ad hoc committee entitled *Investing in health research and development* (*Box 23*).

The basic human rights of people with mental disorders are enshrined in the ***United Nations*** 1948 Universal declaration of human rights, the International covenant on economic, social and cultural rights adopted in 1976 and the 1991 Principles for the protection of persons with mental illness and the improvement of mental health care. In order to focus international efforts on concrete action, WHO initiated in 1996 a major interagency programme of the United Nations called "Nations for mental health". This programme aims specifically at reducing discrimination against people affected by mental disorders, by raising the awareness of governments and the public both about the magnitude of neuropsychiatric and substance abuse problems and about their impact on society, through collaborative strategies with international and nongovernmental organizations.

The drive is now towards implementation of the United Nations systemwide ***Special Initiative on Africa***. With the participation of regional organizations, an implementation strategy for health sector reform was elaborated through a series of interagency technical consultations, organized by WHO. Expected outcomes for Member States are: improved equity; strengthened management; increased sustainability and cost-effectiveness of health services; a measurable reduction in the burden of disease; and increased and better use of resources for health. A collaborative meeting of WHO and Emory University in the United States brought together high-level government representatives of 11 African countries, two African universities, the World Bank, nongovernmental organizations and other institutions, to discuss collaborative support, particularly capacity building for health development in Africa. Similar partnership arrangements in support of health development programmes in Africa and in Asia-Pacific countries were discussed in November 1996 with the University of California, Los Angeles. These developments suggest that, at a time of so-called financial aid "fatigue" for development, intellectual capacity could be harnessed to a greater extent than hitherto, with WHO providing a platform to facilitate this process across countries and continents.

Currently under way in collaboration with ***UNCTAD***, the project on trade in health services is examining the difficulties that developing countries face in that domain and the openings it can offer. On the basis of a global analysis and of specific case studies in a number of countries, which will be followed by an expert meeting in June 1997, the project aims to help build up countries' competence and to identify commercial opportunities. WHO is contributing its expertise to the project in order to provide national health authorities with appropriate advice and guidance on handling the impact of an expansion of trade in services. It will ensure that both the social advantages and disadvantages are adequately analysed, so that developing countries will be in a position to maximize the benefits stemming from such trade, while minimizing any potential cost. WHO's concern is to guard against the risk of financial interests taking precedence over people's health.

The fiscal year 1996 saw the highest lending to the health sector in the history of the ***World Bank***, with $2.3 billion in *new* commitments. The Bank's increasing country focus emphasizes closer involvement of the client, and attention to quality and results at country level. Initiatives to facilitate WHO/World Bank partnership in the health sector included consultations between Bank representatives and WHO staff at regional level. To facilitate this cooperation in a systematic manner a document, *Procedural strategies for implementation of the recommendations for health development*, was issued.

Following the 1992 International Conference on Nutrition, WHO and **FAO** have facilitated the preparation of over 140 national plans of action. The international community's commitment to eliminate hunger and malnutrition was reaffirmed at the World Food Summit in Rome in November 1996. WHO for its part is currently assessing the worldwide prevalence of malnutrition and monitoring global progress towards reducing and eliminating it.

The ***European Union*** is increasingly becoming an instrument for cooperation among its 15 Member States in all aspects of public policy which, since the end of 1993, has included public health. The Union is already the largest provider of development assistance and humanitarian aid. It sets norms and standards in a variety of health-related fields, from the marketing of pharmaceuticals to the quality of drinking-water. It is therefore of legitimate concern to Member States that the activities of WHO and the European Union do not conflict with or duplicate each other but rather that the greatest degree of coherence exists for the sake of efficacy, while the two bodies continue to respect each other's mandate.

WHO has prepared for the European Commission the first report on the state of health in the European Community.

WHO has prepared for the European Commission the first report on the state of health in the European Community, has developed on request country health profiles within and outside the Union, and has provided up-to-date, validated scientific information on transmissible spongiform encephalopathies, on plague and Ebola virus outbreaks, and on the risks for human health of pesticide residues in drinking-water, allowing the European institutions to determine the most appropriate course of action. Under the umbrella of the Transatlantic

WHO regularly organizes meetings with potential donors, at which a "menu" of WHO activities is presented. This enables donors to select those which are consistent with their priorities.

Agenda currently developed between the European Union and the United States, WHO will be called upon to contribute to the networking and alert system on infectious diseases. The joint organization, with IAEA, of the conference "One decade after Chernobyl: summing up the radiological consequences of the accident", has been the most visible element of a collaboration on nuclear risks.

WHO works with all the major ***development banks***. For example, WHO collaborated with the African Development Bank to revise the health sector policy paper for its lending programme and provided technical inputs to two studies by the Asian Development Bank on its health sector policy priorities and on Emerging Asia. Inputs were also made to health projects financed by the Asian Development Bank in Cambodia, Mongolia, Pakistan, Thailand and Vanuatu. WHO and the European Bank for Reconstruction and Development confirmed the main principles of their mutual cooperation, including the promotion of environmentally sound and sustainable development. WHO met with the Inter-American Development Bank and the Islamic Development Bank to identify issues of common interest and expand cooperation at country level within existing collaborative frameworks.

In the context of its work with ***regional groups*** , WHO met in June 1996 with the secretariat of the Association of South-East Asian Nations to establish a broader cooperation framework in support of national socioeconomic development processes. WHO made a first contact with the Asia-Pacific Economic Cooperation secretariat to identify potential collaborative areas of mutual interest. Other partners include the League of Arab States and the Organization of the Islamic Conference, including the Islamic Educational Scientific and Cultural Organization; the Organization of African Unity (for the African regional nutrition strategy, the Dakar and Tunis declarations on HIV/AIDS, and capacity building of African nongovernmental organizations); and the Southern African Development Community (to establish a health sector). Collaboration was resumed with the Common Market for Eastern and Southern Africa in the area of pharmaceuticals.

In its efforts to mobilize resources, WHO concentrates on enhancing collaboration with those Member States which have committed themselves to devoting a part of their gross national products to ***external development goals***. The health sector continues to be a prominent feature of government and organizational consultations. In 1996 two potential new contributors (the Republic of Korea and Singapore) to WHO's Voluntary Fund for Health Promotion were approached to explore the possibility of their cooperation with the Organization. WHO regularly organizes meetings with potential donors, at which a "menu" of WHO activities is presented. This enables donors to select those which are consistent with their priorities.

Consultation and collaboration with ***nongovernmental organizations*** on an informal basis are ways in which WHO is able to seek the advice and opinions of different groups, whether from the professions, medical and clinical sciences, or users of health services (*Box 24*). These informal contacts with nongovernmental organizations sometimes culminate, when it has been possible to establish regular and ongoing collaboration, in their admission into official relations. At its meeting in January 1996, the Executive Board brought to 184 the number of nongovernmental organizations in official relations with WHO by admitting the following organizations into official relations: the Thalassaemia International Federation, the European Centre for Ecotoxicology and Toxicology of Chemicals (ECETOC), Alzheimer's Disease International, and the World Federation for Ultrasound in Medicine and Biology (WFUMB). These nongovernmental organizations had worked on, for example, community education to improve public knowledge and understanding of the hereditary disease thalassaemia and of Alzheimer disease and other forms of dementia and related disorders, and advocacy for the development of thalassaemia control programmes in countries where they are most needed. ECETOC contributed to WHO's work in evaluating the risk posed by specific chemicals to human health and the environment. Ultrasound machines are ubiquitous; however, resource constraints mean that in many countries, doctors, nurses and midwives do not have ready access to expert advice and, in order to overcome this situation, WFUMB and WHO developed a manual of diagnostic ultrasound to provide guidance on the use of ultrasound in the diagnosis of a wide variety of common conditions at the primary and first-referral levels of health care.

Information exchange

To make partnerships effective and mutually supportive, WHO collects, analyses and publishes scientific information and the practical health experiences of countries at all levels of development. The Organization facilitates the exchange of this information to enable appropriate strategies to be formulated to improve the health of populations. The efficient dissemination of information and its management are crucial to this task. They provide a vital means of ensuring that new knowledge is put to good use, and that past lessons guide future action.

Taking full advantage of the economies of time and money offered by advances in ***information technology***, WHO uses the services available via the Internet. The audience reached is vast: the WHO home pages attract an average 1.7 million "hits" each month. From these pages, users can access a wealth of constantly updated statistical, technical and practical information, including weekly alerts to disease outbreaks, daily countdowns on cases of specific diseases, country and global statistics, advice on the risks to health and the environment posed by hundreds of industrial chemicals, and vaccinations required for

Box 24. How NGOs build awareness of the value of international health cooperation

Nongovernmental organizations (NGOs) in the United States are increasingly persuading the public and policy-makers that sustained support and leadership in international health is important to their country. WHO has many NGO partners in the United States committed to building this greater awareness of the need for and advantages of international cooperation in health activities. WHO also works closely with many United States Government agencies such as CDC, NIH and FDA.

New political leaders who are the successors of those who created the United Nations system and WHO 50 years ago need to learn about the complex ways in which domestic and international health are intertwined, and about the budgetary savings to be gained from global health cooperation.

NGOs and scientific bodies in the United States now realize that they can play a unique role as partners in international health work, with WHO and with each other. Their contribution is invaluable in building community awareness and support for WHO's work, including its normative, technical and operational functions, which otherwise would remain poorly understood outside narrow technical and scientific circles. They also explain how WHO's activities relate to trade, economic opportunity and human well-being in their own country and elsewhere.

For example, Rotary International, WHO's partner in polio eradication activities worldwide, now acknowledges each year the outstanding commitment of individual legislators to the eradication effort. Industry groups explain to United States politicians how international organizations such as WHO provide the scientifically-based framework of norms and standards that underpin the international rule of law and orderly trade opportunities. The American Medical Association and the American Public Health Association have resolved to work closely with WHO in technical areas. The United States Institute of Medicine has prepared a report from the scientific community explaining the vital interests of the country in global health and the need to support WHO. In June 1996, the National Council on International Health provided the public forum where Vice President Al Gore announced the decision of the President of the United States to direct policy priority towards global and national action on emerging diseases. University-based WHO collaborating centres in the country work together to develop strategies for building local awareness of international health linkages. Students at Brown University have launched a student-led International Health and Development Association to raise awareness among university students.

All these activities in the United States help to educate new generations of voters and policy-makers so that interest and support for international collaboration in health can be sustained for the benefit of all. As new health challenges emerge worldwide in an era of stagnant public resources and increasing public expectations, grass-roots and professional groups everywhere can decide to help shape the global health future. Recognizing and responding appropriately to these contributions is part of the challenge faced by national governments and by WHO in building strong partnerships that will sustain and renew the health-for-all strategy into the 21st century.

Global electronic networks, maintained by WHO, monitor such critical developments as the spread of antibiotic resistance, levels of air and water pollution, toxic reactions to chemicals, and adverse reactions to medicinal drugs.

international travel through the popular *International travel and health*, issued annually. Users can find the conclusions reached by experts and consult a host of press releases and fact sheets (almost 150 in 1996 alone).

To facilitate the search for appropriate health information, WHO also offers access to the 60 000 items in its library database, as well as full descriptive and bibliographic details for over 700 recent publications. To date, the full texts of over 12 000 technical documents, ranging in nature from profiles of health conditions in eastern European countries to reports of WHO consultations on bovine spongiform encephalopathy, are stored in the WHO library on optical disks. To enhance its ability to serve as the collective memory for the Organization, the library is collaborating with the *Institut Louis Jeantet d'Histoire de la Médecine* in Geneva in setting up a resource centre for the study of the history of public health in general and of WHO in particular, a project which aims to offer the catalogue of this important collection over Internet to the international community of researchers in the history of public health. In 1996 WHO also established the first Internet e-mail network of African health librarians. Response was enthusiastic, with over 80 regular participants. Other activities include the launch of the *bibliothèques bleues*, ready-to-use mini-libraries packaged in a blue tin trunk for use at the district level in Africa. The reach of the 150 WHO depository libraries was extended by a growing network of public reference points – some 900 libraries where comprehensive collections of WHO publications are available for public consultation.

Global electronic networks, maintained by WHO, monitor such critical developments as the spread of antibiotic resistance, levels of air and water pollution, toxic reactions to chemicals, and adverse reactions to medicinal drugs. These and other rapidly-changing databases are increasingly made available in electronic form.

As part of its ***publications*** programme, WHO brought out in 1996 a second edition of the highly successful guidelines on *Cancer pain relief* and an interagency report on *Trace elements in human nutrition and health*. As it updated its mortality database with the latest available and validated data on causes of death, WHO published the *World health statistics annual 1995*, with data covering the newly independent States of the former USSR. Volume 3 of the tenth revision of the International Classification of Diseases (ICD-10) was published in French and Spanish; Volume 2 was published in Spanish. *Teaching health statistics*, a set of lessons and seminar outlines to guide teachers of health statistics, first published by the Organization in 1986, was revised and expanded for publication. To facilitate the carrying out by countries of the third round of evaluation of progress in the implementation of their health-for-all strategies, WHO prepared a common framework which was distributed to all Member States.

Most of the books published by WHO in 1996 were designed in-house, as well as hundreds of brochures, newsletters, posters, maps, charts, graphs and slides for most WHO technical programmes. The demand for WHO publications remained high, as reflected in the sales results for 1996, amounting to $4.2 million. WHO's public health policy, with its reliance on community participation and self-help orientation, underlies its language service activities. Some WHO publications have been translated into over 60 languages – from Akan and Bengali to Samoan, Serbian and Swahili – in support of primary health care initiatives and to meet the demand for WHO's knowledge and experience at the country level.

In support of its advocacy role, WHO's health communication and ***public relations*** activities during 1996 were marked by a shift towards producing material for the media. Apart from preparing a range of press kits covering events of global interest such as the international conference on mental health in Madrid, hundreds of telephone requests for interviews or information were handled during the year and many press conferences and special briefings were organized. The *World Health Report 1996* was launched in Washington, London, Brussels and Geneva. The briefing on bovine spongiform encephalopathy and Creutzfeldt-Jakob disease was particularly well attended, with more than 200 journalists and 20 different television crews coming specially to Geneva to hear the latest information on this new health problem from the international experts convened by WHO.

Emergency relief and humanitarian assistance

As outlined in the *World Health Report 1995*, WHO's policy of emergency management for sustainable development provides a bridge between relief work and development proper, the aim being to provide a long-term solution for reducing human suffering and avoiding economic loss due to epidemics, complex emergencies and mass population displacements.

In 1996 WHO supported 58 Member States in activities such as control of infectious diseases and epidemiological surveillance and investigations. Most of WHO's response programmes focused on coordination and provision of technical support to national and international implementing partners, as well as provision of emergency vaccines, laboratory supplies and equipment for control of epidemics, and training of health workers.

In the light of resolutions adopted by the United Nations Commission on Narcotic Drugs and the World Health Assembly, and to ensure proper implementation of the international drug control system, WHO has taken the lead in developing an international consensus for simplifying the current export-import control procedures to allow timely provision of controlled medicines in emergency situations. It procured pharmaceuticals worth $9 million which were shipped to 37 different destinations. Connected tendering procedures, warehousing and transport constituted an exceptional challenge for the WHO units concerned. The number of types of health kits for use in emergency relief operations was increased to more than 20 and most of them are kept ready for shipment within 48 hours. The first catalogue covering medical supplies with generic specifications for use by field offices in emergency situations was completed in 1996.

Because of the high prevalence of mental health problems and injuries as a result of armed conflicts, WHO implemented integrated mental and physical rehabilitation programmes based on public health principles, notably in Bosnia and Herzegovina, Croatia and Rwanda. WHO also assisted health professionals in these countries in training, categorizing mental health problems, and data collection. Emphasis was placed on community-based care rather than costly hospital services. This also applied to services for victims of physical injuries, who received prostheses, physical therapy, and counselling.

In the context of current international efforts to give priority to the needs of underserved populations, WHO established a programme in 1996 to target the health needs of refugees and displaced persons, as well as those affected by wars and disasters. To complement support provided by UNHCR and other nongovernmental organizations, it prepared special guidelines, entitled *Mental health and refugees*, for use by those with no special training in psychology or mental health .

The WHO Panafrican Emergency Training Centre in Addis Ababa, Ethiopia, continued to focus on three main areas: training in disaster management, promoting emergency preparedness, and research into health and complex emergencies in Africa. In 1996 training and workshops were organized in Ethiopia, Lesotho, Namibia and Zimbabwe, and a programme for health emergency management training in Africa was designed, strategies and materials prepared, and

WHO has taken the lead in developing an international consensus for simplifying the current export-import control procedures to allow timely provision of controlled medicines in emergency situations.

WHO developed a roster of staff and experts who could provide technical assistance to countries in response to epidemics at 24 hours' notice.

external funding secured. Partners in these activities include the Organization of African Unity, the United Nations Disaster Management Training Programme, UNHCR, the United Nations Economic Commission for Africa, the International Committee of the Red Cross and the major regional nongovernmental organizations.

Guidelines for ***epidemic preparedness and response*** to cholera and epidemic diarrhoeal diseases, diphtheria, epidemic meningitis, Ebola fever, measles, rabies, typhoid fevers, viral hepatitis and viral haemorrhagic fevers were issued, as well as a manual on universal precautions, including barrier nursing. Ready-to-use kits of key equipment and supplies for rapid response to epidemics were stockpiled at WHO headquarters and regional offices. So as to ensure a rapid response to epidemics, the Organization developed a roster of regional and headquarters staff and external experts who could provide technical assistance to countries in response to epidemics at 24 hours' notice. This roster currently includes over 50 WHO staff and 20 external experts.

During 1996, WHO cooperated in the assessment and control of epidemics in Angola (meningococcal meningitis and anthrax), Indonesia (dengue haemorrhagic fever), Iraq (Crimean-Congo haemorrhagic fever), Japan (*E. coli* O157:H7 enteritis), and Sudan (epidemic febrile syndrome). At a meeting coordinated by WHO of ministers of health and the interior of West African countries, Angola and Chad, countries signed a protocol and a cooperation plan for combating epidemics in the subregion.

The process of revising the *International health regulations* was initiated in 1996. The revisions, and practical guidelines based on them, will be validated and field-tested in several countries in different regions, to assess their validity and applicability before submission to the Committee on International Surveillance of Communicable Diseases for its consideration and subsequent publication.

WHO, in its capacity as health and medical adviser to the World Food Programme (WFP), participated in WFP interagency evaluation and/or appraisal missions for ***food aid*** development projects in Africa. For example, four of them were aimed at increasing health services utilization among food-insecure households, in particular pregnant women, nursing mothers and preschool children; and four were in support of school feeding programmes intended to improve attendance and performance of primary school children. A statement of guiding principles for infant and young child feeding in emergencies was drawn up, and a manual on management of nutrition in major emergencies finalized.

Programme development and management

Since 1993, WHO has focused on adapting its programme development and management to the profound political and economic changes which took place in the early 1990s, in order to make a more effective contribution to global health work, and in Member States. The task before the Organization is to enhance its comparative advantages, increase responsiveness and improve effectiveness.

Management ***reform*** in 1996 took place in the areas of budgeting and accounting, planning and priority-setting, performance measurement, and rationalization of the work of the governing bodies, leading to substantial savings (*Box 25*). WHO is currently upgrading the existing elements of its management information system to permit rapid flow and feedback of information relevant for programme management at all levels of the Organization. A totally new desktop environment is being introduced, based on powerful workstations and servers using a standard graphical user interface, with Windows NT as the client operating system. This will be supported by the new local area network at headquarters, which should provide high-speed transmission to desktop workstations and modern telephone capacity. A new videoconferencing service was launched at headquarters in

1996, with sessions taking place between universities, ministries of health and organizations located in Geneva, Washington, Bangkok and Barcelona.

The ***financial situation*** of the Organization, owing to a shortfall in the collection of contributions, remained a central concern. The question of available resources to enable the further development and implementation of approved programmes was a key subject of discussion throughout 1996. A number of governments, however, continued to provide extrabudgetary funds to many WHO programmes both globally and regionally. The long-standing and constructive dialogues with government officials continued in 1996. Finland, Ireland, Luxembourg, the Netherlands, Norway, Sweden, and the United Kingdom held formal policy and programme reviews with the WHO secretariat showing the importance attached to WHO's work and the efforts being made by each government to ensure that additional funds are made available to various programmes for the attainment of agreed targets.

In the face of a substantially reduced staffing level, continued and sustained efforts were made in seeking efficiency improvements in the ***general administration*** support provided to WHO's technical programmes. These efforts have resulted in the elimination of certain services and a significant reduction in the levels of others. Economic opportunities are being explored for further contracting out of certain maintenance services, and for taking advantage of the intense competition prevailing in the global telecommunications market.

During 1996 far-reaching reforms in the Organization's ***personnel policy***, aimed at better responding to global change and the needs of Member States, were either implemented or under study. Significant changes were made with regard to staffing patterns, types of contract, staff development and performance appraisal. While the total number of posts in the professional and higher-graded categories decreased from 1558 in 1994 to 1345 in 1996, the proportion of women in these categories remained at 26%.

Box 25. Reform of WHO's governing bodies

The World Health Assembly, in approving programme budgets for recent years, has consistently emphasized the need to shift resources from the allocation for governing bodies to priority programmes. The expenditure for governing bodies has, therefore, been closely scrutinized with a view to making economies. The result in 1996:

- the duration of Executive Board and Health Assembly sessions has been shortened;
- the number of pages of documentation for sessions of the governing bodies has been reduced;
- support provided to the sessions has been rationalized.

Regional offices have instituted similar measures to reduce the cost and rationalize the work of regional committees.

Shorter sessions. In the programme budget for the financial period 1996-1997 the duration of the Health Assembly in 1996 was cut from 9 days to $5^1/_2$, and that of the January 1997 session of the Executive Board was cut by two days, as was the 1997 Health Assembly. Shortening the sessions has been accomplished by:

- compressing formalities;
- limiting the number of items on the agenda;
- establishing timetables for completion of the work programme;
- starting meetings earlier; and
- limiting time allowed to speakers.

The shorter Health Assembly in 1996 was generally judged a success – it adopted 29 resolutions and completed its work on time. Delegates used the time available judiciously, holding informal discussions on resolutions prior to formal discussions in main committees and convening drafting groups during breaks.

Documentation. The number of pages of documentation for Executive Board and Health Assembly sessions in 1996-1997 has been reduced to 60% of the 1994-1995 level. The cost of editing, translation, word-processing, printing and mailing has been reduced, and participants in the governing bodies have also appreciated the sharper focus given to the documents by the shorter format. In order to ensure timely receipt despite the end-of-year holidays, documents for the January 1997 session of the Executive Board were sent by electronic mail to members of the Board who had provided electronic mail addresses.

Support services. Overtime paid to support services for governing body sessions was identified as a significant item of expenditure. In order to economize, a larger number of headquarters secretariat staff are now requested to provide support. Most staff work on shifts but where overtime is necessary, it is compensated with time off rather than payment.

Regional highlights

A characteristic feature of WHO is its decentralization. It has "regional organizations", of which there are six, each consisting of a regional committee and a regional office. The regions vary widely in size, socioeconomic development, epidemiological characteristics, culture and history. Highlights are presented in the following pages.

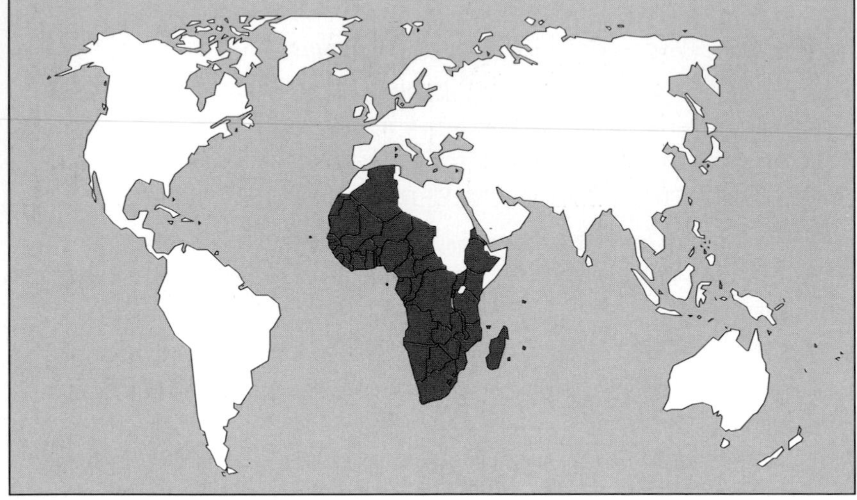

46 Members
Population (1996): 602 million

GNP per capita
- Regional average (1994) $598
  minimum: Rwanda $80
  maximum: Seychelles $6 680
- Annual average growth rate (1985–1994)
  minimum: Cameroon -6.9%
  maximum: Botswana 6.6%

Algeria	Liberia
Angola	Madagascar
Benin	Malawi
Botswana	Mali
Burkina Faso	Mauritania
Burundi	Mauritius
Cameroon	Mozambique
Cape Verde	Namibia
Central African Republic	Niger
Chad	Nigeria
Comoros	Rwanda
Congo	Sao Tome and Principe
Côte d'Ivoire	Senegal
Equatorial Guinea	Seychelles
Eritrea	Sierra Leone
Ethiopia	South Africa
Gabon	Swaziland
Gambia	Togo
Ghana	Uganda
Guinea	United Republic of Tanzania
Guinea-Bissau	Zaire
Kenya	Zambia
Lesotho	Zimbabwe

Tabular material concerning population, health indicators and GNP is based on United Nations and World Bank estimates. Data given in the text are from regional sources.

Africa

Although some countries in the African Region continue to experience political and social unrest, WHO has made every effort to minimize disruption in its work. Improvements in telecommunications and electronic mail systems have facilitated contact within and outside the Region.

Like other parts of the world, Africa is going through rapid social changes and new lifestyles are emerging, some of which lead to hazardous behaviours, including an increase in alcohol and tobacco abuse, affecting mainly the young. Awareness of the health risks of smoking is still low, and powerful and well-organized antismoking organizations do not exist. Tobacco is becoming a public health problem in the Region and deserves the attention of all countries, especially in the form of involvement of top-level policy-makers and a firm political will. African countries need the support of the United Nations agencies if these efforts are to succeed. They are willing to consider the diversification of their crops and to eventually replace tobacco cultivation by other commercial crops if they have a guarantee that it will not lead to more economic hardship. All Member States have now appointed a national focal point to manage their control programme, developed an education programme designed to sensitize the public to the health risks associated with tobacco use, and introduced teaching modules into their school curricula.

Cancer in the Region is often associated with infection, e.g. hepatitis B (liver cancer) and *Schistosoma haematobium* infection (bladder cancer). In order to combat these cancers, countries have started to incorporate hepatitis B vaccination in their immunization programmes (e.g. the Gambia and Zimbabwe). Countries have also started mass chemotherapy with praziquantel against schistosomiasis, and improvement of water and sanitation in communities at risk.

A number of countries have begun to train health workers in the prevention and control of cardiovascular diseases in the communities. Guidelines for the management of non-insulin-dependent diabetes mellitus (NIDDM) were published as a consensus document for the whole of Africa by IDF and WHO. A review of human resource development for the prevention of blindness was completed in June 1996. More nurses or medical assistants are to be trained as cataract surgeons and plans are at an advanced stage to open another training centre for countries in central Africa.

A study carried out in 1995 showed that 45% of African countries have prepared a national programme on mental health, and 32% on prevention and control of substance abuse; 17% have set up a national coordination mechanism for implementation of mental health

Selected health-for-all (HFA) indicators	1980 Average	1980 Maximum	1980 Minimum	1996 Average	1996 Maximum	1996 Minimum	2000 Average	2000 Maximum	2000 Minimum	HFA targets	No. of Member States which have not met the HFA targets in 1996
Life expectancy at birth (years)	48	66	35	53	71	40	54	72	42	> 60	37
Infant mortality rate (per 1000 live births)	117	191	33	91	158	16	85	148	14	< 50	39
Under-5 mortality rate (per 1000 live births)	188	291	39	142	242	17	131	227	14	< 70	40

activities; 32% have integrated mental health into primary health care services; and 25% have a community-oriented programme. WHO sponsored the seventh technical meeting of the African group for action in mental health, which discussed mental health among children and adolescents in the Region. In the next few years, priority will be given to the elaboration of national mental health policies, training of health workers in mental interventions, particularly in countries which have suffered war, and promotion of violence prevention. Mental health activities will be included in the minimum district package of health activities.

In the field of oral health, two countries have initiated preventive oral health care programmes as part of community primary health care and in schools, using non-oral health personnel in selected districts. A major achievement is the preparation of models of oral health education and promotion materials which countries can adapt for use in health centres, schools and outreach campaigns. This reflects the need for emphasis on preventive and promotive measures to control oral disease. For the next years, regional priorities will include the development of a regional oral health strategy and plan of action. Research activities on oral diseases of regional interest will be promoted as well as appropriate training programmes for oral health workers, particularly at the district level.

Further progress was achieved in the eradication of poliomyelitis and dracunculiasis, malaria control and tuberculosis prevention and control. An intensification of advocacy, such as the "Kick polio out" campaign in South Africa, has resulted in increased financial support for various interventions, notably from Rotary International, USAID and several nongovernmental organizations. Other achievements include the extension of the implementation of directly-observed short-course chemotherapy for tuberculosis, more vigorous promotion of the use of insecticide-impregnated bednets and closer monitoring of resistance to antimalarial drugs. Priority was given to interventions aimed at reducing infant and child mortality. The implementation of the Integrated Management of Childhood Illnesses (IMCI) has already begun in six countries. In 1996, WHO organized a coordination meeting with the interested partners and a consensus was reached on the strategy for its implementation. The prevention and control of HIV/AIDS remain major concerns, and a new regional strategy was launched in September 1996.

Remarkable progress was made in the area of emergency and humanitarian action. The Regional Office is now equipped to address the emergency and humanitarian problems that have been on the increase in the Region, and its activities are closely guided by a standing committee on emergency situations. Training was organized for WHO Representatives in dealing with emergency and humanitarian problems.

In view of the critical role that nurses and midwives play in the implementation of primary health care programmes, a training needs assessment was undertaken, and the information generated will be used to develop appropriate programmes. There were major changes in the management of the WHO fellowships programme, so that most countries of the Region now have a fellowship selection committee, and in 1996 84% of the fellows were placed in African training institutions.

WHO's advocacy efforts centre on assisting Member States to consolidate their capacity and to create an informed public opinion and empower individuals, families and communities to take full responsibility for the promotion of their own health and that of their environment. Action plans covering the period 1996-1998 were elaborated for several countries.

Thus, the various problems or constraints that arose were taken as challenges, and appropriate strategies were developed to cope with them. Past experience makes the Region look to the future with hope. Despite all odds, with prudent and transparent management, sincerity of purpose, genuine and effective collaboration among the various partners, effective leadership from WHO, and more peace and stability in Member States, remarkable health development in the Region will not be the illusion that it may seem to many.

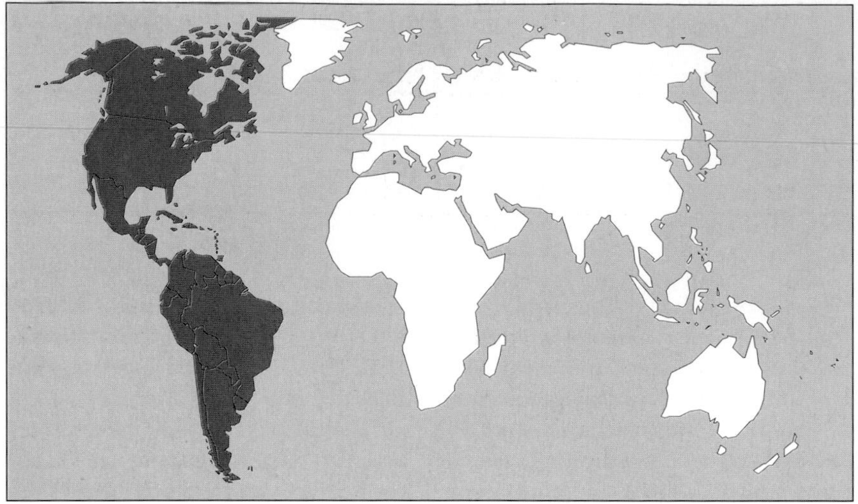

35 Members
1 Associate Member
Population (1996): 785 million

GNP per capita

- Regional average (1994) $11 739
  minimum: Haiti $230
  maximum: United States $25 880

- Annual average growth rate (1985–1994)
  minimum: Nicaragua -6.1%
  maximum: Chile 6.5%

Antigua and Barbuda
Argentina
Bahamas
Barbados
Belize
Bolivia
Brazil
Canada
Chile
Colombia
Costa Rica
Cuba
Dominica
Dominican Republic
Ecuador
El Salvador
Grenada
Guatemala
Guyana
Haiti
Honduras
Jamaica
Mexico
Nicaragua
Panama
Paraguay
Peru
Saint Kitts and Nevis
Saint Lucia
Saint Vincent and the Grenadines
Suriname
Trinidad and Tobago
United States of America
Uruguay
Venezuela

Associate Member:
Puerto Rico

Tabular material concerning population, health indicators and GNP is based on United Nations and World Bank estimates. Data given in the text are from regional sources.

The Americas

The economic situation of the Region of the Americas during 1996 was characterized by modest inflation and modest growth rates, and the economic crises suffered by two major contributors did not spread to the other countries as feared. In spite of continued widespread poverty and inequality that pose a potential threat to political stability, stable democracy is the norm.

The Pan American Health Organization and WHO (PAHO/WHO) have devoted substantial efforts in the Americas to establishing relations with new partners, including public sectors other than health, the private health sector, nongovernmental organizations and the media, as well as working towards providing ministers of health with arguments to support the view that investments in health have a positive effect on subsequent economic growth. The Inter-American Development Bank and ECLAC are joining PAHO/WHO in a study which will attempt to demonstrate the relationship between investments in health and economic growth, as well as how investments in health can contribute to reducing income inequality and improving such traditional health indicators as life expectancy and infant mortality rates.

In order to advocate for a different perception of health and to try to put health higher in the public agenda and the public debate, the Organization has actively supported the health aspects of the subregional integration movements in the Southern Cone (MERCOSUR), the Caribbean (CARICOM), the Andean region, and in Central America, giving advice and help as required in the firm belief that health as a critical aspect of functional cooperation can be a common platform for productive discussion and understanding.

As part of the process of reviewing its work, the Organization launched an initiative on "Rethinking International Technical Cooperation in Health" (RITCH) to re-examine different aspects of technical cooperation within a process aimed at improving effectiveness.

One of the critical components of technical cooperation is the mobilization of resources. PAHO/WHO has worked hard to establish partnerships with the major multilateral funding institutions such as the World Bank and the Inter-American Development Bank in order to establish complementarity of expertise to the benefit of countries and not necessarily seeking grants from these institutions.

In Latin America and the Caribbean, mortality from all causes was recently estimated at about 3 million. Of this, communicable, maternal and perinatal causes accounted for 966 000 (32.3%) and injuries for 293 000 (9.8%). Noncommunicable diseases accounted for more than 1.7 million

Selected health-for-all (HFA) indicators	1980 Average	1980 Maximum	1980 Minimum	1996 Average	1996 Maximum	1996 Minimum	2000 Average	2000 Maximum	2000 Minimum	HFA targets	No. of Member States which have not met the HFA targets in 1996
Life expectancy at birth (years)	68	75	52	72	78	58	73	78	59	> 60	1
Infant mortality rate (per 1000 live births)	50	120	10	33	80	6	31	72	6	< 50	4
Under-5 mortality rate (per 1000 live births)	65	171	13	41	104	8	38	93	7	< 70	3

deaths (57.9%), almost 800 000 of which were due to cardiovascular disease (45.4%), 340 000 to cancers (19.7%) and 85 000 to diabetes (4.9%).

Unlike Canada and the United States, where reductions of around 15% in the proportional mortality from diseases of the circulatory system have been seen since 1980, many countries in Latin America and the Caribbean are experiencing an increase attributable to these causes, in all adult age groups. The underlying risk factors such as high fat diets, sedentary way of life and smoking are established at a young age, and require lifestyle modification. Nonetheless, secondary interventions are also effective, including a more active role for clinical preventive medicine throughout life.

Most countries have not yet developed population data on cardiovascular disease risk factors, but those surveys which have been carried out generally reveal high prevalence rates. The prevalence of hypertension in the English-speaking Caribbean is generally in the range 20-30%. Some countries are developing national strategies for the prevention of ischaemic heart disease and stroke (e.g. Argentina, Chile, Costa Rica, Cuba, Uruguay), while others have not yet systematically assessed their impact and potential for control.

The impact of cancer throughout the Americas has greatly increased (by 73% overall from the early 1960s to the late 1980s), as shown in a recent 25-year analysis. Proportional mortality from this cause has increased in virtually every country. The leading cancers in Latin America and the Caribbean are: cervix, stomach, mouth-pharynx, oesophagus, breast, lung, liver, colon-rectum, lymphoma and leukaemia. The rates for cervical cancer, the leading cancer site, are among the highest in the world. While stomach cancer rates are steadily declining, those for breast cancer are increasing. Unlike North America, where a decline in lung cancer is now being experienced, rates are still rising throughout Latin America and the Caribbean. Programme priorities in most countries include tobacco control, while an increasing number are considering more cost-effective screening strategies for cervical cancer. A major unmet need in these countries is palliative care for persons with terminal cancer at all ages.

The recently established CARMEN project (integrated action for the multifactoral reduction of noncommunicable diseases) focuses particularly on cardiovascular disease prevention, but also aims to address the priority areas of cervical cancer prevention, diabetes management and injury prevention. Diabetes is the leading cause of blindness in the Americas, the leading cause of nontraumatic amputations and the leading cause of renal failure. The Declaration of the Americas on Diabetes, proclaimed in Puerto Rico in 1996, is being used as a launching pad for programme development in the Region.

The newly adopted regional plan of action on violence and health is expected to strengthen the commitment of the governments to act forcefully and intersectorally to attack the causes and diminish the consequences of violence.

As of March 1997, the total number of confirmed cases of measles in Latin America and the Caribbean was 1464, compared with 6489 cases reported in 1995. Neonatal tetanus is decreasing. The cooperative efforts of the ministries of health of Argentina, Bolivia, Brazil, Chile, Paraguay and Uruguay to eliminate Chagas disease are bearing fruit and in the countries with good surveillance there has been a dramatic reduction.

A major achievement for 1996 was the establishment of the mechanisms for defining and collecting a basic set of core data for each country, ensuring that these data are accessible and interchangeable throughout the Americas via Internet.

The intersectoral action needed for genuine health development must take place at the local level – hence PAHO/WHO's work in stimulating healthy "spaces", communities, work places, schools, etc. This movement is helped by information, and to this end a non-technical publication, *Perspectives in health*, was launched in 1996.

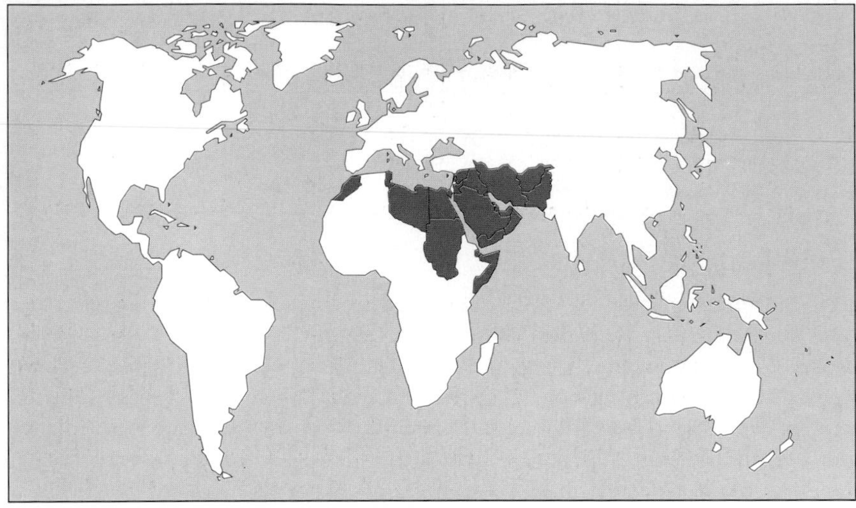

22 Members
Population (1996): 466 million

GNP per capita

- Regional average (1994) $1 249
  minimum: Yemen $280
  maximum: Kuwait $19 420
- Annual average growth rate (1985–1994)
  minimum: Jordan -5.6%
  maximum: Cyprus 4.6%

Afghanistan	Morocco
Bahrain	Oman
Cyprus	Pakistan
Djibouti	Qatar
Egypt	Saudi Arabia
Iran (Islamic Republic of)	Somalia
Iraq	Sudan
Jordan	Syrian Arab Republic
Kuwait	Tunisia
Lebanon	United Arab Emirates
Libyan Arab Jamahiriya	Yemen

Tabular material concerning population, health indicators and GNP is based on United Nations and World Bank estimates. Data given in the text are from regional sources.

Eastern Mediterranean

1996 has been a year of great variety with occasional setbacks. Progress in public health has been steady. Countries that had already achieved reasonably good levels of health have managed to climb even higher with some of them reaching their targets before the target dates. Other countries with less favourable circumstances, and those caught in the grip of strife and upheavals, have also managed to show some progress albeit uneven, and the after-effects of the 1990-1991 Gulf War are still affecting the lives of millions of people.

Among the significant achievements in 1996, 11 countries continued to report no new cases of poliomyelitis during the year and seven of them have reported no cases for three or more consecutive years; 17 countries reported immunization coverage of 90% and above. National immunization days were held in 20 countries during 1996, including war-torn Afghanistan, and considerable progress is being seen in countries whose immunization coverage has been inadequate. However, the situation in Afghanistan and Somalia is not conducive to proper planning; efforts and initiatives continue to be made in these countries so that the whole Region will achieve the poliomyelitis eradication target.

Another disease on its way to being eradicated from the Region is dracunculiasis. Pakistan has been certified by the Global Commission on Dracunculiasis Eradication to have eradicated the disease. National efforts to achieve eradication in Sudan and Yemen are progressing and it is hoped that the disease will be completely eradicated from the Region in the near future.

Various elements of the regional strategic plan in response to emerging and re-emerging diseases, adopted by Member States in 1996, are being implemented at both national and regional levels.

Special efforts were made during 1996 in the fight against tuberculosis. These efforts were directed specifically towards introducing the strategy of directly-observed therapy, short-course (DOTS) and at collaboration between countries in important areas, such as tuberculosis control among high-risk groups, particularly refugees and displaced persons.

Demographic and socioeconomic changes in the Region over the last two decades have resulted in changing disease patterns in many countries and a consequent rise in lifestyle-related diseases. Reliable data on the magnitude of noncommunicable diseases are lacking but evidence suggests that cancer is now the leading cause of death in several Member States. Smoking, which appears to have increased in the Region faster than in most others, and newly acquired dietary habits, are among the most important lifestyle factors that appear to be responsible for a substantial

Selected health-for-all (HFA) indicators	1980 Average	1980 Maximum	1980 Minimum	1996 Average	1996 Maximum	1996 Minimum	2000 Average	2000 Maximum	2000 Minimum	HFA targets	No. of Member States which have not met the HFA targets in 1996
Life expectancy at birth (years)	55	74	40	63	78	45	65	78	46	> 60	5
Infant mortality rate (per 1000 live births)	113	183	18	69	157	7	62	150	7	< 50	10
Under-5 mortality rate (per 1000 live births)	160	280	21	97	248	9	86	228	7	< 70	9

number of cancers. Discussions in 1996 highlighted the need to initiate comprehensive cancer control activities, including prevention, early detection and screening, treatment and palliative care, as well as to develop a regional database on cancer. Member States adopted a regional plan for tobacco control which will have a considerable impact on health in the Region, including on cancer prevention. Diabetes and cardiovascular diseases are similarly increasing in prevalence and regional plans have been developed to tackle them.

Genetic blood disorders are a problem of considerable magnitude in the Region, linked to the high rate of consanguineous marriage. Blindness rates also remain high.

Control of micronutrient deficiencies, especially iodine and iron deficiency, continued to receive the priority it deserves. Efforts to promote iodization of salt continued through both national authorities and the Regional Association of Iodized Salt Producers. A joint WHO/UNICEF consultation, held in 1995 in the Islamic Republic of Iran, to develop regional strategies for control of iron deficiency suitable for the countries of the Region, was followed up in 1996 by a strategy development workshop, held jointly with several partners including UNICEF in Oman, on food fortification with special reference to iron fortification of flour. The use of effective food-inspection systems, built around preventive food control methodologies, such as the hazard analysis critical control point (HACCP), is also being vigorously promoted as one of the focal points of the regional food safety programme.

The regional programme on essential drugs is placing increasing emphasis on promoting local drug industries and strengthening national quality assurance systems. A regional plan for quality assurance of biologicals has been formulated and the programme is also supporting the publication of national documents covering various areas of special importance to the national drug formulary. The development of blood transfusion services in the Region has continued according to plan, and is being strengthened through collaboration with the Arab Gulf Programme for United Nations Development Organizations (AGFUND). Provision of safe blood and blood products based on regular voluntary nonremunerated donation remains the target.

It is now widely recognized that the health priorities of countries are not matched by the curricula of medical education institutions. 1996 saw a significant response to the recommendations of a ministerial consultation on medical education and health which was held at the end of 1995.

The basic development needs (BDN) initiative has met with considerable success to date. Through this approach, villagers in undeveloped and underserved communities have been encouraged to become self-reliant, receiving support in initiating income-generating projects, improving water availability and access to safe water and sanitation, and raising levels of nutrition, female literacy and community participation. The loans they received have been returned before time, and remarkable progress has been achieved in a comparatively short period. This is an appropriate approach for all communities, whether urban or rural, poor or comparatively well-off, and one that can incorporate many of the initiatives advocated by WHO.

The basic development needs/quality of life concept is gaining ground in the region. At present, 11 countries have embarked on BDN programmes, albeit at different rates. Replicability – the potential to expand, extend or transfer model or pilot schemes to wider applications – is crucial to these programmes; and replication of BDN schemes is increasing. Somalia, despite its civil strife, is one of the countries where BDN activities have been expanding.

Basic development needs replication has taken place in urban settings (for example, in Egypt) as well as rural ones. The BDN partners that have contributed to such replication are many and varied: local nongovernmental organizations; organizations within the United Nations system, such as UNICEF (in Egypt and Jordan), IFAD (in Somalia) and UNDP (in Morocco); and universities and medical schools.

A spirit of reform permeated the annual round of joint government/WHO programme review missions, which monitor and formulate programmes of collaboration. Measurable targets set on the basis of national priorities aimed at producing identified products through clearly defined activities. Other health-related sectors began to be involved in the process of health policy and planning.

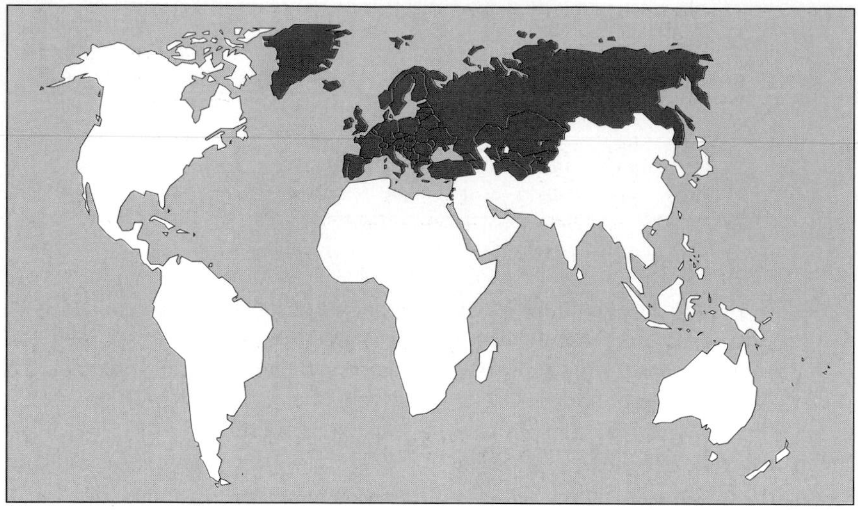

50 Members
Population (1996): 858 million

GNP per capita

- Regional average (1994) $10 766
  minimum: Tajikistan $360
  maximum: Luxembourg $39 600

- Annual average growth rate (1985–1994)
  minimum: Armenia -13%
  maximum: Malta 5.1%

Albania
Armenia
Austria
Azerbaijan
Belarus
Belgium
Bosnia and Herzegovina
Bulgaria
Croatia
Czech Republic
Denmark
Estonia
Finland
France
Georgia
Germany
Greece
Hungary
Iceland
Ireland
Israel
Italy
Kazakstan
Kyrgyzstan
Latvia
Lithuania
Luxembourg
Malta
Monaco
Netherlands
Norway
Poland
Portugal
Republic of Moldova
Romania
Russian Federation
San Marino
Slovakia
Slovenia
Spain
Sweden
Switzerland
Tajikistan
The Former Yugoslav Republic of Macedonia
Turkey
Turkmenistan
Ukraine
United Kingdom of Great Britain and Northern Ireland
Uzbekistan
Yugoslavia

Tabular material concerning population, health indicators and GNP is based on United Nations and World Bank estimates. Data given in the text are from regional sources.

Europe

Economic development has been extremely varied in the Region. In western European countries, slow economic growth of about 2-4% per annum continued. The countries of central and eastern Europe as a whole managed to reverse the previous trend, achieving average growth rates of about 4%, although there were considerable variations between individual countries. For most of the newly independent States the situation continued to be bleak, although in some countries certain signs of recovery in gross domestic product have been observed recently.

Overall, health improved in many western European countries; notably, the reported number of new cases of AIDS dropped for the first time. Trends in life expectancy and infant mortality showed signs of improvement in central and eastern Europe. For the first time since the late 1980s life expectancy increased slightly in the Baltic States and the Russian Federation. However, the situation in the newly independent States in general was poor, and has deteriorated considerably with regard to noncommunicable diseases. Equally alarming in these countries were the steep increases in mortality from external causes of injury and poisoning, particularly homicide in relative terms. Mortality trends in central, eastern and western Europe were fairly stable or slightly declining.

The devastation caused by armed conflicts in the Region reached levels not experienced for the past 50 years. The end of war in Bosnia and Herzegovina in 1996 was welcomed, although the task of reconstruction will doubtless require the combined efforts of the whole international community for many years ahead. WHO has been involved from an early stage, contributing to setting up a framework to rebuild the country's health system and chairing the sectoral task force on health. In Croatia, the Organization has been working very closely with the Government in its efforts to draw up a master plan (in line with its updated health-for-all policy) for reconstruction of its war-damaged health care facilities.

WHO has been operating in the area around Chechnya, for example by helping to implement a project which included provision of vitally needed laboratory kits, drugs, vaccines and medical equipment. Humanitarian assistance was also provided to Armenia, Azerbaijan, Georgia and Tajikistan.

The catastrophic socioeconomic development for the hundreds of millions of people in the more eastern part of the Region has created rapidly growing health inequity, rising criminality, changing cultural and social norms and increasing health problems. In many cases, health services lack essential drugs, equipment and often even the

Selected health-for-all (HFA) indicators	1980 Average	1980 Maximum	1980 Minimum	1996 Average	1996 Maximum	1996 Minimum	2000 Average	2000 Maximum	2000 Minimum	HFA targets	No. of Member States which have not met the HFA targets in 1996
Life expectancy at birth (years)	71	77	61	73	79	66	73	79	68	> 60	0
Infant mortality rate (per 1000 live births)	33	111	7	21	56	5	19	48	5	< 50	2
Under-5 mortality rate (per 1000 live births)	36	119	9	26	66	4	24	60	4	< 70	0

funds to pay personnel. In addition to the long-term trend of increasing cardiovascular diseases and cancer, the people in the newly independent States in particular, but to some extent also those of central and eastern European countries, face a rapidly increasing rate of accidents and homicides, as well as suicides and other consequences of severe stress.

In order to help reduce the public health problem of alcohol abuse, WHO has produced a series of nine technical documents providing an up-to-date review of major international developments in that area.

In 1996, the Organization published the conclusions of the 1995 Pan-European consensus conference on stroke management, which identified a series of quality indicators.

A quality of care model developed by WHO was also successfully used to improve the health of people with diabetes, not only in western Europe but also in eastern Europe in the EUROHEALTH countries that have adopted this new approach.

The diphtheria epidemic that broke out in the Russian Federation in 1990 has since affected all 15 newly independent States, with over 50 000 cases reported. On the basis of the difference between projected and reported cases, an estimated 100 000 cases appear to have been prevented as a result of the combined efforts of the Member States involved, with international cooperation.

A new and rapidly increasing threat was the reappearance of malaria in Azerbaijan and Tajikistan. In Tajikistan, the threat grew particularly serious in 1996, with some 100 000 cases occurring, including cases of the deadly falciparum form of the disease. In 1996, with assistance from WHO experts, plans for malaria control in Azerbaijan, Tajikistan and Turkey were elaborated and submitted to the international donor community for financial support. Countries bordering Tajikistan will receive assistance in preventing malaria spread and in treating imported cases.

In most newly independent States and some countries of central and eastern Europe, morbidity and mortality rates for tuberculosis have increased sharply since 1995, with two-thirds of notified cases in young adults. The lack of antituberculosis drugs in most of these countries results in inadequate treatment, increased mortality and greater prevalence of the disease. Furthermore, multidrug resistance is hampering control efforts. Because of migration, the decreasing trends of tuberculosis that were earlier seen in western Europe and parts of central and eastern Europe are now levelling off.

Particularly disturbing in recent years has been the very fast rise of syphilis, particularly in the newly independent States but also in central and eastern Europe; Lithuania, for example, has shown a six-fold increase in the last three years. This development is not only a grave problem in itself, but it also represents a great risk for increasing AIDS transmission in this part of Europe. A sharp rise in the incidence of HIV infection is now occurring in Belarus, the Russian Federation and Ukraine.

The sudden discovery in March 1996 of a new variant of Creutzfeldt-Jakob disease and its possible link to bovine spongiform encephalopathy has given rise to much concern. WHO responded to this new threat by organizing several technical meetings, and by planning a surveillance system.

Analysis of the outcome of 4.5 million births in the European Region indicated that some countries of central and eastern Europe might have more cost-effective quality of care programmes than many western European countries. When gathering information for such comparative analyses, it was essential that data were internationally accepted – a WHO task – and that the confidentiality of both the patient and the care provider was respected.

WHO in Europe has stepped up its effort to spread knowledge about its activities, in order to create a better understanding of its role, by issuing a new quarterly newsletter and intensifying public relations activities in connection with significant events.

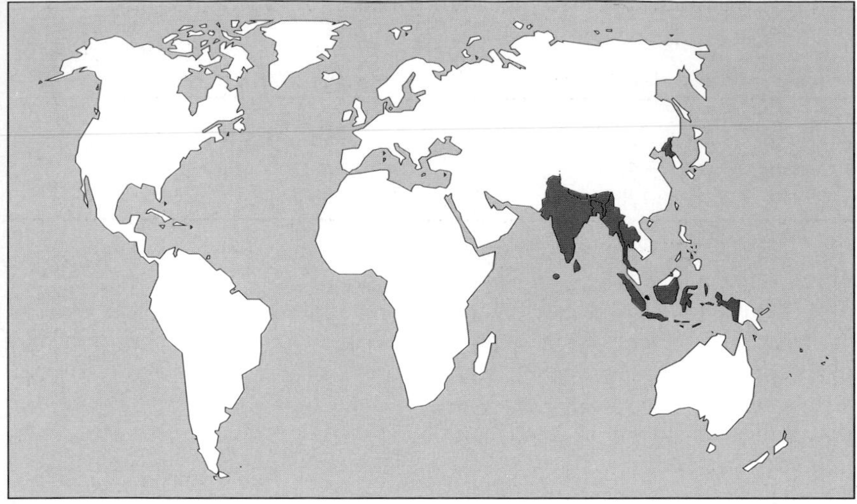

10 Members
Population (1996): 1.5 billion

GNP per capita

- Regional average (1994) $487
  minimum: Nepal $200
  maximum: Thailand $2 410
- Annual average growth rate (1985–1994)
  minimum: Bangladesh 2%
  maximum: Thailand 8.6%

Bangladesh
Bhutan
Democratic People's Republic of Korea
India
Indonesia
Maldives
Myanmar
Nepal
Sri Lanka
Thailand

South-East Asia

The Region is undergoing a profound transition: economic reforms, growing urbanization and political, social and cultural changes. In countries dominated by poverty and illiteracy and a heavy burden of disease, more change also needs to take place in an area that touches the lives of all: health. In today's global village, any breakthrough achieved in this populous region is bound to have an impact on the health status of the world. The health scenario has altered significantly in recent years. With changing lifestyles and demographic patterns, the health needs of the people are also changing. The size, population, literacy levels and economic status of the countries of the Region vary considerably. Literacy rates range from 41% and 14% for males and females respectively in Nepal to 100% for both sexes in the Democratic People's Republic of Korea.

The decline in crude birth and fertility rates, together with the increase in life expectancy, have resulted in the progressive ageing of populations. While poverty, malnutrition and infectious diseases are still prevalent, diseases associated with affluent countries, such as ischaemic heart disease, cancer and diabetes, have also taken hold. The declining crude death rate and increasing life expectancy, together with unfavourable lifestyles, have resulted in a substantial rise in chronic diseases, even among the younger generation. In India alone, nearly 800 000 people die from ischaemic heart disease and more than 600 000 from stroke each year, while the overall prevalence of rheumatic fever/rheumatic heart disease is of 11 per 1000 population. Oral cancer attributable to tobacco use is also of concern.

More than 50% of all deaths in Thailand are attributable to noncommunicable diseases (including accidents and other forms of violent death). According to the most recent estimates, the incidence of cancer was 154 per 100 000 in males and 129 per 100 000 in females, while cardiovascular diseases accounted for 17% of all deaths. Moreover, the prevalence of hypertension was found to be 10% in urban areas, 14-17% in slum areas and 3-4% in rural populations.

The death rate from cancer in some countries is almost 40 per 100 000 population per year. The number of new cases of cancer in 1992 in respect of a few cities in India was about 80 per 100 000 population, and in Thailand it was about 130 per 100 000. Cancer of the breast, cervix, mouth and pharynx dominated the clinical picture in India, while in Thailand, liver cancer is the most frequent malignancy among males, with lung cancer second. These two cancers account for 44% of all new malignancies in men. In women, cervical cancer is the most frequent, followed by liver cancer, breast cancer and lung cancer. These account for 52% of all new malignancies in women. Accidents and injuries constitute 9-10% of the total mortality in India.

Tabular material concerning population, health indicators and GNP is based on United Nations and World Bank estimates. Data given in the text are from regional sources.

Selected health-for-all (HFA) indicators	1980 Average	1980 Maximum	1980 Minimum	1996 Average	1996 Maximum	1996 Minimum	2000 Average	2000 Maximum	2000 Minimum	HFA targets	No. of Member States which have not met the HFA targets in 1996
Life expectancy at birth (years)	54	68	44	63	73	52	64	74	54	> 60	4
Infant mortality rate (per 1000 live births)	113	160	31	73	112	15	66	99	14	< 50	7
Under-5 mortality rate (per 1000 live births)	153	219	38	97	145	19	85	130	17	< 70	5

It is estimated that there are a total of 11.5 million blind persons in the Region – almost one-third of the world total. Cataract accounts for an average of nearly 70% of the blindness. The cataract backlog needing surgical intervention is estimated to be 8 million.

A prolonged epidemiological transition seems under way, and its course and outcome will depend largely on trends and interactions in four key areas: population growth, urbanization, environmental degradation and poverty. The double burden of chronic and infectious diseases is stretching the resources of countries in the Region as never before. Tuberculosis claimed 1.2 million lives in 1995; for children under 5, pneumonia and diarrhoea remain major killers (1.4 million and 1 million deaths respectively every year). To further complicate matters, drug-resistant strains of tuberculosis and malaria have appeared. The surveillance and epidemiological analysis of infectious diseases show that some of them (e.g. poliomyelitis, neonatal tetanus and leprosy) are on the verge of eradication or elimination, while others (e.g. plague and malaria) that had almost disappeared by the 1970s, have reappeared. In addition, there are new diseases such as cholera caused by strain O139 and HIV/AIDS.

There are sharp inequities within countries that broad statistics do not reveal. The rich are getting richer while the poor are getting poorer. There is a growing number of speciality hospitals offering the most advanced and sophisticated treatment, while in many areas safe drinking-water is not available and primary health care services are lacking. A large percentage of the people live in abject poverty, sometimes so extreme that even a severe bout of malaria puts a family into debt for years. Women's status in the Region has not improved markedly even though it is widely acknowledged that women's full participation is essential for sustainable development. Maternal mortality ratios are unnecessarily high and unsafe abortions cause a large number of deaths. Female literacy continues to be low in several countries.

To effectively integrate health into the development process, the government health sector has to move beyond its present confines and interact with other sectors such as environment, education and housing, to define health-related responsibilities. A partnership between the government and community will foster participatory relationships that will not only make programme implementation more effective but also facilitate local problem-solving. Although it is now realized that health measures are crucial for economic development, this recognition is not sufficiently translated into adequate political commitment in most countries. Accountability for health must be accepted at the highest level of government.

Sustainability is a key issue, and one of the major challenges that governments will have to face as the countries move into the 21st century. Much of the success of health programmes to date – such as that for immunization – is due to investment in terms of financial and human resources by countries, WHO, other agencies of the United Nations system and bilateral donors. Increasingly, the countries of the Region are now having to meet the challenge of sustaining such programmes on their own.

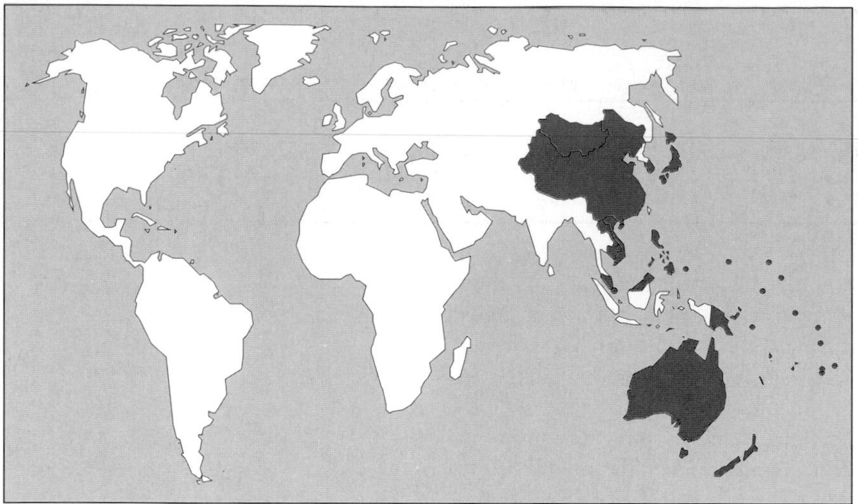

27 Members
1 Associate Member
Population (1996): 1.6 billion

GNP per capita

- Regional average (1994) $3 762
  minimum: Viet Nam $200
  maximum: Japan $34 630

- Annual average growth rate (1985–1994)
  minimum: Mongolia -3.2%
  maximum: China, Republic of Korea 7.8%

Australia
Brunei Darussalam
Cambodia
China
Cook Islands
Fiji
Japan
Kiribati
Lao People's Democratic Republic
Malaysia
Marshall Islands
Micronesia (Federated States of)
Mongolia
Nauru
New Zealand
Niue
Palau
Papua New Guinea
Philippines
Republic of Korea
Samoa
Singapore
Solomon Islands
Tonga
Tuvalu
Vanuatu
Viet Nam

Associate Member:
Tokelau

Tabular material concerning population, health indicators and GNP is based on United Nations and World Bank estimates. Data given in the text are from regional sources.

Western Pacific

Year after year, WHO in the Western Pacific implements its programmes to improve the health and quality of life of the peoples of the Region, yet the size of the task does not get smaller as the problems are dealt with. Each year the population grows, new diseases emerge or old diseases re-emerge, and health systems face new challenges. Meanwhile, the funds available are eroded by inflation and the real cost of operations increases. There is now more need than ever for prioritization exercises affecting all levels, in order to ensure delivery of a compromise programme with reduced funding. Fortunately, support from extrabudgetary partners has allowed WHO to accelerate the conduct and guarantee the success of the priority programmes.

Rapid industrialization and urbanization in the Region, social change and ageing of populations are contributing to increased prevalence of chronic diseases, but prevention and control of infectious diseases also continue to demand close attention.

Over the last decade the epidemiological situation for malaria has significantly improved although it is still a serious concern. The number of cases detected by microscopy in 1994 was more than 50% lower than in 1984. Incidence decreased by 90% in China during the same period, but remains high in Cambodia and the Lao People's Democratic Republic. In the Solomon Islands, a multisectoral "healthy islands" programme has reduced the number of malaria cases in the first 10 months of intensified malaria control efforts in 1996 by 77% compared to the same period in 1995.

The eradication of poliomyelitis has almost been achieved, while routine immunization of infants has been maintained at over 90% regionally. The elimination of leprosy is progressing, with special projects in six countries where the disease is still highly endemic. Among the other infectious diseases, diarrhoeal diseases and acute respiratory infections are the most important causes of death among children under 5. In a number of countries and areas there are now indications of a downward trend in infant and child morbidity and mortality, which can be attributed to improved sanitation and successful health interventions such as better case management.

The notification rate of tuberculosis in the Region has increased by 30% over the last decade. This is partly due to the improved reporting system. Tuberculosis control is being strictly implemented through the WHO policy package known as DOTS, already with promising results. For example, at subnational level in Cambodia, a cure rate of more than 80% has been achieved. The plan is now to implement the programme nationwide.

Selected health-for-all (HFA) indicators	1980			1996			2000			HFA targets	No. of Member States which have not met the HFA targets in 1996
	Average	Maximum	Minimum	Average	Maximum	Minimum	Average	Maximum	Minimum		
Life expectancy at birth (years)	66	76	39	70	80	53	71	80	55	> 60	3
Infant mortality rate (per 1000 live births)	51	212	7	37	106	4	33	96	4	< 50	5
Under-5 mortality rate (per 1000 live births)	59	301	8	43	143	6	38	127	6	< 70	4

A task force for outbreak response was established in April 1996, and dealt with an outbreak of diphtheria in the Lao People's Democratic Republic in July. Governments were supported in controlling outbreaks of cholera in Mongolia and the Philippines in August and September.

The steps being taken to improve reproductive health are already bringing positive results, although improvements in the levels of maternal morbidity and mortality have varied widely between and within countries. In 11 countries of the Region, the maternal mortality ratio remains above 100 per 100 000 live births and 1000 or more per 100 000 live births in some isolated or underserved communities. However, better access to fertility regulation methods resulted in a significant decline in the total fertility rate in the Region from an average of 5.1 in 1960 to 2.1 in 1995. This has contributed considerably to reductions in maternal morbidity and mortality. In Malaysia and the Republic of Korea, for example, the maternal mortality ratio has dropped by two-thirds since 1960.

At the other end of life, cancer is among the leading causes of adult mortality in 24 countries/areas. Cardiovascular disease is one of the three leading causes of adult mortality in 28 countries/areas. Behaviour changes are necessary to reduce the incidence of these degenerative diseases. The principal approaches are promotion of healthy lifestyles and health-supportive environments, and advocacy on avoidance of risk factors provided through various settings, such as the home, the school and the workplace. Regional guidelines on the development of health-promoting workplaces will be available in 1997.

There is much more still to be done. All over the Region, governments have endorsed and are working with WHO to implement the concepts and directions of the policy document *New horizons in health*. Healthy islands and healthy cities activities are becoming very popular. These activities represent a change in emphasis from what can be done at the national level, to how municipal authorities, community organizations and individual households can best be supported in developing and implementing community-based initiatives.

Serious and far-reaching changes have been made in the health services and the scope of work of health personnel. Health systems reform continues to be a priority. Issues being faced include delivery of health care services, rising costs, equity of access, quality assurance and efficiency. WHO has worked with countries to reorient both basic training and continuing education of health professionals towards current and future needs. Postgraduate education in the Pacific is a priority and is progressing rapidly.

The question facing WHO in the Region now is not the ability to achieve significant results in health, but how it can be done with continually diminishing funding. WHO must act decisively to provide support to the areas where real progress can be made, and be seen to be made.

Chapter 3

Charting the future

During the period 1975-1995 there were overall improvements in the living standards of most populations worldwide: smallpox was eradicated, the proportion of children immunized against the six major childhood diseases increased from less than 5% in 1974 to over 80% in 1995.

Disease trends

Of every 100 babies born alive during 1955, more than 75 survived 20 years to enter the economically productive workforce in 1975; life expectancy at birth was 48 years in 1955. Of every 100 babies born alive in 1975, more than 85 survived to join such a workforce in 1995; life expectancy at birth was 59 years in 1975 and 65 years in 1995. This substantial improvement was the result of many factors, including progress in public health, enhanced application of scientific knowledge already available and marked improvements in infectious disease prevention and control, particularly in the domain of environmental sanitation and immunization. During the period 1975-1995 there were overall improvements in the living standards of most populations worldwide: smallpox was eradicated, the proportion of children immunized against the six major childhood diseases increased from less than 5% in 1974 to over 80% in 1995. The percentage of the population in rural areas with access to safe water increased from 13% in 1970 to 61% in 1990, and with access to adequate sanitation from 11% to 36%. Because of the experience gained in the process it has been possible to target many other infectious diseases for eradication, elimination and control, and there has been perceptible progress in achieving these targets.

The continued emergence of infectious diseases is, however, a worrying trend but, as shown in *The World Health Report 1996 – Fighting disease, fostering development*, workable solutions exist for dealing with many of these diseases. With renewed commitment at global and national levels to combat them, the challenges that they pose can be overcome (*Box 26*). HIV/AIDS is, however, an exception because of its ever-changing character and the increasingly complex role of the factors that influence the progression from HIV infection to full-blown AIDS. Though the overall prevalence of the disease is low, it has spread to every inhabited continent, and kills and incapacitates young and middle-aged adults, disproportionately affecting skilled and managerial workers (*Box 27*, *Map 5*). Even so, there is heartening evidence that some preventive campaigns are slowly but definitely influencing its spread. Increasing emphasis is being given to AIDS research, to the development of vaccines and topical microbicides, and to finding treatment regimens that are simpler, more economical and accessible for most of those infected or vulnerable to HIV, due consideration being given to long-term survival possibilities and ethical issues.

Rising life expectancy, resulting primarily from declines in child mortality and in fertility, and from the prevention of deaths from fatal infectious diseases, is increasing the risks of developing chronic and debilitating diseases such as heart disease, cancer, diabetes and mental disorders. It is estimated that the elderly population (aged 65 and above) will increase globally by more than 80% during the next 25 years; in 10 countries at least, one out of every five persons will be "elderly" by the year 2020 (*Map 6*). Most deaths among the elderly will be due to cancer, lung and heart diseases. Meanwhile, because of profound changes in working methods and environments, and lifestyles associated with modernization, conditions such as diabetes and premature disability related to ergonomic factors are increasing among young adults and in the working population. In addition, an increasing

Box 26. Progress in infectious disease control

Among the main issues examined in *The World Health Report 1996* were the control of "old" and "new" infectious diseases, and the spread of antimicrobial resistance. On both these fronts there were significant advances in 1996.

The campaign for the global eradication of ***poliomyelitis*** has progressed with continued vigour; 116 countries have already conducted national immunization days (NIDs) and the number of reported cases in 1996 was down by over 90% since the eradication effort was launched in 1988. In India about 120 million children under 5 were immunized against polio in a single day during each round of NIDs held in December 1996 and January 1997.

The ***leprosy*** elimination campaign also progressed. The global prevalence of registered cases fell from 2.3 to 1.7 per 10 000 population during 1995-1996. Over the past 11 years, the leprosy problem has been reduced by 82% worldwide. With a donation of $10 million received from the Nippon Foundation, WHO supplied drugs for multidrug therapy (MDT) free of cost to a large number of countries; in 1996, over 90% of all registered cases in the world were receiving MDT.

The ***Onchocerciasis*** Control Programme which began in West Africa in 1974 has since protected an estimated 36 million people from the disease, which has been eliminated as a public health problem from Benin, Burkina Faso, Ghana, Niger and Togo and large areas of south-eastern Mali and northern Côte d'Ivoire. An area of 25 million hectares of previously-infected arable land has been made available for cultivation – enough to support 17 million people. The African Programme for Onchocerciasis Control began in January 1996 and covers 19 additional countries. The Onchocerciasis Elimination Programme in the Americas was started in 1991 in six Latin American countries and aims to eliminate severe pathological manifestations of the disease and to reduce morbidity in the Americas through the distribution of ivermectin.

Dracunculiasis (guinea-worm disease) is a debilitating parasitic disease that appears likely to be eradicated in the near future. Between 1992 and 1996, the number of endemic villages around the world was reduced from 23 000 to 9900 and global incidence declined from 3.5 million cases in 1986 to 130 000 cases in 1996. Already, the International Commission for the Certification of Dracunculiasis Eradication has certified 21 endemic countries as "being free of dracunculiasis transmission".

Within the framework of the Initiative of the Southern Cone Countries, the elimination of transmission of ***Chagas disease*** – a chronic and incurable disease which can cause disability and death, was achieved during 1996 in Brazil, which accounts for over 40% of prevalence of the disease in Latin America.

Trachoma is an infectious disease that has caused irreversible blindness in about 6 million people; another estimated 147 million people suffer from the active disease and are in need of treatment, if blindness is to be prevented. WHO has launched an alliance consisting of a number of international nongovernmental development organizations, the Edna McConnell Clark Foundation and the philanthropic section of Pfizer International Inc. – the company that has developed azithromycin, a new long-acting antibiotic that may be used to fight trachoma. The target is the elimination of the disease by the year 2020.

In 1957, when the world's population was 2.9 billion, ***malaria*** incidence was estimated at 200 million, with 2 million deaths annually. Forty years later the world population has more than doubled to over 5.8 billion people, and malaria cases increased to 300-500 million, with 1.5 to 2.7 million deaths annually. In 1992, the Ministerial Conference in Amsterdam adopted the Global Malaria Control Strategy, which aims to reduce malaria mortality by at least 20% in at least 75% of affected countries by the year 2000, compared to the 1995 data. At present, the great majority of endemic countries have completed malaria control plans in accordance with the Global Strategy, and 93 countries are implementing the plans. A new initiative for research and development of antimalarial drugs – Tropical Diseases R&D Alliance (TDRA), has been launched to forge new partnerships with the private sector. Field trials in Africa suggest that insecticide-treated bednets can, in certain epidemiological conditions, reduce overall childhood mortality by 15-35%. Research and field trials of several possible malaria vaccines are progressing.

There were at least 42 million cases of ***measles*** and 1 million deaths due to the disease in 1995 worldwide. As of March 1997, the total number of confirmed cases of measles in Latin America and the Caribbean was 1464, and there is hope of certifying the Region of the Americas free of measles in the year 2000.

Epidemic ***meningitis*** is a recurrent problem in the "meningitis belt" of Africa stretching from Senegal to Ethiopia and including all or part of at least 15 countries with an estimated population of 300 million people. In 1996, more than 150 000 cases and 16 000 deaths, mostly children, were reported, and WHO launched an initiative that resulted in an international coordination group of various United Nations agencies, nongovernmental organizations and other technical partners meeting with manufacturers of vaccines and injection material and securing their commitment to reserve for WHO 14 million doses of vaccine for epidemic control in 1997.

The largest outbreak of foodborne infection ever recorded involving the ***E. coli*** pathogen occurred in Japan, affecting more than 6300 schoolchildren and causing two deaths. In Scotland, an outbreak of

Box 26. Progress in infectious disease control (continued)

food poisoning due to *E. coli* killed almost 20 people and affected several hundred others; the source was cooked and processed meat products. Both outbreaks were the subject of major public health investigations which resulted in the strengthening of international and national capability for early detection and rapid response.

To test the hypothesis that the cluster of cases of the new variant form of ***Creutzfeldt-Jakob disease*** (CJD) identified in the United Kingdom in 1996 may be a consequence of exposure of humans to the bovine spongiform encephalopathy (BSE) agent, international experts reviewed scientific evidence concerning possible transmission of BSE to humans and are carrying out studies in laboratory animal models; methods to characterize human agents including the agent of the new variant form of CJD and to compare them to animal agents especially the BSE agent have been developed. WHO is organizing a consultation on medicinal products and other products in relation to human and animal transmissible spongiform encephalopathy (TSE) in March 1997.

To combat ***newly emerging*** infectious diseases and the spread of pathogens that are resistant to antibiotics, WHO is electronically linking more than 200 collaborating centres, 190 health ministries, 142 WHO country offices and six WHO regional offices, together with almost 100 national laboratories, for the rapid international exchange of information on disease outbreaks.

In November 1996, WHO and the pharmaceutical industry, represented by the International Federation of Pharmaceutical Manufacturers Associations, agreed on a framework for future collaborative efforts to contain the spread of ***antibiotic-resistant*** bacteria. This is expected to improve opportunities for successful, cost-effective treatment of infections, and to encourage research and development of new antibiotics.

number of persons are likely to suffer from psychiatric and neurological conditions. Possible trends in respect of some of the major chronic diseases are given below.

The burden of ***cancer*** is predicted to increase over the next decades both in absolute numbers of cases and deaths, and as a proportion of the overall burden of disease. This increase is ascribed to population growth and ageing, and more particularly to an increasing incidence rate of cancer, especially due to smoking, which already accounts for one in seven cases worldwide. Though the risk of developing a cancer is increasing for individuals of a given age, the increase is not uniform for all types of cancer; for instance, the risk of developing stomach cancer appears to be falling almost everywhere, while there are rising trends for many of the more common cancers such as lung cancer linked to tobacco smoking; and colorectal, breast and prostate cancer linked to the so-called "Western lifestyle" (a relatively sedentary way of life with a diet low in fibre and fresh fruit and vegetables but rich in calories, meat, fat, salt, additives and alcohol). Increasing incidence of these cancers has been observed, although the death rate has not increased to the same extent, because of improvements in therapy.

It is projected that, even if incidence rates remain the same as in 1995, the annual number of new cases of cancer will increase by more than 30% to 13.6 million by the year 2010, and by 45% to 14.7 million by the year 2020. Based on present knowledge, it is anticipated that for the countries of the European Union the increase during 1995-2005 may range from 11% for colorectal cancer in women to 40% for prostate cancer in men; there is likely to be 33% more lung cancer in women, two-thirds of which will be the result of their increased risk of developing the disease.

Increases in the annual number of new cases of cancer in the developing world will probably be higher because of the rapidly increasing incidence of cancers such as those of the lung, breast, colon, prostate and ovary; for example, in the last two decades the incidence rates of the last four have approximately doubled in Singapore. Based on available information, the total number of new cases of cancer is expected to double by the year 2020 in the developing world, compared to an increase of about 40% in the developed world.

In most countries for which time-trend data are available, mortality rates from ***circulatory diseases*** have been declining in recent decades in people aged over 65 as well as in younger age groups.

Map 5. AIDS deaths and HIV/AIDS prevalence among adults aged 15–49, 1996

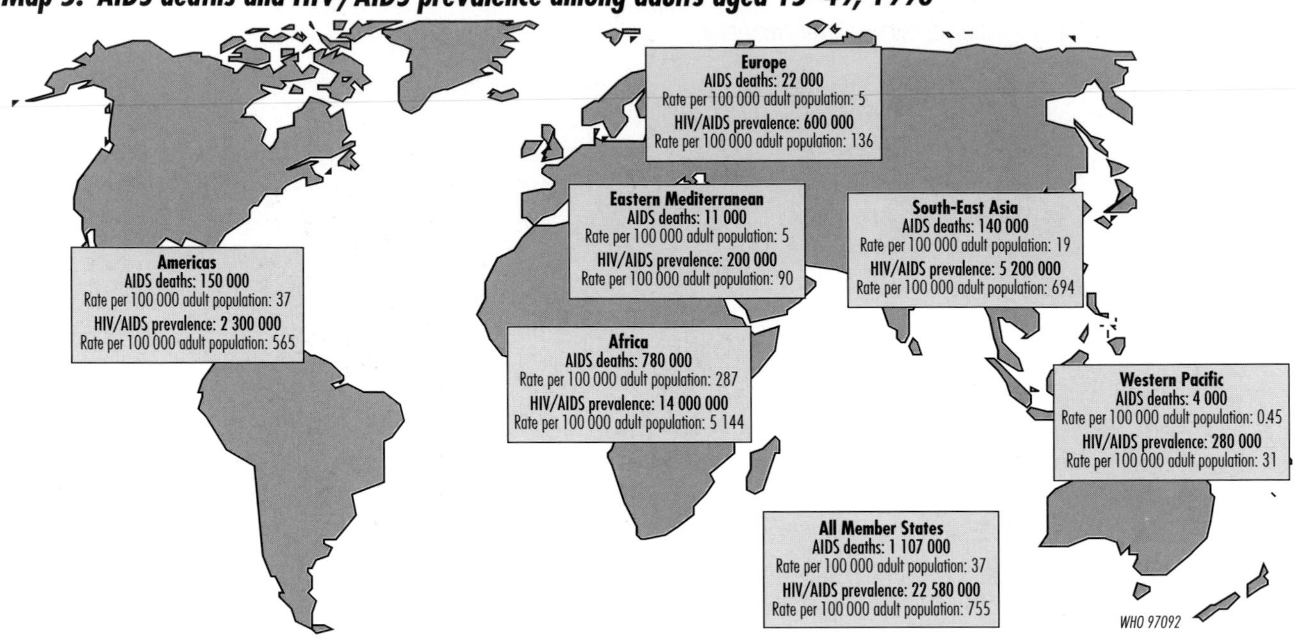

Box 27. The HIV/AIDS situation, 1996

The latest estimates show that there were more than 3.1 million new HIV infections in 1996, and that about 1.5 million people, including 350 000 children, died of HIV/AIDS-associated illnesses. Some 22.6 million people are now living with HIV infection or AIDS, including 21.8 million adults and 830 000 children. Since the start of the epidemic, an estimated 5 million adults and 1.4 million children have died.

Worldwide, 75-85% of HIV infections in adults have been transmitted through unprotected sexual intercourse, with heterosexual intercourse accounting for more than 70%. Mother-to-child transmission accounts for more than 90% of global infections in infants and children. Sharing HIV-infected injection equipment by drug users accounts for 5-10% of all adult infections, and transfusion of HIV-infected blood or blood products represents 3-5%.

Currently, 14 million people are living with HIV/AIDS in sub-Saharan Africa – about 63% of the world's total of infected persons. Surveys in seven African countries show that more than 10% of women attending antenatal clinics in urban areas are HIV-infected. Rates have been as high as 40% in some surveillance sites.

In Asia, HIV infection is spreading explosively in some parts of India, particularly to rural areas through migrant workers and truck drivers.

Rates are climbing rapidly among sex workers in Malaysia, Myanmar and Viet Nam. There has been an estimated tenfold growth in the number of people with HIV infection in China between 1993 and 1995, from 10 000 to 100 000. In Thailand, HIV infection rates in men have been declining, but prevalence continues to rise among women attending antenatal clinics.

In central and eastern Europe, spread is occurring, sometimes quite rapidly, to communities and countries that were hardly affected by the epidemic only a few years ago. Ukraine reported a dramatic increase in newly infected drug users in cities bordering the Black Sea. In the Russian Federation, 190 out of 46 000 drug injectors tested were HIV-positive, compared to none among more than 84 000 tested in 1994.

In the United States, although the overall number of new HIV infections has decreased over the past few years, studies suggest that a new generation of homosexual and bisexual men are becoming infected in some cities. In the United Kingdom, male-to-male transmission, which was declining in the late 1980s, seems to have been increasing again since 1990.

In Latin America and the Caribbean, epidemics are increasingly occurring among women and adolescents. Recent studies in Haiti have shown high HIV infection rates among pregnant women aged 14-24.

In the area of prevention, a study in one region of the United Republic of Tanzania has strengthened evidence that treating STDs diminishes HIV transmission. Prevalence among women attending antenatal clinics in Uganda has declined. Condom use in commercial sex transactions is now the norm in Thailand. A recent international study has shown that HIV infection among drug injectors is preventable through the early and vigorous implementation of prevention activities such as community outreach and needle exchange programmes.

Since 1 January 1996, when a new joint United Nations Programme on HIV/AIDS (UNAIDS) was launched, WHO's main focus has been to ensure a coordinated global, regional and country-level response to STDs and HIV/AIDS including in areas such as surveillance, blood safety, STD treatment and HIV/AIDS care.

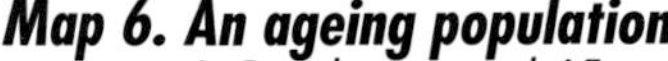

Map 6. An ageing population

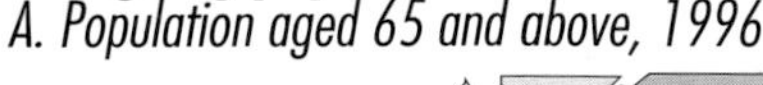

A. Population aged 65 and above, 1996

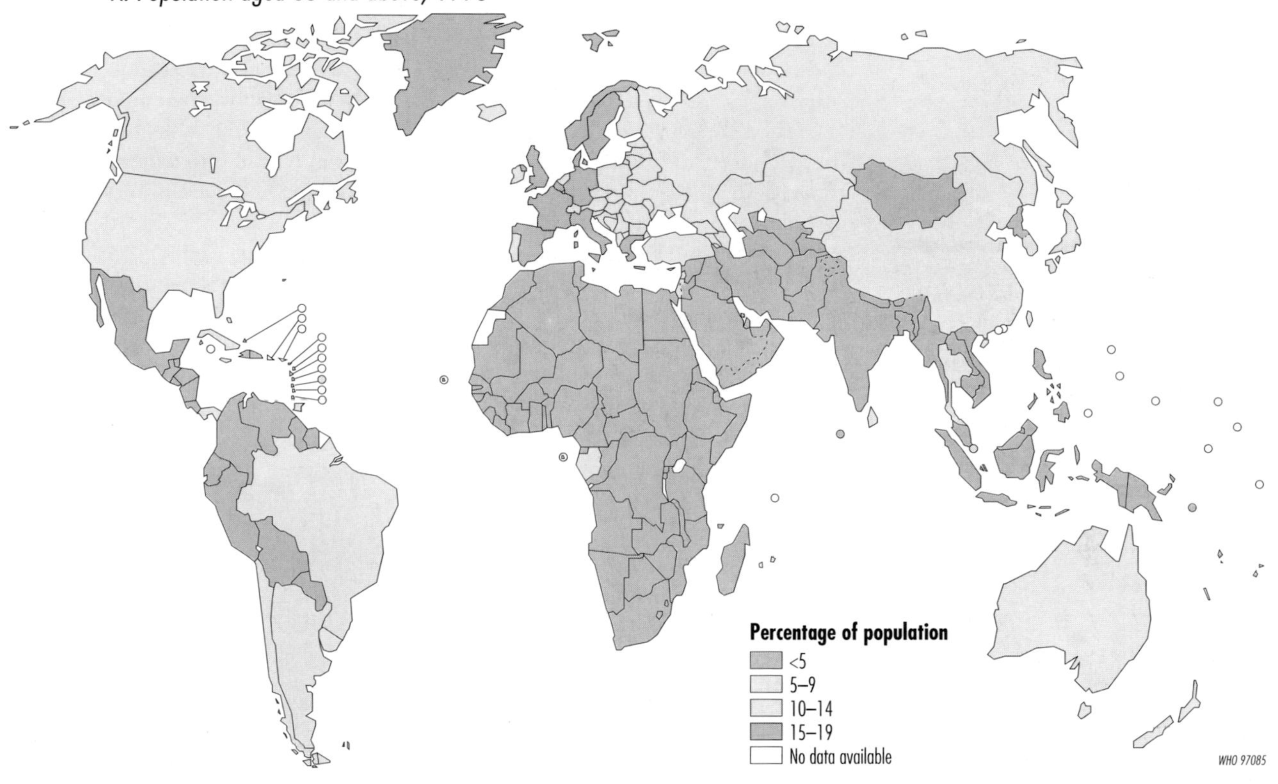

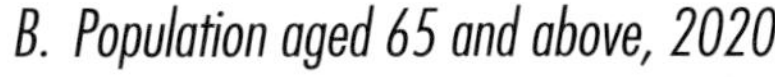

B. Population aged 65 and above, 2020

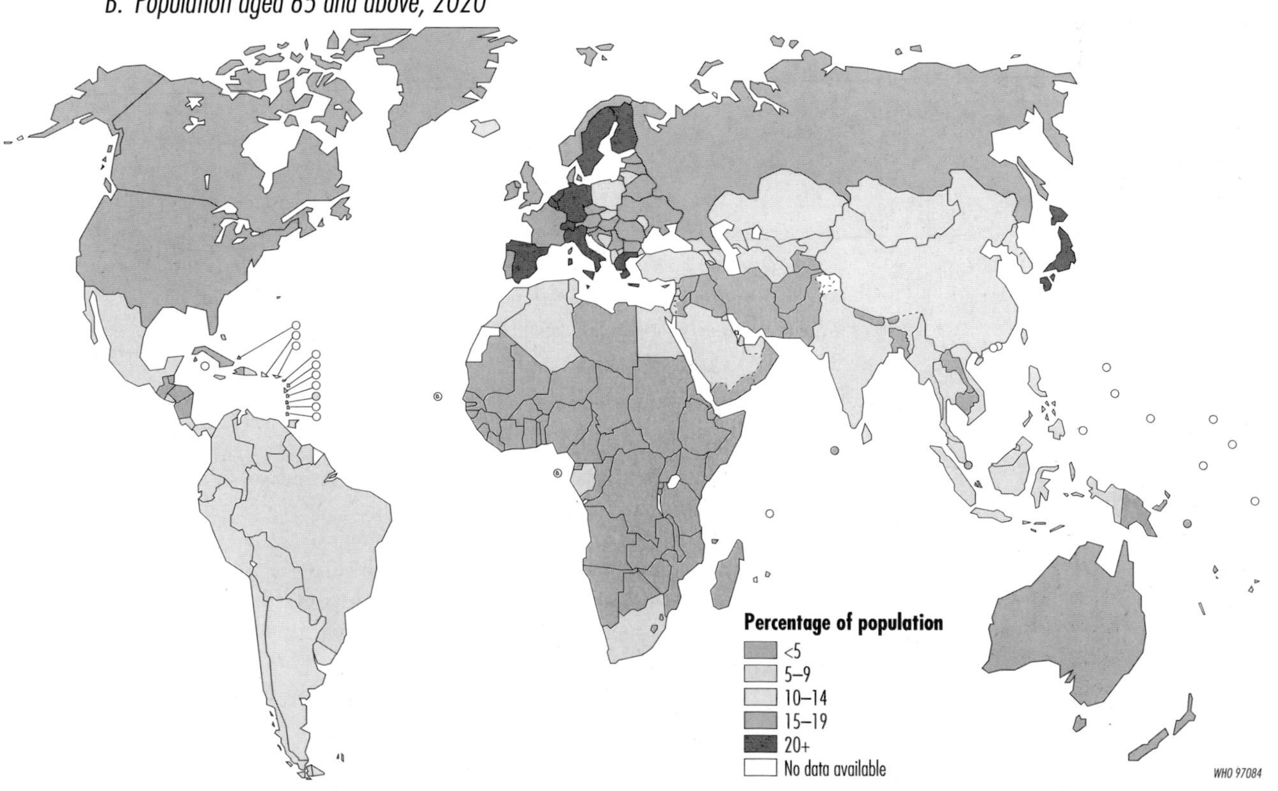

Since the International Conference on Health Promotion in 1986 in Ottawa, only a few countries in the developing world have introduced measures that encourage healthy public policies, promote healthy lifestyles and improve the human environment.

Many questions remain unanswered about the exact causes of these large reductions in mortality, which have occurred in countries with very different baseline levels of the diseases, different patterns of the well-established risk factors, and diverse medical care systems. The decline in mortality may be due to a reduction in incidence (fewer new events) or to a reduction in case-fatality rates (i.e. a higher survival rate) either because of reduced severity of the disease or because of better management in the acute phase, such as with angioplasty and bypass surgery. There is some evidence that the decline in mortality from coronary heart disease in elderly people has been associated both with a decline in the incidence rates of the condition and with a more substantial decline in hospital case-fatality rates for acute myocardial infarction primarily due to significant reductions in the time-lag between the onset of a heart attack and admission to hospital. It is likely that favourable trends in some risk factors, for example reduced smoking and improved diet, are involved in the decline in incidence of coronary heart disease.

However, the rapid mechanization of everyday life (when due consideration is not given to its health impact) brings with it hazards related to changing behaviour (sedentary living; excessive or ill-balanced diets rich in calories, cholesterol and salt; smoking) and to a deteriorating environment (air pollution, exposure to chemicals, contamination of soil and water, hazards to food safety and exposure to biological agents). As a consequence, global ill-health attributable to diseases such as coronary heart disease, stroke and hypertension has been increasing. Since the launching of a global initiative on promotion of health at the International Conference on Health Promotion in 1986 in Ottawa, only a few countries in the developing world have introduced measures that encourage healthy public policies, promote healthy lifestyles (beginning with the young) and improve the human environment (beginning with housing and better working conditions). It is therefore expected that cardiovascular diseases will continue to increase significantly in the next few decades, particularly among young adults and the middle-aged.

Rheumatic fever/rheumatic heart disease (RF/RHD) is decreasing only slowly, but with improvement in standards of living and accessibility to effective medical care, the decline can be continued and even accelerated. Though there is no safe and effective antirheumatic streptococcal vaccine or genetic marker to identify people at high risk of developing rheumatic fever, methods for the secondary and primary prevention of RF/RHD have proved cost-effective. There are effective methods for the diagnosis and treatment of acute attacks of rheumatic fever and also clinical and surgical methods for the palliative care of rheumatic heart disease and also for rehabilitation.

It is estimated that ***diabetes*** will affect more than 150 million people in the year 2000 and 300 million in the year 2025, compared to about 135 million in 1995. Increases in the numbers of cases will not be uniform between 1995 and 2025. Prevalence is expected to triple in Africa, the Eastern Mediterranean and South-East Asia; to double in the Americas and the Western Pacific; and to rise by less than 50% in Europe. The major factor contributing to these trends is increased longevity associated with rapid modernization, particularly in the newly industrialized and developing countries. Rapidly increasing incidence of new cases, and growing disability due to diabetes mellitus, may result in premature mortality and substantial economic cost if appropriate preventive action is not taken.

In many parts of the world economic progress and gains in overall longevity have been accompanied by an increase in mental, behavioural and social health problems. According to recent studies, ***mental health*** problems (including self-inflicted injuries) are one of the most frequent causes of lost years of good-quality life. Hundreds of millions of women, men and children suffer from mental illnesses; other behavioural problems affect the lives of countless adolescents, young adults and the elderly.

Greater longevity and economic progress have been accompanied by an increasing burden of chronic disease and associated social and behavioural health problems. More people live to a later age, when heart disease, cancer, arthritis, stroke and dementia are more common. The result has been personal suffering and impairment in role functioning and social relations, leading to diminished quality of life, and substantial monetary costs to the individual and to society.

Of course, these problems are not new. But some are more common than they were a century ago, and some have become especially important in recent years. The number of persons with major mental illnesses is likely to increase substantially in the decades to come, for two reasons. First, the numbers of men and women living on to the ages of higher risk for some of these illnesses are increasing because of demographic changes. Thus, the number of persons with schizophrenia will rise by 30% between 1985 and the year 2000 because of a 30% increase in the global population between the ages of 15 and 45. There will be a substantial rise in the senile dementias, including Alzeimer disease, again by virtue of the increase in the numbers of people living to the age of 65 and beyond. Second, rates of depression have risen in recent years due to high unemployment, stressful work conditions, gender discrimination, etc. Depression is now being seen at younger ages and more frequently in several countries, both developed and developing. The relative risk of depression has increased from one ten-year birth cohort to the next in some countries.

Health prognosis

Health conditions are likely to continue to change in the future with the rapid ageing of the global population and modifications in working methods and conditions, and leisure activities.

The demographic changes now taking place are creating an unprecedented imbalance between the young and the old. In the next 25 years, the population aged 65 and above is likely to grow by 82% compared to an increase of 46% in the working-age population (20-64 years) and of only 3% in newborns. For every child born today in an industrialized country, there are 10 people aged 65 years or over. By the year 2020 there will be 15 such elderly persons for every baby. Meanwhile, in developing countries, for every baby born today there are two people over 65. By the year 2020 there will be four people over 65 for every newborn.

One result of this situation with socioeconomic implications for many countries will be the imbalance between the elderly and the working populations. Increasingly, relatively fewer people of productive age will have to provide for an expanding number of dependants, not merely in the form of direct support to elderly relatives, but also through taxation, the provision of health and social services, social security, etc.

It follows that the longer the elderly population can be helped to remain in good health, disability-free and productive, the smaller the social cost to the younger generation in particular and to society in general. It is equally clear that the longer the health of the working population can be sustained without disability, the more productive it will be and the more able to support the elderly dependants of society.

It is also obvious that with increased life expectancy, together with the ability of medical technologies to postpone death without always restoring health, individuals are saved from death due to certain diseases, but are subsequently exposed to other risks of death, that is, a decrease in mortality from one cause leading to an increase in mortality from another – "substitute mortality". While later death is in itself a benefit, the question of quality of life during the additional years needs to be considered.

The independent life expectancy reflecting the quality of life for various

In the next 25 years, the population aged 65 and above is likely to grow by 82% compared to an increase of 46% in the working-age population (20-64 years) and of only 3% in newborns.

Table 5. Independent life expectancy at age 65, in years

Selected countries	Male		Female	
	Life expectancy	Disability-free life expectancy	Life expectancy	Disability-free life expectancy
Canada, 1986	14.9	8.1	19.2	9.4
Finland, 1986	13.4	2.5	17.4	2.4
Indonesia, 1989	11.5	11.4	12.8	12.4
Myanmar, 1989	12.0	11.1	13.5	12.8
Netherlands, 1990[a]	14.4	9.3	19.0	9.1
Thailand, 1989	12.6	12.4	14.2	13.6
United Kingdom, 1991	14.3	13.6	18.1	16.9

[a] Life expectancy in good perceived health.
Source: Network on Health Expectancy and the Disability Process (REVES).

Box 28. Prevention of blindness and deafness

Much disability is ageing-related, reflecting a situation either of a cumulating risk for disease leading to impairments, such as for the increase of cataract by age, or of the evolution of disease and resulting complications over time, as in the case of diabetes complications or eyelid scarring from trachoma. Disability from trauma is also generally age-related, with a cumulative risk throughout life, even if there are particularly vulnerable and/or exposed population groups.

Sensory impairments, for example vision and hearing problems, are very often ageing-related and the resulting disability is of great importance in terms of social dependency, ill-health and quality of life of the elderly. This is a matter of considerable concern, given the demographic trends, with a rapidly increasing proportion of elderly worldwide. It is thus possible to project the expected increase of impairments and resulting disability for the coming generations for those disorders which are particularly related to ageing. *Fig. 9* shows that the number of elderly blind will *double* over the 25-year period up to the year 2020.

There are several similar examples of ageing-related, usually noncommunicable, disorders leading to disability in the elderly; this is likely to become a major global issue of health and social care for coming generations.

Fig. 9. Eye and ear problems in the elderly population, worldwide, 1995–2020

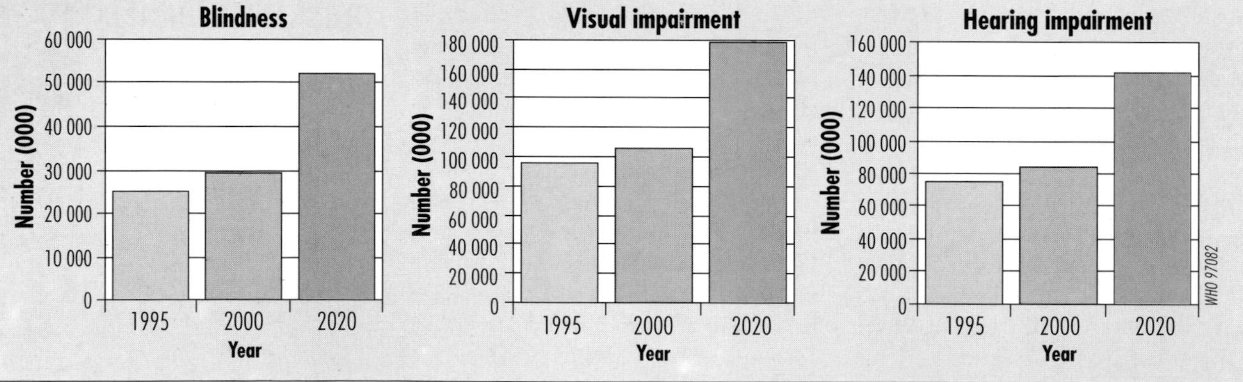

countries is given in *Table 5*. Increasingly, a substantial share of the number of unhealthy years of life is attributable to debilitating conditions associated with chronic diseases and disorders as they replace acute illnesses in the same population. Several of these conditions, such as arthritis, osteoporosis, dementia and reduced vision and hearing, are manifestations of the natural ageing processes in that they can occur in every member of the population, are progressive and generally irreversible; they cause pain, suffering and disability and with an ageing population the worldwide burden of ill-health will increase (*Box 28*, *Fig. 9*). However, many other conditions, such as cancer, heart and lung diseases, diabetes and mental and neurological disorders, are age-associated in that their incidence increases with age, and ageing aggravates the progression of the disease or condition.

With rapid industrialization, mechanization and modernization associated with global mass media communication, individuals in many developing countries are exposed to numerous risk factors such as pollution and food contamination, limited physical activity, increased intake of dietary fat, smoking, excessive alcohol consumption, drug abuse and unsafe sex, which singly and in combination lead to many health problems and diseases. It is increasingly observed that adolescents and young adults are also victims of premature morbidity and mortality due to many of these diseases.

Priorities for action

Increasing life expectancy provides the potential for better health expectancy, but steps towards fulfilling that potential can only be taken if the pathways are clearly marked. In terms of controlling chronic noncommunicable diseases, this means defining realistic priorities for international action.

It is not a simple task. A wide variety of diseases affect both physical and mental health. The impaired individual well-being and socioeconomic burdens that they impose vary greatly. There is a diversity of health infrastructures (and resources) to deal with them in Member States. There are differing perceptions and degrees of political will to respond to them.

Currently, in the majority of countries the problem of ill-health is addressed primarily by medical services through traditional disease-specific vertical programmes, in most cases aimed at diagnosis and treatment of the established disease or condition. This approach may be quite successful under certain circumstances, given the sophisticated technology now available. However, almost inevitably its high cost creates a barrier and precludes its availability to the whole population even in developed countries, to say nothing about those in greater need.

On the other hand, it is clear from the analysis made in this report that major chronic diseases share a relatively small number of common and crucial risk factors which enable the development of an integrated strategic approach to the prevention of a number of these diseases.

Although the major thrust must be towards the prevention of noncomunicable diseases – a hitherto almost neglected area in their control – assessing and applying cost-effective methods in disease detection and case management should remain an important component of the control process. The time has now come to develop integrated packages for controlling these diseases based on best experiences and good practices; these can serve as a framework for intervention at different levels of public health services (as applicable in different local contexts), including primary health care and referral institutions.

In addition, there is an urgent need to develop and incorporate activities that raise awareness of, and motivation for, healthy lifestyles and the environments to support them. A major, intensified and sustained global campaign to encourage healthy lifestyles is vital. To succeed, such a campaign requires high-level international collaboration and multisectoral cooperation.

This demands a new relationship in which specialists, experts and leaders in various fields look beyond their own professional boundaries. They need to recognize that many diseases have common risk factors, and to share their skills and experience so as to tackle them together. This risk factor recognition must be communicated clearly to the public at large.

Greater attention should be paid to the integration of primarily clinical and public health functions to enable better development and utilization of human resources, and to ensure effective cooperation of the family and community at local levels.

Major chronic diseases share a relatively small number of common and crucial risk factors which enable the development of an integrated strategic approach to the prevention of a number of these diseases.

For the treatment of coronary heart disease, low-cost and effective medical interventions have been identified, which are simple to administer.

identifying and controlling hypertension, and to a lesser extent, raised blood cholesterol levels. Hypertension is the most important risk factor for stroke, and one of the most important in heart disease. Even modest blood pressure reduction in hypertensive people could reduce half of the stroke events worldwide. Well-established methods exist for controlling or lowering high blood pressure and elevated blood cholesterol levels.

Primary prevention strategies can be supplemented by a strategy for dealing with high-risk groups in the population, by identifying and helping individuals in need of special protection. This will include treatment with or without drugs to control hypertension and reduce serum cholesterol levels.

In preventing ***rheumatic heart disease***, early detection and correct treatment of streptococcal sore throat or pharyngitis are necessary to avoid the first attack of acute rheumatic fever.

Prevention and control of ***diabetes*** must be integrated into broader programmes for the prevention of major noncommunicable diseases at the community level. A diabetes strategy should focus on the early identification and management of the disease, based on an active partnership between health professionals and diabetic individuals. Early detection of hypertension, high cholesterol and vision-threatening retinopathy are crucially important. Retinopathy screening should be routine in people with diabetes. Evaluation of different options for primary, secondary and tertiary prevention of diabetes is necessary.

A number of ***hereditary disorders*** can be detected by genetic screening, which needs to be supported by appropriate counselling services for individuals and families at risk. Genetic studies are becoming increasingly important in the understanding of many major noncommunicable diseases, including some mental disorders. Genetics services are cost-effective in view of the great social and financial burden of the chronic disease avoided. About 50% of congenital abnormalities, around 10% of inherited diseases and about 2% of chromosomal disorders can be successfully treated or corrected. Within the next five years, genetic counselling based on a family-oriented approach will be further developed. The genetic influences on health-related behaviour deserve further, preferably interdisciplinary, research.

Treatment

In ***cancer*** therapy, advances have been made for cancers at some specific organ sites, which can now be successfully treated in more than 60% of cases (e.g. some malignant lymphomas, (including Hodgkin disease), childhood leukaemia) and more than 90% in testicular cancer. Similarly, though less dramatically, improvements have been made in the treatment of breast cancer (the use of tamoxifen) and in therapy of childhood tumours (including those of the nervous system). In the case of cancers for which available evidence indicates that radiotherapy is an essential component of treatment, the acquisition of appropriate equipment and the training of personnel in their use, are recommended.

For patients suffering from ***circulatory diseases***, the priority should be to avoid the recurrence and progression of the disease. Improved methods for the management of acute stroke are available and have contributed to the decline in mortality from cerebrovascular disease in industrialized countries. For the treatment of coronary heart disease, low-cost and effective medical interventions have been identified (the use of aspirin, streptokinase), which are simple to administer. Surgical and nonsurgical invasive technologies are widely practised in industrialized countries and are increasingly used in developing ones. Simple, low-cost measures for the rehabilitation of patients with a wide range of circulatory diseases are available for use in even severely disabled, medically complex cases in all age groups, and could be integrated into existing health care delivery systems in all countries.

For the control of hypertension, effective and low-cost pharmacological and nonpharmacological methods have been developed. There are cost-effective drugs (e.g. penicillin) and surgical methods available for the management of patients with rheumatic heart disease, which lends itself to prevention through the treatment of underlying infections.

In the case of ***diabetes***, effective treatment can considerably improve the outcome, by reducing the incidence or progression of long-term complications. However, insulin, which is considered as an essential drug, is still unavailable in many parts of the world. In the case of people with non-insulin-dependent diabetes, the condition may be adequately controlled by diet, physical exercise or oral hypoglycaemic agents. Noninvasive laser therapy is now available for the early stages of diabetic retinopathy. Treatment of hypertension may reduce the incidence of diabetic kidney disease. Education of the person with diabetes in the self-management of the condition is also a cornerstone of modern treatment of the disease.

Many ***mental disorders*** can be treated easily and cheaply, but it is vital to ensure that essential medications are available at affordable cost at the point of contact of the patient with the health care system. Help is needed to ensure that treatment for such disorders is integrated within the first health contact level.

Palliative care

Individual suffering from cancer is a burden that goes far beyond the statistics on incidence and mortality, and is borne by the patient's entire family and friends. Relief from unnecessary pain should be higher on the public health agenda in both developing and developed countries. WHO has in the past advocated the use of suitable measures to palliate pain in terminal illness, but has often found itself in conflict with laws primarily designed to control the use of illicit drugs. There are those with some mental disorders for whom humane and loving care is all that can be offered, preferably by families supported by the health sector. Good models of care need to be designed and descriptions of existing good practice disseminated to countries.

Policies

Health promotion

Health promotion calls for countrywide community-based programmes supported by national or federal and local economic and social policy. The active participation of the community and the involvement of the mass media are essential. Several countries have adopted comprehensive approaches and their experience should be built upon.

Legislative action and financial measures should be considered in support of disease prevention programmes, such as: reducing the availability of tobacco to children; labelling all packages with a health warning; controlling the advertising of tobacco products and restricting smoking in public places, schools and workplaces; taxing products known to increase risk; subsidizing healthy nutritional items; and providing facilities for recreational physical exercise.

Changes in the structure and practices of the health sector are also necessary, involving a reallocation of resources, stronger emphasis on prevention, and new approaches to training primary health care workers.

Modern medicine is confronted with vast opportunities provided by a proliferation of diagnostic and therapeutic technology. Their application, however, leads to spiralling health care costs, while their net benefits are unclear. It is thus imperative that all dimensions of their benefits should be evaluated objectively in order to guide the decisions of health personnel. Methods for the evaluation of quality of care should be developed for use in both the public and private health care sector.

Healthy environment

Socioeconomic development should be carried out in such a way as to protect, and where possible enhance, human health and well-being. There is a need for improvements in the existing human environment, including the upgrading of housing, the reduction of long-standing pollution, and the provision of better working conditions.

Changes in the structure and practices of the health sector are necessary, involving a reallocation of resources, stronger emphasis on prevention, and new approaches to training primary health care workers.

Such measures involve many aspects of government at central, regional and local levels, and require well-integrated, multisectoral planning and management. Because many of the problems, such as air and water pollution and the transportation of potentially harmful materials, may affect more than one country, there is a need for international collaboration on surveillance and control measures.

Table 6. Cancer deaths, selected countries, latest available year

	France 1993	Mexico 1993	Republic of Korea 1994	Russian Federation 1994	United States of America 1992
Life expectancy at birth (in years)	77	71	71	68	76
Cancer sites	**Average age at death (in years)**				
All sites	**69**	**61**	**61**	**63**	**69**
Breast (female)	67	57	53	62	66
Colon-rectum	73	65	63	67	71
Liver	68	64	59	...	66
Lung	67	67	65	64	69
Prostate	76	74	70	69	75
Stomach	73	66	63	65	70
	Percentage of deaths under age 55				
All sites	**12**	**29**	**28**	**20**	**13**
Breast (female)	19	48	57	30	23
Colon-rectum	6	23	25	13	9
Liver	9	19	38	...	16
Lung	14	15	17	16	10
Prostate	1	3	7	5	1
Stomach	7	20	23	17	12
	Total number of deaths (000)				
All sites	**143**	**45**	**49**	**300**	**521**

The development of new technologies, for instance in the areas of energy production and chemical manufacture, must be such as to minimize the potential adverse effects on human health, and this requires the establishment of systematic mechanisms for risk assessment and the study of alternatives.

Caring society

Too often the high-technology care used in an effort to prolong life in fact reduces the quality of life. It may prevent patients from dying with dignity in a situation of their choice. There is a need to develop well-integrated community-based programmes that are sufficiently tailored to the circumstances of individuals with special needs. The time has come for a caring society to do what cannot be done by a curing profession. This is illustrated by data available for both industrialized and developing countries which show few differences between life expectancy at birth and average age at death due to some cancers (*Table 6*).

Research

Research is continuing to develop new therapeutic drugs and treatments for a number of noncommunicable diseases. Some have recently been marketed, others are at an advanced stage of development (*Box 30*).

Within the next five years, gene therapy for common disorders including cancer, coronary heart disease, diabetes and autoimmune disorders will become available.

Research will not only help further to refine knowledge of the environmental and lifestyle factors which increase the risk of cancer in a population. It will permit identification of the specific individuals at highest personal risk from exposure to these factors, probably in terms of genetic endowment which renders them more susceptible. The search continues for chemopreventive agents which can reduce cancer risk. Although the initial enthusiasm for micronutrients (e.g. vitamins) has waned, other approaches (the use of nonsteroidal anti-inflammatory drugs, tamoxifen-like anti-estrogens and calcium-fibre preparations) are being investigated for possible benefits, inconvenience or side effects.

Research into the genetic basis of circulatory diseases, especially hypertension, should be encouraged. The use of molecular genetics may in the near future make it possible to identify and pay more specific attention to susceptible individuals. Hypertension in pregnancy is a major cause of premature birth and perinatal death; more research efforts should therefore concentrate on studying its mechanisms in order to facilitate prevention and develop suitable treatment. The problem of coronary heart disease in women is causing increasing concern. Knowledge of the natural history of this disease before, during and after the menopause is inadequate and more research is needed on menopause-related pathobiological and metabolic changes.

More detailed information is required on the genetics of diabetes as a means of identifying persons at risk. Studies on asthma prevalence in different areas and population groups are needed to identify environmental risk factors, as are studies on cost-effectiveness in asthma management and prevention programmes.

Research aimed at uncovering the determinants of nonfatal disability, and designing interventions to avoid their consequences, should be given high priority.

Emerging ethical issues

Identifying priorities in the prevention of disease, the relief of pain and suffering, caring and curing, and the avoidance of premature death, cannot be achieved without recognizing the many ethical and human rights issues associated with them. The goals of health care are being reoriented towards quality of life and health expectancy as well as life expectancy. Equity and ethics are becoming of ever-greater importance at a time when societies are witnessing both the ageing of their populations and increasing strains on their resources. Longer life has often come at the price of greater suffering, disability and higher costs.

Balancing the advantages against the disadvantages of advanced medical technology is an increasingly important priority for policy-makers. People want the benefits of science and technology. But they also want to be consulted about them and reassured that these advances are properly harnessed to protect rather than endanger human dignity, health, well-being and diversity.

Advances in the fields of genetics, screening and organ transplantation are only a few examples of the many complex ethical challenges facing all concerned – scientists, physicians, health workers, economists and politicians – on behalf of the wider public.

The danger that some of the advances in biomedical sciences have potentially adverse consequences for the integrity, dignity and human rights of the individual has been recognized. Recent research work involving the cloning of animals appears to have exciting potential, but may be inappropriate or dangerous if applied before the implications for society are fully investigated and explained. Such issues are reflected in the latest draft of a Universal Declaration on the Human Genome and Human Rights, formulated under the auspices of UNESCO, with input from WHO.

Box 30. New drugs and treatments for chronic diseases

Promising research initiatives are under way in the development of new and innovative products for the prevention and cure of noncommunicable diseases; extensive comparative clinical trials of a variety of treatments are also taking place, in order to show which are the most beneficial and cost effective. Some of them are listed below.

Prophylactic vaccines to prevent infection and also vaccines to reduce or eliminate established infection leading to specific ***cancers*** are being developed, most notably a vaccine against the human papilloma virus that is a causative agent in the majority of cases of cervical cancer. Monoclonal antibodies, armed with toxins or radioisotopes and genetically-manipulated components of the immune system, have also reached early stages of clinical trials (see also *Box 7*).

In the area of ***circulatory diseases***, a range of drugs is available for effective treatment of conditions such as hypertension, hypercholesterolaemia, cardiac arrhythmias, myocardial infarction and chronic angina. Thrombin inactivators and fibrinogen receptor antagonists are found to improve considerably the efficacy and safety of antithrombotic therapy.

New human insulin analogs, new routes of insulin delivery, organ transplantation and gene therapy are improving the effectiveness of ***diabetes*** treatment. Evidence is also accumulating on their preventive effect.

In ***osteoporosis***, for example, the experience of hormone replacement therapy has been encouraging. So too have the first results of studies on the use of antiresorptive agents including a nasal spray form of calcitonin. Transforming growth factor B and insulin-like growth factor are promising candidates for increasing bone formation in older people.

With new agents such as cytokine inhibitors, improvements are also indicated in the treatment of ***arthritis***; the genetically-engineered human interleukin-1 receptor antagonist has been shown in studies to relieve rheumatoid arthritis, reducing inflammation and joint tissue destruction. The drug appears to slow the autoimmune disease process without seriously affecting other functions of the immune system.

Conclusion

Inevitably, each human life reaches its end. Ensuring that it does so in the most dignified, caring and least painful way that can be achieved deserves as much priority as any other.

Priority areas for international action in health should be:

1. Integration of disease-specific interventions in both physical and mental health into a comprehensive chronic disease control package that incorporates prevention, diagnosis, treatment and rehabilitation, and improved training of health professionals.
2. Fuller application of existing cost-effective methods of disease detection and management, including improved screening, taking into account the genetic diversity of individuals.
3. A major intensified but sustained global campaign to encourage healthy lifestyles, with an emphasis on the healthy development of children and adolescents in relation to risk factors such as diet, exercise and smoking.
4. Healthy public policies, including sustainable financing, and legislation on pricing and taxation, in support of disease prevention programmes.
5. Acceleration of research into new drugs and vaccines, and into the genetic determinants of chronic diseases.
6. Alleviation of pain, reduction of suffering and provision of palliative care for those who cannot be cured.

The World Health Report 1997 indicates priorities for action that are intended to improve humanity's ability to prevent, treat, rehabilitate and where possible, cure major noncommunicable diseases, and to reduce the enormous suffering and disability that they cause.

Inevitably, each human life reaches its end. Ensuring that it does so in the most dignified, caring and least painful way that can be achieved deserves as much priority as any other. This is a priority not merely for the medical profession, the health sector or the social services. It is a priority for each society, community, family and individual.

Annex 1

Members and Associate Members of WHO

As of 31 December 1996, WHO had 190 Members and two Associate Members. They are listed below with the date on which they became a party to the constitution or were admitted to associate membership.

Afghanistan 19 April 1948
Albania 26 May 1947
Algeria* 8 November 1962
Angola 15 May 1976
Antigua and Barbuda* 12 March 1984
Argentina* 22 October 1948
Armenia 4 May 1992
Australia* 2 February 1948
Austria* 30 June 1947
Azerbaijan 2 October 1992
Bahamas* 1 April 1974
Bahrain* 2 November 1971
Bangladesh 19 May 1972
Barbados* 25 April 1967
Belarus* 7 April 1948
Belgium* 25 June 1948
Belize 23 August 1990
Benin 20 September 1960
Bhutan 8 March 1982
Bolivia 23 December 1949
Bosnia and Herzegovina* 10 September 1992
Botswana* 26 February 1975
Brazil* 2 June 1948
Brunei Darussalam 25 March 1985
Bulgaria* 9 June 1948
Burkina Faso* 4 October 1960
Burundi 22 October 1962
Cambodia* 17 May 1950
Cameroon* 6 May 1960
Canada 29 August 1946
Cape Verde 5 January 1976
Central African Republic* 20 September 1960
Chad 1 January 1961
Chile* 15 October 1948
China* 22 July 1946
Colombia 14 May 1959
Comoros 9 December 1975
Congo 26 October 1960
Cook Islands 9 May 1984
Costa Rica 17 March 1949
Côte d'Ivoire* 28 October 1960
Croatia* 11 June 1992
Cuba* 9 May 1950
Cyprus* 16 January 1961
Czech Republic* 22 January 1993
Democratic People's Republic of Korea 19 May 1973
Denmark* 19 April 1948
Djibouti 10 March 1978
Dominica* 13 August 1981
Dominican Republic 21 June 1948
Ecuador* 1 March 1949
Egypt* 16 December 1947
El Salvador 22 June 1948
Equatorial Guinea 5 May 1980
Eritrea 24 July 1993
Estonia 31 March 1993
Ethiopia 11 April 1947
Fiji* 1 January 1972
Finland* 7 October 1947
France 16 June 1948
Gabon* 21 November 1960
Gambia* 26 April 1971
Georgia 26 May 1992
Germany* 29 May 1951
Ghana* 8 April 1957
Greece* 12 March 1948
Grenada 4 December 1974
Guatemala* 26 August 1949
Guinea* 19 May 1959
Guinea-Bissau 29 July 1974
Guyana* 27 September 1966
Haiti* 12 August 1947
Honduras 8 April 1949
Hungary* 17 June 1948
Iceland 17 June 1948
India* 12 January 1948
Indonesia* 23 May 1950
Iran (Islamic Republic of)* 23 November 1946
Iraq* 23 September 1947
Ireland* 20 October 1947

* Member States that have acceded to the Convention on the Privileges and Immunities of the Specialized Agencies and its Annex VII.

Israel 21 June 1949
Italy* 11 April 1947
Jamaica* 21 March 1963
Japan* 16 May 1951
Jordan* 7 April 1947
Kazakstan 19 August 1992
Kenya* 27 January 1964
Kiribati 26 July 1984
Kuwait* 9 May 1960
Kyrgyzstan 29 April 1992
Lao People's Democratic Republic* 17 May 1950
Latvia 4 December 1991
Lebanon 19 January 1949
Lesotho* 7 July 1967
Liberia 14 March 1947
Libyan Arab Jamahiriya* 16 May 1952
Lithuania 25 November 1991
Luxembourg* 3 June 1949
Madagascar* 16 January 1961
Malawi* 9 April 1965
Malaysia* 24 April 1958
Maldives* 5 November 1965
Mali* 17 October 1960
Malta* 1 February 1965
Marshall Islands 5 June 1991
Mauritania 7 March 1961
Mauritius* 9 December 1968
Mexico 7 April 1948
Micronesia (Federated States of) 14 August 1991
Monaco 8 July 1948
Mongolia* 18 April 1962
Morocco* 14 May 1956
Mozambique 11 September 1975
Myanmar 1 July 1948
Namibia 23 April 1990
Nauru 9 May 1994
Nepal* 2 September 1953
Netherlands* 25 April 1947
New Zealand* 10 December 1946
Nicaragua* 24 April 1950
Niger* 5 October 1960
Nigeria* 25 November 1960
Niue 4 May 1994
Norway* 18 August 1947
Oman 28 May 1971
Pakistan* 23 June 1948
Palau 9 March 1995
Panama 20 February 1951
Papua New Guinea 29 April 1976
Paraguay 4 January 1949
Peru 11 November 1949
Philippines* 9 July 1948
Poland* 6 May 1948
Portugal 13 February 1948
Qatar 11 May 1972
Republic of Korea* 17 August 1949
Republic of Moldova 4 May 1992
Romania* 8 June 1948
Russian Federation* 24 March 1948
Rwanda* 7 November 1962
Saint Kitts and Nevis 3 December 1984
Saint Lucia* 11 November 1980
Saint Vincent and the
Grenadines 2 September 1983
Samoa 16 May 1962
San Marino 12 May 1980
Sao Tome and Principe 23 March 1976
Saudi Arabia 26 May 1947
Senegal* 31 October 1960
Seychelles* 11 September 1979
Sierra Leone* 20 October 1961
Singapore* 25 February 1966
Slovakia* 4 February 1993
Slovenia* 7 May 1992
Solomon Islands 4 April 1983
Somalia 26 January 1961
South Africa 7 August 1947
Spain* 28 May 1951
Sri Lanka 7 July 1948
Sudan 14 May 1956
Suriname 25 March 1976
Swaziland 16 April 1973
Sweden* 28 August 1947
Switzerland 26 March 1947
Syrian Arab Republic 18 December 1946
Tajikistan 4 May 1992
Thailand* 26 September 1947
The Former Yugoslav Republic
of Macedonia 22 April 1993
Togo* 13 May 1960
Tonga* 14 August 1975
Trinidad and Tobago* 3 January 1963
Tunisia* 14 May 1956
Turkey 2 January 1948
Turkmenistan 2 July 1992
Tuvalu 7 May 1993
Uganda* 7 March 1963
Ukraine* 3 April 1948
United Arab Emirates 30 March 1972
United Kingdom of Great Britain
and Northern Ireland* 22 July 1946
United Republic of Tanzania* 15 March 1962
United States of America 21 June 1948
Uruguay* 22 April 1949
Uzbekistan 22 May 1992
Vanuatu 7 March 1983
Venezuela 7 July 1948
Viet Nam 17 May 1950
Yemen 20 November 1953
Yugoslavia* 19 November 1947
Zaire* 24 February 1961
Zambia* 2 February 1965
Zimbabwe* 16 May 1980

Associate Members

Puerto Rico 7 May 1992
Tokelau 8 May 1991

* Member States that have acceded to the Convention on the Privileges and Immunities of the Specialized Agencies and its Annex VII.

Annex 2

Statistics

Notes

... *Data not available or not applicable*

"Billion" means a thousand million

$ denotes United States dollars

Unless specified otherwise, data refer to 1996

Explanatory notes

The *World Health Report 1997 – Conquering suffering, enriching humanity* presents an overview of the global health situation based on an assessment carried out in 1996 using 1996 or latest available data. The content of the report was determined essentially by its theme as well as by the availability of information concerning key health and health-related indicators. The majority of Member States still experience great difficulty in obtaining valid and timely data on many indicators such as disease morbidity and health-care coverage. Official statistics reported to WHO were incomplete, often not comparable among countries, nor up to date. Considerable efforts were made to assemble and validate best available and reasonably reliable data from such sources as national reports and publications, reports and publications of all WHO offices, WHO collaborating centres and personal communications. Reference was also made to publications and documents of other intergovernmental bodies and nongovernmental organizations. The main source of estimates relating to demographic indicators, including life expectancy at birth and infant mortality, was the Population Division, Department for Economic and Social Information and Policy Analysis, United Nations, hereinafter referred to as United Nations Population Division. A number of statistical values such as the under-5 mortality rate were derived from those estimates, but otherwise no attempt was made, for the present report, to refine figures taken from recognized international sources and research publications.

Surveillance data for a number of diseases – communicable and noncommunicable – of major public health concern are lacking; global and regional estimates of prevalence, incidence and even mortality are not available except for a few diseases. Using whatever reliable estimates were available, efforts were made to assess diseases/conditions according to their effect on people's health at different stages of life, i.e. children, school-age children and adolescents, adults and the elderly, in order to provide an overview of the situation and trends.

Because many of WHO's activities in different fields are interdependent, programmes were clustered and their activities, products and other outputs synthesized according to their objectives and target age groups, the aim being to provide a global overview of WHO's work during the year 1996, irrespective of the organizational level at which activities were carried out, i.e. country, regional or interregional.

As of 31 December 1996 WHO had 190 Member States and two Associate Members (see *Annex 1*). The global health assessment relates only to Member States. For analytical purposes they have been grouped according to the United Nations classification (shown below).

Developed market economies. Australia, Austria, Belgium, Canada, Denmark, Finland, France, Germany, Greece, Iceland, Ireland, Italy, Japan, Luxembourg, Monaco, Netherlands, New Zealand, Norway, Portugal, San Marino, Spain, Sweden, Switzerland, United Kingdom, United States of America.

Economies in transition. Albania, Armenia, Azerbaijan, Belarus, Bulgaria, Czech Republic, Estonia, Georgia, Hungary, Kazakstan, Kyrgyzstan, Latvia, Lithuania, Poland, Republic of

Moldova, Romania, Russian Federation, Slovakia, Tajikistan, Turkmenistan, Ukraine, Uzbekistan.

Developing countries – excluding least developed countries. Algeria, Antigua and Barbuda, Argentina, Bahamas, Bahrain, Barbados, Belize, Bolivia, Bosnia and Herzegovina, Botswana, Brazil, Brunei Darussalam, Cameroon, Chile, China, Colombia, Congo, Cook Islands, Costa Rica, Côte d'Ivoire, Croatia, Cuba, Cyprus, Democratic People's Republic of Korea, Dominica, Dominican Republic, Ecuador, Egypt, El Salvador, Fiji, Gabon, Ghana, Grenada, Guatemala, Guyana, Honduras, India, Indonesia, Iran (Islamic Republic of), Iraq, Israel, Jamaica, Jordan, Kenya, Kuwait, Lebanon, Libyan Arab Jamahiriya, Malaysia, Malta, Marshall Islands, Mauritius, Mexico, Micronesia (Federated States of), Mongolia, Morocco, Namibia, Nauru, Nicaragua, Nigeria, Niue, Oman, Pakistan, Palau, Panama, Papua New Guinea, Paraguay, Peru, Philippines, Qatar, Republic of Korea, Saint Kitts and Nevis, Saint Lucia, Saint Vincent and the Grenadines, Saudi Arabia, Senegal, Seychelles, Singapore, Slovenia, South Africa, Sri Lanka, Suriname, Swaziland, Syrian Arab Republic, Thailand, The Former Yugoslav Republic of Macedonia, Tonga, Trinidad and Tobago, Tunisia, Turkey, United Arab Emirates, Uruguay, Venezuela, Viet Nam, Yugoslavia, Zimbabwe.

Least developed countries. Afghanistan, Angola, Bangladesh, Benin, Bhutan, Burkina Faso, Burundi, Cambodia, Cape Verde, Central African Republic, Chad, Comoros, Djibouti, Equatorial Guinea, Eritrea, Ethiopia, Gambia, Guinea, Guinea-Bissau, Haiti, Kiribati, Lao People's Democratic Republic, Lesotho, Liberia, Madagascar, Malawi, Maldives, Mali, Mauritania, Mozambique, Myanmar, Nepal, Niger, Rwanda, Samoa, Sao Tome and Principe, Sierra Leone, Solomon Islands, Somalia, Sudan, Togo, Tuvalu, Uganda, United Republic of Tanzania, Vanuatu, Yemen, Zaire, Zambia.

Throughout the report "developed world" refers to countries classified as "developed market economies" and "economies in transition"; and "developing world" to "least developed countries" (LDCs) and other "developing countries". In some cases the "developed world" has also been referred to as the "industrialized countries" or "developed countries" in the text.

The designations used for groupings of countries in the text and tables are intended solely for statistical and analytical purposes and do not necessarily express a judgement about the stage reached by a particular country in the development process.

As countries are added to or removed from a particular group, revised estimates are computed for the groups and subgroups of countries retroactively to ensure comparability over time. Accordingly, data by WHO region or by the United Nations classification in this report may differ from comparable figures presented in earlier World Health Reports (1995 and 1996).

A major constraint in the assessment of the global health situation relates to data on ***health status***. There are no clear positive measures of health. Even in respect of negative ill-health measures, little information is at present available on disability, and the data on incidence and prevalence of diseases, particularly in the developing world, are notoriously unreliable and enormously variable. Although mortality data are imperfect, they are nevertheless used to illustrate general patterns and orders of magnitude of major health problems. This report, based primarily on four distinct measures of ill-health – mortality, incidence, prevalence and disability (long-term) – uses reasonably reliable data and estimates from a variety of statistical sources. For example, the United Nations Population Division biennially assesses the global demographic situation and makes estimates of numbers of deaths by age and sex for many countries. The report uses the 1994 assessment. While major differences may be considered indicative of actual disparities and trends, caution is necessary in interpreting small differences in values of different groups.

Country data on ***causes of death***, in respect of communicable and noncommunicable diseases and conditions, pose a problem. Underreporting, imprecise listing of causes and inaccurate diagnosis complicate both national and international studies of mortality. Furthermore, attributing death to specific causes often results in epidemiological and clinical judgement in identifying underlying causes. Following the rules and procedures of the *International statistical classification of diseases and related health problems, tenth revision* (ICD-10), unique causes were assigned to deaths and thereby double counting was avoided. Efforts were made to reduce the paucity of data by preparing "guesstimates" in accordance with epidemiological and statistical principles and procedures while ensuring a reasonable degree of reliability, and of international comparability.

Global values for mortality, morbidity and disability from a large number of diseases and conditions were determined following extensive consultation on the quality and consistency of the estimates with experts within the Organization and at WHO collaborating centres. Judicious use was made of available data from a variety of sources and the most recent data were reviewed, interpreted and extrapolated in a global context. Coverage of diseases and conditions is restricted to those of major public health concern and falls far short of the total spectrum of such diseases covered by the ICD-10. The resulting figures relating to 1996 indicate orders of magnitude of health problems associated with these selected diseases, but they lack the degree of precision necessary for any more in-depth disease-specific analysis. In spite of all these efforts, it is to be recognized that the uncertainties associated with the statistical information and the epidemiological assumptions add to the margin of error that would in any event be involved in estimation procedures.

To carry out its *directing* and *coordinating* functions at international and regional levels, WHO has since 1990 been incrementally developing its database on global and regional estimates of mortality and morbidity by diseases/conditions, based on official country data supplemented by reliable national and international estimates. The extensive use, in this report, of data based on estimates and other indirect approaches should not, however, give the mistaken impression that the necessary data are already being collected by all developing and developed countries; rather, it is a matter of concern that use of such estimates may detract from the current efforts being made to compile accurate and timely data on health indicators in the developing world. Empirical data continue to be essential for assessing health situations, identifying problems and working out solutions in the area of health development. It would thus be appreciated if readers would send their comments and suggestions for improving the quality of the estimates used in this report and assist WHO by suggesting more reliable data sources for use in the future.

Primary sources of data

Table A – Basic indicators gives data on key health and health-related indicators relating to the world health situation. It contains data for 1996 or for the latest available year in respect of WHO's 190 Member States.

The following indicators which were used in last year's report have been updated: life expectancy at birth; under-5 mortality rate; infant mortality rate; population (total and growth rate per annum); population aged 65 years and above (percentage and growth rate per annum); age and sex standardized death rate; immunization coverage data (BCG, DPT3, OPV3, measles and tetanus toxoid 2); reported cases of AIDS, tuberculosis, malaria, polio, measles and neonatal tetanus; GNP per capita.

New indicators added this year are: increase in life expectancy at birth (male and female); decrease in under-5 mortality rate (male and female); decrease in infant mortality rate (both sexes); average annual growth rates of the population (all ages and 65+); reported cases of leprosy; diabetes mellitus (prevalence); literate adults: number and increase (both sexes and sex ratio); purchasing power parity (PPP) estimates of GNP per capita; speed of integration index; population below $1 a day; physicians, and nurses and midwives (per 100 000 population).

Data for most of the indicators were assembled by WHO from the various sources listed; data concerning health status and health care were taken from WHO publications or are estimates made by WHO programmes on the basis of information supplied by Member States. Although every effort was made to standardize the data for international comparison, care must be taken in using it for comparative analysis and interpreting the results.

Table B – Analytical tabulations are primarily based on the values given in *Table A*. In addition, the following health-related indicators appear only in *Table B*: age-specific death rates for the age groups 5-19, 20-64 and 65 years and above; HIV incidence; prevalence of: iodine deficiency disorders, vitamin A deficiency and iron deficiency anaemia; adult literacy rate; dentists per 100 000 population; carbon dioxide emissions from industrial processes per capita; average annual growth rates of households. Figures refer to all 190 Member States, which in 1996 had an estimated population of 5789 million, or 99.7% of the world population. The population data are estimates of the United Nations Population Division following the 1994 population assessment. These figures serve as denominators for various rates and weights used for computing the aggregate values in *Table B*. Further details are given in the reference publications and documents listed in each case under *Source*.

All tables, figs and maps are compiled especially for *The World Health Report 1997* on the basis of data provided by WHO technical programmes and the International Agency for Research on Cancer (IARC), except for *Tables 1* & *5*, for which the source is mentioned explicitly.

1. Population and demography

1.1 Population size, growth rate, age and sex distribution.
Sources:
(a) *World population prospects (with supplementary tabulations), 1994 revision*. New York, United Nations, 1995.
(b) *Demographic indicators 1950-2050, 1994 revision* and *Sex and age annual 1950-2050, 1994 revision*. New York, United Nations, 1995 (databases).

2. Health status

2.1 ***Global health situation: mortality, morbidity and disability, selected diseases, all ages, 1996 estimates***.
Source: WHO.

2.2 ***Number of deaths , infant mortality rate and life expectancy at birth***.
Sources: see section 1- Population and demography, above.

2.3 **Under-5 mortality rate** refers to the probability of dying between birth and exactly 5 years of age expressed per 1000 live births.
Source: Office of World Health Reporting, using data given in the *World population prospects, 1994 revision* and the formula provided by the United Nations Population Division.

2.4 ***Age and sex standardized death rate*** is obtained by applying the age- and sex-specific death rates of a given population for a country or group of countries to a standard population, the standard population being the 1990 world population, estimated at 5.3 billion (*sources 1a and 1b*).
Source: WHO.

2.5 **Age-specific death rates** refer to the number of deaths in the age groups 5-19, 20-64 (male), 20-64 (female) and 65 and above, per 100 000 population in the same age and sex groups (*sources 1a and 1b*).
Source: WHO.

2.6 ***Annual number of reported cases*** refers to the number of cases of selected diseases reported by WHO Member States for the year concerned: leprosy, AIDS, tuberculosis, malaria, poliomyelitis, measles and neonatal tetanus. In view of possible delay in the

reporting of these data to WHO, numbers given in this report may differ from national values.
Source: WHO.

2.7 ***Diabetes mellitus.*** Prevalence refers to the number of persons with diabetes in 1995, 2000 and 2025.
Source: WHO.

2.8 ***Acquired immune deficiency syndrome (AIDS)/ human immunodeficiency virus (HIV)***.
Source: WHO.

2.9 ***Iodine deficiency disorders (IDD)***. Iodine deficiency occurs when iodine intakes are less than physiological requirements (about 150 μg daily per person) over a long period, sufficient to produce goitre or other consequences such as cretinism or abortion. The prevalence of IDD among the total population, given in *Map 2* and *Table B*, is estimated from the total goitre rate of school-age children (aged 6-11).
Source: WHO.

2.10 ***Vitamin A deficiency***. Vitamin A deficiency occurs when body stores are depleted to the extent that the physiological functions are impaired. Depletion occurs when the diet contains, over a long time, too little vitamin A (or its precursors) to replace the amount used by tissues or for breast-feeding; the safe intake level being 400-600 μg retinol per day, depending on age of the subject, and 850 μg for lactating women. In *Table B*, Vitamin A deficiency prevalence refers to the number of children under age 5 affected clinically.
Source: WHO.

2.11 ***Iron deficiency anaemia***. Iron deficiency is present when body iron stores are depleted; this is usually assessed by ferritin levels. Anaemia is only a late sign of iron deficiency. Anaemia is present when the haemoglobin level is below 110 g/l in pregnant women or children 0-5 years of age; below 115 g/l in children 6-11 years; below 120 g/l in older children and non-pregnant women; and below 130 g/l in men.
Source: WHO.

2.12 ***Hepatitis C***.
Source: WHO.

2.13 ***Eye and ear problems in the elderly population***.
Source: WHO.

2.14 ***Cancer***.
Sources: International Agency for Research on Cancer (IARC) and WHO.

2.15 ***Independent life expectancy at age 65*** is a measure of severe disability-free life expectancy (DFLE). It represents the average number of years an individual aged 65 is expected to live without restrictions in either (1) certain activities of daily living (ADL) – bathing, dressing, eating, getting in and out of bed, using the toilet, or (2) instrumental activities of daily living (IADL) – preparing own meals, shopping, managing money, using the telephone, doing light housework, if current patterns of mortality and of problems related to ADL/IADL continue to apply. It is an example of handicap-free life expectancy.
Source: REVES. *Global assessment in positive health*. Contribution of the Network on Health Expectancy and the Disability Process. Montpellier, INSERM, 1994 (unpublished document).

3. Health care and environment

3.1 ***Immunization coverage for BCG, DPT3, OPV3 and measles*** refers respectively to the percentages of infants surviving to age 1 who have been fully immunized with BCG, a third dose of diphtheria-pertussis-tetanus vaccine, a third dose of oral polio vaccine and measles vaccine; ***Immunization coverage for TT2*** refers to the percentage of pregnant women immunized with two or more doses of tetanus toxoid given during pregnancy. Data as at 11 March 1997 for 1995.
Source: WHO.

3.2 ***Carbon dioxide (CO_2) emissions from industrial processes*** consists of the sum of CO_2 flux from solid fuels, liquid fuels, gas fuels, gas flaring and cement manufacture.
Source: World Resources Institute/ United Nations Environment Programme/United Nations Development Programme/World Bank. *World resources 1996-97*. New York/Oxford, Oxford University Press, 1996.

3.3 ***Households: annual rate of growth***. A household is a unit reflecting the arrangements made by persons for living together and sharing housekeeping, budget and other essentials. A household may be either a one-person household or a multiperson household.
Source: United Nations Centre for Human Settlements (HABITAT). *An urbanizing world: global report on human settlements, 1996*. Oxford, Oxford University Press, 1996.

3.4 ***Oral health status*** is expressed in terms of decayed, missing, filled permanent teeth (DMFT) for populations aged 12 and 35-44.
Source: WHO.

4. Education

4.1 **Adult literacy**.
Source: World education report 1995. Paris, UNESCO, 1995.

5. Economy

5.1 ***Gross national product (GNP) per capita, purchasing power parity (PPP) estimates of GNP per capita***. The PPP conversion factor is defined as the number of units of a country's currency required to buy the same amounts of goods and services in the domestic market as $1 would buy in the United States. The GNP per capita stated in international dollars is derived by applying the PPP conversion factor to local currency GNP per capita.
Source: World Bank. *World development report 1996*. New York, Oxford University Press, 1996.

5.2 ***Speed of integration index*** measures the participation in the international markets for goods, services and capital. It is the average of changes between the early 1980s and early 1990s of four integration variables (which are expressed as standardized scores), namely: the ratio of real trade to gross domestic product (GDP); the ratio of foreign direct investment to GDP; *Institutional investor* credit ratings; the share of manufactures in exports.
Source: World Bank. *Global economic prospects and the developing countries 1996*. Washington DC, 1996.

5.3 ***Population below $1 a day***. To ensure international comparability, the minimum poverty line is set at $1 (converted with the PPP factor for consumption in 1985) per person per day. Values are for the latest available year in the period 1990-1994.
Source: World Bank. Personal communication.

5.4 ***Foreign direct investment flows as a share of GDP***, given in *Table 1*, reflects the average of the period 1993-1995.
Source: World Bank. *Global economic prospects and the developing countries 1996*. Washington DC, 1996.

6. Human resources

6.1 ***Physicians, nurses and midwives, and dentists.*** "Physicians" refers to all graduates of any faculty or school of medicine, currently working in any medical field (practice, teaching, administration, research, laboratory, etc.). Nurses are those qualified, registered or authorized by a country to provide responsible and competent service for the promotion of health, prevention of illness, the care of the sick, and rehabilitation, and who are currently working in that country. Midwives relate to all personnel who have completed a programme of midwifery education and have acquired the requisite qualifications to be registered in a country and/ or legally licensed to practice midwifery, and are currently working. "Nurses and midwives" includes midwives having prior nursing education. Dentists are graduates of any faculty or school of dentistry, odontology or stomatology, currently working in any dental field.
Source: WHO.

Table A1. Basic indicators

Estimates are obtained or derived from relevant WHO programmes or from responsible international agencies for the areas of their concern

Member States[a]	Life expectancy at birth (years): Both sexes 1996	Life expectancy: Increase Male 1980-95	Life expectancy: Increase Female 1980-95	Under-5 mortality rate: Both sexes 1996	Under-5 mortality rate: Average annual rate of decrease (%) Male 1980-95	Under-5 mortality rate: Average annual rate of decrease (%) Female 1980-95	Infant mortality rate: 1996	Infant mortality rate: Decrease 1980-95	Population: Total (000) 1996	Population: Average annual growth rate (%) All ages 1980-95	Population: Average annual growth rate (%) Age 65+ 1980-95	Population: Age 65+ (%) 1996	Age and sex standardized death rate (per 100 000 population) 1995-2000
WHO Member States with values above all three health-for-all targets[b]													
Africa													
Algeria	68	8	9	54	4.9	5.3	47	51	28 566	2.7	2.1	3.6	794
Botswana	67	8	8	57	3.8	4.1	39	30	1 531	3.4	4.4	2.5	831
Cape Verde	66	6	5	60	2.4	2.0	44	22	403	2.1	-0.4	4.2	911
Mauritius	71	4	6	17	4.4	5.3	16	16	1 129	1.0	4.1	5.9	683
Americas													
Argentina	73	3	3	25	2.9	3.2	22	13	34 995	1.4	2.4	9.5	597
Bahamas	74	5	6	24	2.8	4.2	20	7	280	1.8	3.8	5.4	610
Barbados	76	4	4	15	3.8	5.2	9	13	263	0.3	1.2	11.4	460
Belize	74	3	4	37	2.1	2.4	30	11	221	2.6	2.7	4.1	474
Canada	78	3	2	8	4.3	1.7	6	3	29 784	1.2	2.8	11.9	429
Chile	74	5	5	17	5.1	5.5	15	18	14 478	1.7	2.9	6.7	545
Colombia	70	4	5	40	2.7	3.0	35	13	35 652	1.9	3.1	4.5	704
Costa Rica	77	4	4	14	4.7	4.9	13	10	3 500	2.7	4.6	4.8	461
Cuba	76	2	2	13	2.9	3.2	11	7	11 118	0.9	2.0	9.0	491
Dominican Republic	71	6	7	46	4.2	4.7	35	42	7 961	2.1	3.8	4.1	673
Ecuador	70	6	7	57	3.3	3.6	47	28	11 699	2.5	3.0	4.4	706
El Salvador	68	13	7	64	3.4	4.0	40	41	5 897	1.6	3.6	4.2	774
Guatemala	66	8	9	67	3.6	3.7	42	32	10 928	2.9	4.3	3.5	820
Guyana	66	5	5	60	3.0	3.3	44	19	844	0.6	0.6	4.0	878
Honduras	69	9	9	50	4.6	5.0	37	33	5 816	3.1	4.2	3.2	706
Jamaica	74	3	3	20	3.1	3.7	13	7	2 465	0.9	0.8	6.5	546
Mexico	72	5	5	40	2.6	3.2	34	19	95 470	2.3	3.0	4.3	633
Nicaragua	68	10	8	66	4.4	3.7	47	44	4 584	3.1	4.5	3.1	764
Panama	74	3	4	28	3.0	2.5	22	9	2 677	2.0	3.0	5.3	557
Paraguay	71	4	4	47	2.1	2.3	36	13	5 090	3.1	3.6	3.8	659
Suriname	71	5	5	26	4.0	4.0	25	16	428	1.2	1.9	4.9	680
Trinidad and Tobago	72	4	4	17	4.2	4.4	16	18	1 320	1.3	1.5	5.8	626
United States of America	77	3	2	9	3.7	2.5	7	4	265 765	1.0	1.7	12.6	476
Uruguay	73	2	2	20	4.4	4.2	17	20	3 204	0.6	1.6	12.3	616
Venezuela	72	4	4	25	3.8	4.0	22	14	22 311	2.5	4.1	4.1	604
Eastern Mediterranean													
Bahrain	72	5	5	23	4.7	5.1	17	15	578	3.3	5.2	2.6	637
Cyprus	78	3	3	9	4.1	8.3	7	10	750	1.1	1.1	10.1	429
Iran, Islamic Republic of	69	9	8	59	5.9	5.0	31	57	68 738	3.7	4.7	4.0	727
Jordan	69	6	7	39	4.0	4.6	31	26	5 654	4.2	3.3	2.7	750
Kuwait	76	5	5	16	6.3	7.0	16	13	1 531	0.8	2.1	1.8	494
Lebanon	69	4	4	36	3.2	3.4	30	18	3 084	0.8	1.0	5.6	737
Oman	71	11	12	32	6.7	8.1	26	46	2 251	4.6	4.7	2.6	691
Qatar	71	5	6	23	6.8	8.2	18	22	562	6.0	9.7	1.4	1 072
Saudi Arabia	71	10	10	30	6.6	7.3	25	41	18 426	4.2	4.1	2.8	675
Syrian Arab Republic	68	6	7	43	3.5	4.3	34	26	15 167	3.5	2.6	2.8	791
Tunisia	69	7	8	49	4.6	5.1	39	39	9 057	2.2	3.3	4.5	753
United Arab Emirates	75	8	6	19	8.3	8.0	16	18	1 946	4.3	7.0	1.8	538
Europe													
Albania	73	2	3	38	1.4	2.0	27	20	3 473	1.7	2.1	5.6	609
Armenia	73	1	1	23	0.7	0.7	20	2	3 646	1.1	2.5	7.7	600
Austria	77	4	3	8	6.4	5.0	6	7	8 013	0.4	0.1	14.9	460
Azerbaijan	71	3	3	37	2.2	2.0	26	8	7 642	1.4	1.9	6.1	655
Belarus	70	-1	0	19	-0.2	0.2	17	4	10 122	0.3	1.4	12.9	759
Belgium	77	4	4	7	5.5	4.9	6	6	10 144	0.2	0.8	15.9	453

Updated statistics April 1997

While *The World Health Report 1997* was in press, revised estimates were made available to WHO by the United Nations Population Division, following their 1996 revision of *World Population Prospects*, for population, life expectancy at birth and infant mortality rate. This table updates some of the data presented in ***Table A1. Basic indicators***, pages 144–147.

Member States[a]	1996 Population (000)	1995-2000 Life expectancy at birth (years)	1995-2000 Infant mortality rate
Afghanistan	20 883	45	154
Albania	3 401	71	32
Algeria	28 784	69	44
Angola	11 185	46	124
Antigua and Barbuda	...	...	...
Argentina	35 219	73	22
Armenia	3 638	71	25
Australia	18 057	78	6
Austria	8 106	77	6
Azerbaijan	7 594	71	33
Bahamas	284	74	14
Bahrain	570	73	18
Bangladesh	120 073	58	78
Barbados	261	76	9
Belarus	10 348	70	15
Belgium	10 159	77	7
Belize	219	75	30
Benin	5 563	55	84
Bhutan	1 812	53	104
Bolivia	7 593	61	66
Bosnia and Herzegovina	3 628	73	13
Botswana	1 484	50	56
Brazil	161 087	67	42
Brunei Darussalam	300	76	9
Bulgaria	8 468	71	16
Burkina Faso	10 780	46	97
Burundi	6 221	47	114
Cambodia	10 273	54	102
Cameroon	13 560	56	58
Canada	29 680	79	6
Cape Verde	396	67	41
Central African Republic	3 344	49	96
Chad	6 515	48	115
Chile	14 421	75	13
China	1 232 083	70	38
Colombia	36 444	71	24
Comoros	632	58	82
Congo	2 668	51	91
Cook Islands	...	...	...
Costa Rica	3 500	77	12
Côte d'Ivoire	14 015	51	86
Croatia	4 501	72	10
Cuba	11 018	76	9
Cyprus	756	78	7
Czech Republic	10 251	73	9
Democratic People's Republic of Korea	22 466	72	22
Denmark	5 237	76	7
Djibouti	617	50	106
Dominica	...	...	...
Dominican Republic	7 961	71	34
Ecuador	11 699	70	46
Egypt	63 271	66	54
El Salvador	5 796	70	39
Equatorial Guinea	410	50	107
Eritrea	3 280	51	98
Estonia	1 471	69	12
Ethiopia	58 243	50	107
Fiji	797	73	20
Finland	5 126	77	5
France	58 333	79	7
Gabon	1 106	55	85
Gambia	1 141	47	122
Georgia	5 442	73	23
Germany	81 922	77	6
Ghana	17 832	58	73
Greece	10 490	78	8
Grenada	...	...	...
Guatemala	10 928	67	40
Guinea	7 518	46	124
Guinea-Bissau	1 091	44	132
Guyana	838	64	58
Haiti	7 259	54	82
Honduras	5 816	70	35
Hungary	10 049	69	14
Iceland	271	79	5
India	944 580	62	72
Indonesia	200 453	65	48
Iran, Islamic Republic of	69 975	69	39
Iraq	20 607	62	95
Ireland	3 554	77	6
Israel	5 664	78	7
Italy	57 226	78	7
Jamaica	2 491	75	12
Japan	125 351	80	4
Jordan	5 581	70	30
Kazakstan	16 820	68	34
Kenya	27 799	54	65
Kiribati	...	...	...
Kuwait	1 687	76	15
Kyrgyzstan	4 469	68	40
Lao People's Democratic Republic	5 035	53	86
Latvia	2 504	68	16
Lebanon	3 084	70	29
Lesotho	2 078	59	72
Liberia	2 245	51	153
Libyan Arab Jamahiriya	5 593	65	56
Lithuania	3 728	70	13
Luxembourg	412	76	6
Madagascar	15 353	59	77
Malawi	9 845	41	142
Malaysia	20 581	72	11
Maldives	263	65	49
Mali	11 134	48	149
Malta	369	77	8
Marshall Islands	...	...	...
Mauritania	2 333	53	92
Mauritius	1 129	72	16
Mexico	92 718	72	31
Micronesia, Federated States of	...	...	...
Monaco	...	...	...
Mongolia	2 515	66	52
Morocco	27 021	67	51
Mozambique	17 796	47	111
Myanmar	45 922	60	78
Namibia	1 575	56	60
Nauru	...	...	...
Nepal	22 021	57	82
Netherlands	15 575	78	6
New Zealand	3 602	77	7
Nicaragua	4 238	68	44
Niger	9 465	49	114
Nigeria	115 020	52	77
Niue	...	...	...
Norway	4 348	78	5
Oman	2 302	71	25
Pakistan	139 973	64	74
Palau	...	...	...
Panama	2 677	74	21
Papua New Guinea	4 400	58	62
Paraguay	4 957	70	39
Peru	23 944	68	45
Philippines	69 282	68	35
Poland	38 601	71	13
Portugal	9 808	75	8
Qatar	558	72	17
Republic of Korea	45 314	72	9
Republic of Moldova	4 444	68	27
Romania	22 655	70	24
Russian Federation	148 126	64	19
Rwanda	5 397	42	125
Saint Kitts and Nevis	...	...	...
Saint Lucia	...	...	...
Saint Vincent and the Grenadines	...	...	...
Samoa	166	69	58
San Marino	...	...	...
Sao Tome and Principe	...	...	...
Saudi Arabia	18 836	71	23
Senegal	8 532	51	62
Seychelles	...	...	...
Sierra Leone	4 297	38	169
Singapore	3 384	77	5
Slovakia	5 347	71	12
Slovenia	1 924	74	7
Solomon Islands	391	72	23
Somalia	9 822	49	112
South Africa	42 393	65	48
Spain	39 674	78	7
Sri Lanka	18 100	73	15
Sudan	27 291	55	71
Suriname	432	72	24
Swaziland	881	60	65
Sweden	8 819	79	5
Switzerland	7 224	79	5
Syrian Arab Republic	14 574	69	33
Tajikistan	5 935	67	56
Thailand	58 703	69	30
The Former Yugoslav Republic of Macedonia	2 174	72	23
Togo	4 201	50	86
Tonga	...	...	...
Trinidad and Tobago	1 297	74	14
Tunisia	9 156	70	37
Turkey	61 797	69	44
Turkmenistan	4 155	65	57
Tuvalu	...	...	...
Uganda	20 256	41	113
Ukraine	51 608	69	18
United Arab Emirates	2 260	75	15
United Kingdom	58 144	77	6
United Republic of Tanzania	30 799	51	80
United States of America	269 444	77	7
Uruguay	3 204	73	17
Uzbekistan	23 209	67	43
Vanuatu	174	67	38
Venezuela	22 311	73	21
Viet Nam	75 181	67	37
Yemen	15 678	58	80
Yugoslavia	...	...	...
Zaire	46 812	53	90
Zambia	8 275	43	103
Zimbabwe	11 439	49	68

[a] Data is not available for the less populous Member States (under 150 000 population in 1995).

... Data not available or not applicable.

Member States[a]	Life expectancy at birth (years)			Under-5 mortality rate			Infant mortality rate		Population				Age and sex standardized death rate (per 100 000 population)
	Both sexes	Increase		Both sexes	Average annual rate of decrease (%)				Total (000)	Average annual growth rate (%)		Age 65+ (%)	
	1996	Male 1980-95	Female 1980-95	1996	Male 1980-95	Female 1980-95	1996	Decrease 1980-95	1996	All ages 1980-95	Age 65+ 1980-95	1996	1995-2000
Bosnia and Herzegovina	73	2	3	20	2.5	3.7	14	17	3 524	-0.8	0.8	8.2	634
Bulgaria	71	-1	1	18	-0.5	1.1	14	6	8 726	-0.1	1.3	14.8	689
Croatia	72	1	2	16	1.1	2.7	9	12	4 483	0.2	0.8	13.1	663
Czech Republic	71	1	1	10	1.0	1.1	9	7	10 302	0.0	-0.4	12.4	730
Denmark	76	1	1	8	1.1	0.2	7	1	5 188	0.1	0.4	15.1	511
Estonia	69	-1	0	19	-0.2	1.1	16	5	1 521	0.2	0.3	13.0	793
Finland	76	3	3	6	5.8	3.8	5	2	5 129	0.4	1.5	14.2	490
France	77	3	3	9	4.5	2.0	7	3	58 211	0.5	0.9	15.1	447
Georgia	73	2	3	21	2.6	2.8	18	6	5 466	0.5	2.1	11.7	591
Germany	77	3	3	7	5.5	4.9	6	7	81 777	0.3	0.1	15.3	479
Greece	78	3	4	10	3.6	3.8	9	11	10 483	0.5	1.8	16.3	429
Hungary	69	-1	1	17	-1.5	0.9	16	8	10 073	-0.4	-0.1	14.1	800
Iceland	79	2	2	4	0.4	0.3	3	2	271	1.1	2.1	11.4	395
Ireland	76	3	3	7	4.4	5.1	7	5	3 565	0.3	0.6	11.2	505
Israel	77	3	3	9	3.5	4.5	8	8	5 759	2.5	3.2	9.5	449
Italy	78	4	4	9	4.6	3.0	7	8	57 218	0.1	1.4	16.3	420
Kazakstan	71	5	3	31	3.5	2.7	28	12	17 209	0.9	1.9	7.1	706
Kyrgyzstan	70	5	4	39	3.3	2.8	33	16	4 823	1.8	1.8	5.9	721
Latvia	69	-1	1	20	-0.3	1.4	14	7	2 536	0.1	0.2	13.5	801
Lithuania	70	-1	0	17	-0.6	0.8	13	7	3 696	0.5	1.0	12.4	724
Luxembourg	76	3	4	8	5.2	3.5	6	6	410	0.7	0.9	13.9	476
Malta	77	4	4	11	4.2	5.7	9	5	368	0.8	1.5	10.9	449
Netherlands	78	2	2	8	3.3	1.1	6	2	15 603	0.6	1.5	13.3	430
Norway	77	1	1	9	1.4	0.6	7	0	4 356	0.4	0.9	15.7	455
Poland	71	0	1	18	0.0	1.1	13	8	38 448	0.5	1.1	11.2	705
Portugal	75	4	4	11	4.7	4.9	9	16	9 818	0.0	2.1	14.3	519
Republic of Moldova	68	2	3	28	2.9	3.8	25	8	4 446	0.7	1.9	9.4	856
Romania	70	-1	1	30	-0.1	1.1	23	6	22 770	0.2	1.1	12.1	738
Russian Federation	68	0	0	27	1.3	1.0	20	8	146 677	0.4	1.5	12.3	876
Slovakia	71	0	1	14	0.3	1.9	12	8	5 374	0.5	0.7	10.8	713
Slovenia	73	1	3	12	1.0	3.9	7	8	1 948	0.4	1.0	12.8	612
Spain	78	3	3	8	3.2	2.2	7	6	39 676	0.4	2.6	15.3	423
Sweden	79	3	3	6	3.3	2.0	5	2	8 822	0.4	0.8	17.2	399
Switzerland	78	3	2	7	3.0	1.2	6	2	7 269	0.9	1.1	14.3	414
Tajikistan	71	6	6	56	2.7	2.8	44	21	6 271	2.9	2.6	4.4	660
The Former Yugoslav Republic of Macedonia	72	1	3	37	1.4	3.7	24	28	2 182	1.3	2.4	8.4	615
Ukraine	69	0	0	21	1.2	1.0	16	6	51 298	0.2	1.2	14.1	791
United Kingdom	77	4	2	8	5.2	3.5	7	5	58 424	0.2	0.4	15.4	469
Uzbekistan	70	4	4	47	2.6	2.2	39	15	23 342	2.4	1.5	4.5	705
South-East Asia													
Democratic People's Republic of Korea	72	5	5	26	2.6	2.2	22	8	24 347	1.8	3.8	4.7	659
Sri Lanka	73	4	5	19	3.9	4.8	15	23	18 584	1.4	3.5	6.0	599
Thailand	68	5	6	43	3.4	3.5	35	15	59 414	1.5	3.9	5.1	775
Western Pacific													
Australia	78	4	3	8	4.8	3.6	6	5	18 320	1.5	2.8	11.7	420
Brunei Darussalam	75	4	4	13	4.5	4.5	8	8	291	2.6	3.5	3.4	455
China	69	2	4	43	1.1	1.7	39	10	1 234 338	1.4	3.1	6.2	739
Fiji	72	4	4	23	3.6	4.5	21	11	796	1.4	3.2	3.9	619
Japan	80	3	4	6	2.0	1.3	4	3	125 382	0.5	3.5	14.6	376
Malaysia	72	5	5	22	4.0	4.7	12	19	20 581	2.6	3.0	4.0	648
New Zealand	76	3	3	10	3.4	3.3	8	4	3 616	0.9	1.8	11.3	485
Philippines	68	6	7	45	3.8	4.2	37	22	68 976	2.3	3.7	3.4	804
Republic of Korea	72	6	6	13	7.3	6.0	10	16	45 429	1.1	3.8	5.8	651
Singapore	76	4	4	9	4.1	6.0	6	5	2 874	1.1	3.5	6.9	501
Solomon Islands	71	4	5	29	3.6	4.5	24	17	391	3.5	4.1	2.8	643
Vanuatu	67	8	8	48	4.2	3.9	41	35	174	2.5	2.7	3.4	1 173
Viet Nam	67	9	9	56	4.1	3.6	39	32	76 161	2.2	2.3	4.9	831

Member States[a]	Life expectancy at birth (years)			Under-5 mortality rate			Infant mortality rate		Population				Age and sex standardized death rate (per 100 000 population)
	Both sexes	Increase		Both sexes	Average annual rate of decrease (%)				Total (000)	Average annual growth rate (%)		Age 65+ (%)	
		Male	Female		Male	Female		Decrease		All ages	Age 65+		
	1996	1980-95	1980-95	1996	1980-95	1980-95	1996	1980-95	1996	1980-95	1980-95	1996	1995-2000
WHO Member States with values below all three health-for-all targets[b]													
Africa													
Angola	48	7	7	179	1.8	1.8	116	36	11 469	3.1	2.9	2.9	1 792
Benin	48	5	5	158	1.9	1.9	81	20	5 574	3.0	2.5	2.9	1 772
Burkina Faso	47	3	3	186	1.2	1.2	125	29	10 593	2.7	3.2	3.1	1 937
Burundi	51	4	4	143	1.6	1.7	98	23	6 578	3.0	1.9	2.9	1 641
Cameroon	58	8	8	109	2.6	2.6	57	36	13 609	2.9	2.8	3.6	1 243
Central African Republic	50	4	4	149	1.7	1.7	98	19	3 397	2.4	2.5	4.0	1 696
Chad	49	6	7	172	1.8	1.8	115	31	6 543	2.4	2.4	3.6	1 753
Comoros	57	6	6	111	2.4	2.2	82	31	677	3.6	3.2	2.4	1 280
Congo	50	1	0	133	1.3	1.2	83	5	2 665	3.0	2.8	3.3	1 731
Côte d'Ivoire	50	2	0	137	1.4	1.3	89	20	14 733	3.8	4.3	2.7	1 766
Equatorial Guinea	49	6	6	167	1.8	1.8	110	31	410	4.2	3.6	4.1	1 681
Eritrea	52	7	7	146	2.2	2.2	97	37	3 627	2.7	3.4	3.0	1 537
Ethiopia	49	8	8	170	2.1	2.1	111	45	56 713	2.8	3.3	2.8	1 724
Gabon	55	6	7	130	2.3	2.3	88	28	1 358	3.3	3.3	5.9	1 405
Gambia	46	6	6	190	1.6	1.7	125	33	1 155	3.8	3.9	2.9	1 903
Ghana	57	5	6	111	2.0	2.1	75	24	17 972	3.3	3.5	2.9	1 264
Guinea	46	6	6	196	1.5	1.5	127	33	6 903	2.7	2.7	2.6	1 955
Guinea-Bissau	45	6	6	203	1.5	1.6	132	35	1 096	2.0	2.1	4.1	2 015
Kenya	55	1	0	106	1.8	1.5	67	17	29 137	3.6	2.5	2.9	1 459
Liberia	57	6	6	151	1.9	1.8	117	40	3 140	3.3	3.2	3.6	1 263
Madagascar	58	7	7	121	2.9	2.7	94	47	15 236	3.3	3.1	2.8	1 260
Malawi	45	1	1	212	1.0	0.9	138	31	11 373	4.0	5.3	2.7	2 012
Mali	47	6	6	184	1.6	1.6	152	31	11 134	3.1	3.1	2.6	1 852
Mauritania	53	6	6	142	2.1	2.1	94	24	2 333	2.6	2.7	3.2	1 507
Mozambique	47	3	3	176	1.1	1.1	140	14	16 537	1.9	2.1	3.2	1 930
Niger	48	6	6	182	1.7	1.8	117	33	9 465	3.3	3.3	2.4	1 827
Nigeria	52	6	6	146	1.7	1.7	79	21	115 020	3.0	3.5	2.8	1 563
Rwanda	47	1	1	161	1.2	1.2	107	21	8 160	2.9	3.4	2.5	1 958
Senegal	51	6	6	157	1.9	1.8	64	26	8 532	2.7	3.0	3.0	1 640
Sierra Leone	40	5	5	242	1.1	1.1	158	31	4 617	2.2	2.0	3.0	2 369
Swaziland	59	8	8	99	2.5	2.6	68	30	879	2.9	2.1	2.5	1 170
Togo	56	7	7	118	2.2	2.3	80	30	4 269	3.1	3.0	3.2	1 321
Uganda	44	-3	-4	172	0.3	0.2	112	1	21 963	3.3	3.1	2.4	2 243
United Republic of Tanzania	52	2	2	126	1.6	1.5	82	22	30 536	3.2	3.9	2.6	1 629
Zaire	52	3	3	131	1.7	1.7	88	23	45 281	3.3	3.4	2.9	1 602
Zambia	47	-2	-4	140	1.0	0.7	101	-14	9 715	3.4	3.4	2.4	2 046
Zimbabwe	52	-2	-3	103	1.4	1.3	66	15	11 515	3.1	3.5	2.8	1 708
Americas													
Haiti	58	6	6	104	2.3	2.7	80	32	7 329	2.0	1.1	3.9	1 286
Eastern Mediterranean													
Afghanistan	45	4	5	248	0.7	0.7	157	24	21 472	1.5	2.2	2.8	2 117
Djibouti	50	5	5	164	1.8	1.7	109	28	589	4.9	6.1	3.4	1 671
Somalia	48	5	5	176	1.6	1.6	115	29	9 484	2.2	1.5	2.7	1 796
Sudan	54	6	6	112	2.2	2.2	73	19	28 855	2.8	3.2	2.9	1 436
Yemen	52	6	6	155	1.8	1.7	112	35	15 067	3.9	3.3	2.3	1 635
South-East Asia													
Bangladesh	57	8	9	144	2.4	2.4	100	31	123 136	2.1	1.3	3.1	1 263
Bhutan	52	8	9	145	2.4	2.7	112	45	1 670	1.9	2.4	3.5	1 572
Myanmar	59	7	7	95	2.8	2.9	76	32	47 513	2.1	2.3	4.1	1 182
Nepal	56	8	9	122	2.7	2.7	90	37	22 484	2.6	3.6	3.4	1 377
Western Pacific													
Cambodia	53	14	14	137	4.8	4.9	106	103	10 530	3.1	3.2	2.6	1 505
Lao People's Democratic Republic	53	7	8	143	2.5	2.5	89	38	5 023	2.8	3.3	3.0	1 544
Papua New Guinea	57	6	6	82	2.5	2.2	64	8	4 400	2.2	6.6	3.0	1 368

Member States[a]	Life expectancy at birth (years)			Under-5 mortality rate			Infant mortality rate		Population				Age and sex standardized death rate (per 100 000 population)
		Increase			Average annual rate of decrease (%)					Average annual growth rate (%)		Age 65+ (%)	
	Both sexes 1996	Male 1980-95	Female 1980-95	Both sexes 1996	Male 1980-95	Female 1980-95	1996	Decrease 1980-95	Total (000) 1996	All ages 1980-95	Age 65+ 1980-95	1996	1995-2000
Other WHO Member States													
Africa													
Lesotho	62	8	8	81	3.5	3.8	72	36	2 105	2.9	3.5	3.9	1 024
Namibia	61	8	8	91	2.8	2.8	55	35	1 580	2.7	3.1	3.7	1 096
Sao Tome and Principe	...	...	...	...	...	...	...	...	*135*	*2.3*	...	...	...
Seychelles	...	...	...	...	...	...	...	...	*74*	*1.0*	...	...	...
South Africa	65	7	7	73	3.2	3.8	49	18	42 388	2.4	3.3	4.4	925
Americas													
Antigua and Barbuda	...	...	...	...	...	...	...	...	*66*	*0.5*	...	...	...
Bolivia	61	9	8	88	4.2	4.0	68	50	7 593	2.2	2.8	3.9	1 097
Brazil	67	4	4	69	2.0	2.1	55	18	164 424	1.9	3.7	5.3	783
Dominica	...	...	...	...	...	...	...	...	*71*	*-0.3*	...	...	...
Grenada	...	...	...	...	...	...	...	...	*92*	*0.2*	...	...	...
Peru	67	8	8	71	3.4	3.4	60	30	24 233	2.1	3.1	4.2	821
Saint Kitts and Nevis	...	...	...	...	...	...	...	...	*41*	*-0.5*	...	...	...
Saint Lucia	...	...	...	...	...	...	...	...	*144*	*1.4*	...	...	...
Saint Vincent and the Grenadines	...	...	...	...	...	...	...	...	*113*	*0.9*	...	...	...
Eastern Mediterranean													
Egypt	65	9	9	70	4.7	4.7	58	64	64 200	2.5	2.8	4.3	897
Iraq	67	5	6	59	2.8	3.5	50	30	21 035	3.1	3.8	3.0	805
Libyan Arab Jamahiriya	65	7	8	80	3.5	3.7	60	40	5 593	3.9	5.0	2.7	919
Morocco	65	7	8	76	3.4	3.6	59	41	27 563	2.2	2.3	4.1	907
Pakistan	63	7	9	104	3.2	3.4	78	44	144 517	3.4	3.6	3.0	978
Europe													
Monaco	...	...	...	...	...	...	...	...	*32*	*1.1*	...	...	...
San Marino	...	...	...	...	...	...	...	...	*25*	*1.2*	...	...	...
Turkey	68	7	6	65	3.8	3.5	56	53	63 120	2.2	2.6	5.1	770
Turkmenistan	66	4	3	66	1.8	1.8	53	13	4 188	2.4	2.3	4.2	861
Yugoslavia	...	...	...	...	...	...	...	...	...	...	...	...	...
South-East Asia													
India	62	7	8	99	2.8	2.6	75	41	952 969	2.1	2.9	4.6	1 029
Indonesia	64	9	10	63	4.5	5.0	51	46	200 596	1.8	3.5	4.4	948
Maldives	64	7	8	68	4.1	3.3	52	45	263	3.2	2.4	3.8	1 025
Western Pacific													
Cook Islands	...	...	...	...	...	...	...	...	*19*	*0.4*	...	...	...
Kiribati	...	...	...	...	...	...	...	...	*80*	*1.7*	...	...	...
Marshall Islands	...	...	...	...	...	...	...	...	*55*	*2.9*	...	...	...
Micronesia, Federated States of	...	...	...	...	...	...	...	...	*128*	*2.7*	...	...	...
Mongolia	65	7	7	68	3.3	3.1	54	28	2 458	2.5	3.4	3.5	900
Nauru	...	...	...	...	...	...	...	...	*11*	*3.1*	...	...	...
Niue	...	...	...	...	...	...	...	...	*2*	*-2.7*	...	...	...
Palau	...	...	...	...	...	...	...	...	*17*	*2.3*	...	...	...
Samoa	69	6	6	71	2.2	2.5	60	23	174	0.5	2.7	3.4	...
Tonga	...	...	...	...	...	...	...	...	*99*	*0.4*	...	...	...
Tuvalu	...	...	...	...	...	...	...	...	*10*	*1.5*	...	...	...

[a] Italics indicate less populous Member States (under 150 000 population in 1990).
[b] The three targets in WHO's strategy for health for all by the year 2000 relating to health status are: life expectancy at birth above 60 years; under-5 mortality rate below 70 per 1000 live births; infant mortality rate below 50 per 1000 live births.
... Data not available or not applicable.

Table A2. Basic indicators

Estimates are obtained or derived from relevant WHO programmes or from responsible international agencies for the areas of their concern

Member States[a]	Immunization coverage (%) 1995[b]					Reported cases of selected diseases during the specified year						
	Children immunized by age 12 months				Pregnant women							
	BCG	DPT 3	OPV 3	Measles	Tetanus toxoid 2	Leprosy[c] 1996	AIDS 1995	Tuberculosis 1995	Malaria 1994	Polio 1995	Measles 1995	Neonatal tetanus 1995
WHO Member States with values above all three health-for-all targets[d]												
Africa												
Algeria	...	...	...	...	...	...	34	...	206	4	8 204	15
Botswana	58	76	77	68	56	...	535	5 655	29 586	0	232	0
Cape Verde	80	73	73	66	...	...	21	303	21	0	10	4
Mauritius	...	...	...	...	...	436	7	153	31	0	6	...
Americas												
Argentina	100	82	88	95	...	3 396	1 634	13 433	948	0	655	3
Bahamas	...	87	86	90	...	...	390	57	...	0	0	0
Barbados	...	93	93	92	...	...	95	20	...	0	0	0
Belize	92	83	83	87	...	...	28	61	9 957	0	4	0
Canada	...	...	...	...	...	...	1 180	...	305	0	2 357	...
Chile	80	98	98	95	...	...	267	...	...	0	0	0
Colombia	100	94	95	80	...	4 738	896	9 912	127 218	0	410	35
Costa Rica	99	85	84	94	...	195	198	321	4 445	0	35	0
Cuba	99	100	95	100	...	684	107	1 607	12	0	1	0
Dominican Republic	76	83	80	85	...	528	385	4 053	1 670	0	0	0
Ecuador	100	74	89	73	...	518	69	7 893	30 006	0	919	50
El Salvador	100	100	94	93	...	...	380	2 422	2 803	0	0	3
Guatemala	79	80	80	83	...	106	104	3 368	22 057	0	23	9
Guyana	93	86	87	77	...	...	96	296	39 566	0	0	0
Honduras	100	96	96	90	...	...	909	4 984	52 110	0	0	3
Jamaica	98	90	90	89	...	...	505	109	3	0	15	0
Mexico	98	92	92	90	...	6 106	4 310	11 329	12 864	0	244	67
Nicaragua	100	85	96	81	...	...	9	2 842	41 490	0	5	4
Panama	99	86	86	84	...	...	203	1 316	684	0	19	1
Paraguay	92	79	79	75	...	828	23	1 773	583	0	73	16
Suriname	...	84	81	79	...	264	20	...	4 704	0	0	0
Trinidad and Tobago	...	89	90	90	...	...	340	178	23	0	0	0
United States of America	...	...	...	...	...	640	40 051	22 860	1 229	0	309	...
Uruguay	90	87	87	84	...	...	127	625	...	0	5	0
Venezuela	92	68	85	67	...	3 954	619	5 554	13 727	0	172	17
Eastern Mediterranean												
Bahrain	...	98	98	95	49	...	8	115	...	0	3	0
Cyprus	...	96	96	83	...	...	3	36	...	1	0	0
Iran, Islamic Republic of	98	99	98	96	45	1 389	9	20 012	51 089	101	263	13
Jordan	...	100	99	92	24	...	2	504	...	0	318	2
Kuwait	...	100	100	98	22	...	4	336	876	0	12	0
Lebanon	...	94	94	85	...	...	8	983	...	0	3	3
Oman	96	100	100	100	54	...	7	224	7 215	0	68	1
Qatar	96	92	92	86	...	...	5	304	398	0	0	0
Saudi Arabia	94	96	96	94	62	952	37	...	10 032	3	2 574	25
Syrian Arab Republic	100	92	92	90	66	230	6	4 404	558	4	1 362	106
Tunisia	89	92	92	91	48	181	61	2 383	...	0	676	7
United Arab Emirates	98	90	90	90	...	...	0	...	...	0	671	0
Europe												
Albania	97	97	98	91	...	...	3	641	...	0	0	2
Armenia	...	...	...	...	...	...	0	1 000	...	3	187	0
Austria	...	...	...	...	...	...	191	1 399	...	0	...	...
Azerbaijan	...	...	...	...	...	...	1	1 429	667	5	432	...
Belarus	...	...	...	...	...	...	3	4 854	...	0	1 516	...
Belgium	...	...	...	...	...	...	216	1 380	...	0	32	...

Member States[a]	Immunization coverage (%) 1995[b]					Reported cases of selected diseases during the specified year						
	Children immunized by age 12 months				Pregnant women							
	BCG	DPT 3	OPV 3	Measles	Tetanus toxoid 2	Leprosy[c] 1996	AIDS 1995	Tuberculosis 1995	Malaria 1994	Polio 1995	Measles 1995	Neonatal tetanus 1995
Bosnia and Herzegovina	...	...	...	...	...	...	6	2 132	...	0	125	...
Bulgaria	...	...	...	...	...	...	1	3 245	...	0	172	0
Croatia	...	...	...	...	...	...	15	2 114	...	0	697	0
Czech Republic	...	96	98	96	...	...	13	1 834	...	0	5	0
Denmark	...	...	...	...	...	...	214	448	...	0	20	0
Estonia	99	84	89	81	...	...	3	624	...	0	17	0
Finland	100	100	100	98	...	...	40	661	...	0	6	0
France	...	...	...	...	...	...	4 877	8 723	...	1	...	...
Georgia	...	...	...	...	...	...	1	1 625	...	0	109	0
Germany	...	...	...	...	...	...	1 391	12 198	...	0	...	...
Greece	...	...	...	...	...	...	176	...	...	0	112	0
Hungary	100	100	100	100	...	...	31	4 339	...	0	19	0
Iceland	...	...	...	...	...	...	3	12	...	0	1	...
Ireland	...	...	...	...	...	...	43	...	...	0	231	...
Israel	...	...	...	...	...	...	54	...	...	0	25	...
Italy	...	50	98	50	...	...	5 467	5 627	782	0	37 054	0
Kazakstan	...	...	...	...	...	...	0	11 310	...	1	284	...
Kyrgyzstan	...	...	...	...	...	...	0	3 393	...	0	17	...
Latvia	100	65	70	85	...	...	3	1 541	...	0	2	...
Lithuania	97	96	89	94	...	...	3	2 362	...	0	188	0
Luxembourg	...	...	...	...	...	...	15	...	...	0	1	0
Malta	...	...	...	...	...	...	3	11	...	0	27	...
Netherlands	...	...	...	...	...	...	477	1 619	236	0	184	...
Norway	...	...	...	...	...	...	64	236	...	0	18	0
Poland	...	...	...	...	...	...	106	15 958	...	0	759	0
Portugal	94	93	95	94	...	...	649	5 577	...	0	190	0
Republic of Moldova	98	96	99	98	...	...	2	2 925	...	0	1 175	0
Romania	100	98	94	93	...	...	650	23 271	...	0	2 188	1
Russian Federation	...	...	...	...	...	...	36	84 980	523	152	6 630	0
Slovakia	98	99	98	99	...	...	2	1 540	...	0	2	0
Slovenia	...	...	...	...	...	...	16	525	...	0	402	...
Spain	...	...	...	...	...	...	6 227	8 764	...	0	8 845	...
Sweden	...	...	...	...	...	...	186	564	...	0	...	...
Switzerland	...	...	...	...	...	...	449	831	...	0	30	0
Tajikistan	...	...	...	...	...	...	0	2 029	2 400	0	160	...
The Former Yugoslav Republic of Macedonia	...	...	...	...	...	...	18	786	...	0	217	0
Ukraine	...	...	...	...	...	...	38	21 459	...	1	1 923	0
United Kingdom	...	...	...	...	...	...	1 527	6 176	1 887	0	7 763	...
Uzbekistan	...	...	...	...	...	...	1	9 866	...	1	295	...
South-East Asia												
Democratic People's Republic of Korea	99	96	99	98	95	...	0	...	...	7	0	3
Sri Lanka	89	91	91	88	81	1 852	17	5 956	273 434	0	112	1
Thailand	98	94	94	89	...	3 015	17 949	45 428	102 119	2	11 153	33
Western Pacific												
Australia	...	86	86	87	...	...	690	1 073	692	0	1 198	0
Brunei Darussalam	...	...	...	...	...	...	0	...	37	0	...	...
China	92	92	94	93	11	4 833	52	357 829	68 612	189	53 232	...
Fiji	100	97	99	94	...	...	0	203	...	0	414	0
Japan	...	...	...	...	...	...	265	43 078	...	0	...	...
Malaysia	...	...	...	...	...	1 561	142	11 988	58 958	0	654	...
New Zealand	...	89	87	84	...	...	50	307	...	0	...	0
Philippines	91	86	86	86	48	11 410	50	235 496	229 059	39	3 913	288
Republic of Korea	...	100	100	93	...	1 126	14	33 196	26	0	71	...
Singapore	97	95	93	88	...	464	56	1 889	277	0	185	0
Solomon Islands	77	69	69	68	71	...	0	352	131 687	0	0	3
Vanuatu	67	73	74	60	18	...	0	79	3 771	0	27	0
Viet Nam	96	94	94	96	82	5 111	181	55 739	860 999	138	6 171	330

Member States[a]	Immunization coverage (%) 1995[b]					Reported cases of selected diseases during the specified year						
	Children immunized by age 12 months				Pregnant women							
	BCG	DPT 3	OPV 3	Measles	Tetanus toxoid 2	Leprosy[c] 1996	AIDS 1995	Tuberculosis 1995	Malaria 1994	Polio 1995	Measles 1995	Neonatal tetanus 1995
WHO Member States with values below all three health-for-all targets[d]												
Africa												
Angola	40	21	23	32	14	2 199	321	7 982	667 376	152	635	101
Benin	94	87	87	81	80	560	214	2 400	546 827	7	10 469	30
Burkina Faso	78	47	47	55	39	726	1 682	1 463	472 355	12	5 669	18
Burundi	69	57	54	44	30	...	494	...	831 481	0	14 782	12
Cameroon	62	48	50	51	13	1 668	2 766	...	136 705	8	2 463	57
Central African Republic	67	40	43	70	13	2 450	649	3 339	82 057	4	902	45
Chad	...	...	...	...	...	3 238	592	3 186	...	192	657	27
Comoros	...	...	...	...	...	...	2	129	...	0	0	2
Congo	58	50	50	39	...	1 053	2 450	3 615	35 957	0	2 185	0
Côte d'Ivoire	48	40	40	57	22	2 168	6 727	11 988	...	117	30 039	311
Equatorial Guinea	...	...	...	...	...	...	98	306	14 827	0	44	0
Eritrea	44	35	35	29	12	...	727	21 453	...	10	185	1
Ethiopia	65	47	47	38	22	9 627	3 867	14 406	...	199	562	...
Gabon	...	...	...	...	...	2 363	334	1 115	...	9	...	...
Gambia	...	...	...	...	...	...	62	1 023	...	0	130	6
Ghana	67	51	50	54	20	2 076	2 578	4 131	...	34	40 276	159
Guinea	...	...	...	...	...	3 873	610	3 465	607 560	27	1 085	120
Guinea-Bissau	...	...	...	...	...	177	79	1 748	...	0	528	5
Kenya	45	40	33	35	40	738	8 232	28 142	6 103 447	12	3 322	30
Liberia	...	...	...	...	...	483	67	1 393	...	0	56	24
Madagascar	82	67	66	59	35	6 130	6	11 828	...	0	11 731	7
Malawi	...	...	...	...	...	1 000	5 261	19 155	4 736 974	0	4 218	6
Mali	75	46	46	49	19	4 605	454	3 087	...	26	3 306	33
Mauritania	...	...	...	...	...	413	33	3 849	...	5	195	1
Mozambique	78	57	57	71	36	11 072	1 180	17 882	...	0	4 166	19
Niger	43	19	19	38	30	2 804	621	1 980	817 204	40	67 986	61
Nigeria	...	...	...	...	...	17 371	...	13 423	...	439	12 393	388
Rwanda	...	...	...	...	...	...	...	3 054	...	1	28 046	1
Senegal	90	80	...	80	39	754	396	7 561	...	1	...	...
Sierra Leone	...	...	...	...	...	561	29	1 955	...	0	344	25
Swaziland	100	96	96	94	...	...	154	2 055	...	0	171	1
Togo	81	73	71	65	43	460	1 710	1 520	328 488	5	6 144	13
Uganda	...	...	...	...	...	1 045	2 192	25 476	...	100	42 659	307
United Republic of Tanzania	86	79	78	75	31	3 924	28 341	39 847	7 976 590	21	3 160	29
Zaire	51	35	36	41	20	6 082	1 875	40 040	...	735	5 443	83
Zambia	90	76	75	78	53	1 296	4 287	12 744	3 514 000	6	8 533	24
Zimbabwe	...	...	...	...	...	118	13 356	30 831	324 188	1	5 619	13
Americas												
Haiti	...	...	...	...	...	689	...	...	23 140	0	...	...
Eastern Mediterranean												
Afghanistan	...	...	...	...	...	658	...	...	...	...	...	...
Djibouti	76	63	63	58	37	...	231	...	6 140	...	8	0
Somalia	...	...	...	...	...	1 084	0	2 883	...	...	...	...
Sudan	92	77	79	77	68	5 718	257	11 084	...	22	841	21
Yemen	60	53	53	53	23	606	11	14 428	37 201	45	225	12
South-East Asia												
Bangladesh	99	91	92	96	94	12 434	6	42 610	166 564	49	4 995	735
Bhutan	98	87	86	85	70	117	0	1 299	38 901	...	120	0
Myanmar	90	84	84	82	61	21 071	618	18 229	701 043	7	1 170	28
Nepal	76	65	66	71	...	12 764	16	19 804	9 442	9	4 810	511
Western Pacific												
Cambodia	95	79	80	75	36	2 886	91	14 599	85 012	114	2 038	8
Lao People's Democratic Republic	59	54	64	68	35	694	4	1 227	52 601	11	3 174	6
Papua New Guinea	78	50	55	63	30	1 318	43	8 041	629 525	1	3 730	150

Member States[a]	Immunization coverage (%) 1995[b]					Reported cases of selected diseases during the specified year						
	Children immunized by age 12 months				Pregnant women							
	BCG	DPT 3	OPV 3	Measles	Tetanus toxoid 2	Leprosy[c] 1996	AIDS 1995	Tuberculosis 1995	Malaria 1994	Polio 1995	Measles 1995	Neonatal tetanus 1995
Other WHO Member States												
Africa												
Lesotho	...	...	...	...	...	...	341	4 846	...	0	304	0
Namibia	77	61	60	57	52	...	1 836	1 540	407 863	15	1 723	75
Sao Tome and Principe	...	...	...	...	...	...	4	...	....	0	23	3
Seychelles	100	97	97	99	100	...	6	9	...	0	0	0
South Africa	...	...	...	...	...	367	2 805	86 924	10 298	0	1 425	9
Americas												
Antigua and Barbuda	...	...	...	...	...	...	5	...	...	0	0	0
Bolivia	77	88	89	83	...	864	11	9 614	34 749	0	76	20
Brazil	100	83	83	88	...	137 908	9 695	88 109	564 406	0	793	85
Dominica	...	...	...	...	...	...	5	8	...	0	0	0
Grenada	...	95	77	88	...	...	18	2	...	0	3	0
Peru	95	94	92	97	...	240	908	45 310	122 039	0	353	97
Saint Kitts and Nevis	...	99	99	99	...	...	5	4	...	0	1	0
Saint Lucia	98	98	98	94	...	...	10	12	...	0	2	0
Saint Vincent and the Grenadines	99	97	97	100	...	...	6	24	...	0	0	0
Eastern Mediterranean												
Egypt	93	91	91	89	66	3 404	16	23 444	...	71	1 833	790
Iraq	99	91	91	95	71	...	6	26 950	98 222	34	7 650	64
Libyan Arab Jamahiriya	99	96	96	92	...	390	2	1 440	29	0	...	...
Morocco	93	90	90	88	78	851	57	29 829	206	0	2 380	14
Pakistan	69	58	57	56	42	2 629	9	9 605	108 586	508	1 720	1 580
Europe												
Monaco	...	...	...	...	...	...	3	...	...	...	...	0
San Marino	...	...	...	...	...	...	...	...	...	0	...	...
Turkey	68	66	67	65	29	...	26	22 981	84 345	28	13 463	127
Turkmenistan	...	...	...	...	...	...	0	1 939	...	8	393	0
Yugoslavia	...	...	...	...	...	...	...	...	...	...	...	...
South-East Asia												
India	93	86	87	79	...	542 511	1 078	1 214 876	2 222 869	3 263	37 077	1 761
Indonesia	99	92	93	92	...	41 649	20	31 908	...	12	22 005	212
Maldives	99	94	97	96	...	...	0	231	16	0	3 070	0
Western Pacific												
Cook Islands	96	93	93	96	...	...	0	...	...	0	7	0
Kiribati	47	60	58	47	38	...	0	...	...	0	4	0
Marshall Islands	71	70	64	57	58	...	0	...	...	0	...	...
Micronesia, Federated States of	50	83	81	90	...	368	0	...	...	0	0	0
Mongolia	94	88	86	85	...	...	0	3 010	...	0	555	0
Nauru	78	56	56	...	...	...	0	...	...	0	0	0
Niue	92	100	100	34	0	...	0	2	...	0	0	0
Palau	...	100	100	100	...	...	0	19	...	0	0	0
Samoa	98	94	94	96	98	...	1	51	...	0	0	0
Tonga	99	95	93	94	83	...	0	20	...	0	0	0
Tuvalu	88	87	91	94	52	...	...	36	...	0	1	0

[a] Italics indicate less populous Member States (under 150 000 population in 1990).
[b] Figures refer to BCG, diphtheria-pertussis-tetanus (third dose), oral poliovirus (third dose), measles and tetanus toxoid (second dose).
[c] Data are provided only for countries with more than 100 registered cases (1996 or latest available information).
[d] The three targets in WHO's strategy for health for all by the year 2000 relating to health status are: life expectancy at birth above 60 years; under-5 mortality rate below 70 per 1000 live births; infant mortality rate below 50 per 1000 live births.

Table A3. Basic indicators

Estimates are obtained or derived from relevant WHO programmes or from responsible international agencies for the areas of their concern

Member States[a]	Diabetes mellitus prevalence (000)			Adult literacy			GNP per capita		Speed of integration index[b]	Population below US $ 1 a day (%)[b]	Ratio (per 100 000 population) around 1993[b]	
	1995	2000	2025	Number (000) 1995	Both sexes increase (%) 1980-95	Sex ratio of increase female /male 1980-95	US $ 1994	PPP[b,c] $ 1994		1990-94	Physicians	Nurses and midwives
WHO Member States with values above all three health-for-all targets[d]												
Africa												
Algeria	606	764	1 937	10 543	169	0.8	1 650	...	-1.5	...	83	...
Botswana	7.2	9.2	25.9	590	128	0.9	2 800	5 210	-0.9	...	...	...
Cape Verde	1.9	2.5	6.8	162	111	1.2	930	1 920	...	...	29	57
Mauritius	9.3	10.6	18.7	670	46	1.1	3 150	12 720	2.4	...	85	241
Americas												
Argentina	1 578	1 714	2 641	23 715	30	1.1	8 110	8 720	0.6	...	268	54
Bahamas	6.9	8.6	19.7	192	53	1.1	11 800	15 470	...	...	141	258
Barbados	8.2	8.7	17.2	195	17	0.8	6 560	11 210	...	...	113	323
Belize	4.2	5.0	14.4	...	...	...	2 530	5 600	...	...	47	76
Canada	1 532	1 701	2 618	...	...	...	19 510	19 960	0.5	...	221	958
Chile	539	624	1 154	9 565	41	1.1	3 520	8 890	0.7	15.0	108	42
Colombia	977	1 171	2 581	21 495	55	1.1	1 670	5 330	-0.5	7.4	105	49
Costa Rica	88	107	257	2 112	65	1.0	2 400	...	0.7	...	126	95
Cuba	416	470	797	8 154	38	1.1	...	...	...	...	518	752
Dominican Republic	165	202	491	4 171	70	1.0	1 330	3 760	-0.04	...	77	20
Ecuador	277	338	791	6 568	76	1.0	1 280	4 190	-0.5	30.4	111	34
El Salvador	120	142	347	2 447	59	1.2	1 360	2 410	0.1	...	91	38
Guatemala	195	235	640	3 286	80	0.9	1 200	3 440	-0.2	...	90	30
Guyana	15	18	48	554	30	1.1	530	2 750	...	...	33	88
Honduras	84	104	306	2 310	97	1.1	600	1 940	-0.1	46.5	22	17
Jamaica	53	60	155	1 439	46	1.0	1 540	3 400	1.2	4.7	57	69
Mexico	3 847	4 654	11 684	53 804	71	1.0	4 180	7 040	1.4	14.9	107	40
Nicaragua	84	106	297	1 574	76	1.3	340	1 800	-0.3	43.8	82	56
Panama	72	85	194	1 592	71	1.0	2 580	5 730	-0.7	...	119	98
Paraguay	106	131	347	2 726	72	1.0	1 580	3 550	-0.3	...	67	10
Suriname	8.9	9.6	25.2	256	37	1.1	860	2 470	...	...	40	227
Trinidad and Tobago	34	39	86	866	28	1.2	3 740	8 670	-0.2	...	90	168
United States of America	13 853	15 009	21 892	...	...	...	25 880	25 880	-0.3	...	245	878
Uruguay	172	179	226	2 343	16	1.2	4 660	7 710	-0.3	...	309	61
Venezuela	646	784	1 775	12 685	68	1.1	2 760	7 770	-0.2	11.8	194	77
Eastern Mediterranean												
Bahrain	29	37	84	325	99	0.8	7 460	13 220	...	...	11	289
Cyprus	65	74	118	...	...	...	10 260	14 800	...	...	231	425
Iran, Islamic Republic of	1 692	1 977	5 215	26 064	146	0.9	...	...	0.2	...	...	...
Jordan	272	338	944	2 669	163	0.9	1 440	4 100	-0.4	2.5	158	224
Kuwait	61	86	237	732	34	8.7	19 420	24 730	-0.5	...	178	468
Lebanon	232	262	555	1 832	33	1.3	...	...	...	...	191	122
Oman	59	75	217	...	...	...	5 140	8 590	-1.0	...	120	290
Qatar	34	44	75	317	192	0.4	12 820	19 100	...	...	143	354
Saudi Arabia	745	944	2 334	6 521	155	0.6	7 050	9 480	-3.4	...	166	348
Syrian Arab Republic	579	718	2 253	5 467	127	0.8	...	...	0.4	...	109	212
Tunisia	229	272	622	3 858	125	0.8	1 790	5 020	0.2	3.9	67	283
United Arab Emirates	109	141	260	1 036	104	0.6	...	...	-0.2	...	168	321
Europe												
Albania	58	65	131	...	...	...	380	...	...	...	141	423
Armenia	155	177	298	...	...	...	680	2 160	...	...	312	831
Austria	123	130	178	...	...	...	24 630	19 560	0.3	...	327	530
Azerbaijan	285	325	627	...	...	...	500	1 510	...	...	390	1081
Belarus	641	696	854	7 911	...	...	2 160	4 320	...	...	379	1160
Belgium	164	171	221	...	...	...	22 870	20 270	2.2[e]	...	365	...

Member States[a]	Diabetes mellitus prevalence (000) 1995	2000	2025	Adult literacy: Number (000) 1995	Both sexes increase (%) 1980-95	Sex ratio of increase female /male 1980-95	GNP per capita: US $ 1994	PPP[b,c] $ 1994	Speed of integration index[b]	Population below US $ 1 a day (%)[b] 1990-94	Ratio (per 100 000 population) around 1993[b]: Physicians	Nurses and midwives
Bosnia and Herzegovina	82	114	131	...	...	...	...	...	...	...	...	...
Bulgaria	286	290	311	...	...	...	1 250	4 380	-1.7	2.6	333	652
Croatia	145	150	167	...	...	...	2 560	...	...	...	201	470
Czech Republic	307	314	373	...	...	...	3 200	8 900	...	3.1	293	944
Denmark	329	335	428	...	...	...	27 970	19 880	0.9	...	283	...
Estonia	49	49	55	1 212	...	...	2 820	4 510	...	6.0	312	636
Finland	300	322	454	...	...	...	18 850	16 150	0.03	...	269	2 184
France	881	935	1 234	...	...	...	23 420	19 670	0.9	...	280	392
Georgia	293	310	414	...	...	...	...	...	...	...	436	863
Germany	1 359	1 434	1 770	...	...	...	25 580	19 480	-0.1	...	319	...
Greece	607	650	772	8 419	...	...	7 700	10 930	0.1	...	387	278
Hungary	326	329	352	8 214	...	...	3 840	6 080	1.0	0.7	337	...
Iceland	13	14	23	...	...	...	24 630	19 210	...	...	...	...
Ireland	156	165	231	...	...	...	13 530	13 550	0.6	...	167	...
Israel	297	327	566	...	...	...	14 530	15 300	0.7	...	459	671
Italy	3 369	3 592	4 365	47 630	...	...	19 300	18 460	0.3	...	...	...
Kazakhstan	389	436	791	...	...	...	1 160	2 810	...	...	360	874
Kyrgyzstan	70	79	182	...	...	...	630	1 730	...	18.9	310	879
Latvia	83	84	89	2 025	...	...	2 320	3 220	...	...	303	628
Lithuania	110	115	137	2 876	...	...	1 350	3 290	...	2.1	399	977
Luxembourg	6.2	6.8	9.3	...	...	...	39 600	35 860	...[e]	...	213	...
Malta	4.8	5.3	7.7	...	...	...	...	...	...	...	250	1 189
Netherlands	222	242	354	...	...	...	22 010	18 750	1.1	...	...	...
Norway	276	280	363	...	...	...	26 390	20 210	-0.5	...	...	...
Poland	1 041	1 103	1 425	29 531	...	...	2 410	5 480	0.6	6.8	...	...
Portugal	513	538	674	7 144	...	...	9 320	11 970	1.9	...	291	304
Republic of Moldova	107	113	154	3 230	...	...	870	...	...	6.8	356	1 020
Romania	654	675	817	17 779	...	...	1 270	4 090	0.3	17.7	176	430
Russian Federation	8 894	9 579	12 240	115 508	...	...	2 650	4 610	...	1.1	380	659
Slovakia	138	148	202	...	...	...	2 250	...	...	12.8	325	...
Slovenia	61	65	77	...	...	...	7 040	6 230	...	...	219	686
Spain	2 156	2 303	2 952	32 132	...	...	13 440	13 740	1.1	...	400	...
Sweden	614	631	827	...	...	...	23 530	17 130	0.7	...	299	1 048
Switzerland	109	118	170	...	...	...	37 930	25 150	0.1	...	301	...
Tajikistan	71	84	235	...	...	...	360	970	...	...	210	738
The Former Yugoslav Republic of Macedonia	50	56	87	...	...	...	820	...	...	...	219	334
Ukraine	3 576	3 801	4 389	40 568	...	...	1 910	2 620	...	...	429	1 211
United Kingdom	912	934	1 186	...	...	...	18 340	17 970	0.3	...	164	...
Uzbekistan	343	402	1 026	...	...	...	960	2 370	...	...	335	1 032
South-East Asia												
Democratic People's Republic of Korea	443	527	1 038	...	...	...	...	...	...	...	...	...
Sri Lanka	275	318	617	11 480	40	1.3	640	3 160	1.0	4.0	23	112
Thailand	863	1 017	1 923	39 539	64	1.0	2 410	6 970	2.1	0.1	24	99
Western Pacific												
Australia	330	367	610	...	...	...	18 000	18 120	-0.7	...	...	...
Brunei Darussalam	5.0	6.0	12.2	166	80	1.0	14 240	...	...	...	...	...
China	16 016	18 637	37 555	732 780	72	1.0	530	2 510	-0.3	29.4	115	88
Fiji	43	52	119	469	47	1.0	2 250	5 940	...	...	38	215
Japan	6 269	6 905	8 543	...	...	...	34 630	21 140	-0.4	...	177	641
Malaysia	300	362	807	10 440	90	1.0	3 480	8 440	1.8	...	43	160
New Zealand	63	68	103	...	...	...	13 350	15 870	-0.6	...	210	1 249
Philippines	942	1 137	2 519	39 478	57	1.0	950	2 740	1.0	...	11	43
Republic of Korea	1 099	1 256	1 958	33 677	43	1.1	8 260	10 330	0.6	...	127	232
Singapore	85	98	136	2 005	37	1.3	22 500	21 900	3.5	...	147	416
Solomon Islands	12	15	45	...	...	...	810	2 100	...	...	...	141
Vanuatu	5.3	7.0	19.0	...	...	...	1 150	2 370	...	...	...	...
Viet Nam	870	1 015	2 454	43 707	70	1.1	200	...	...	...	...	...

Member States[a]	Diabetes mellitus prevalence (000) 1995	2000	2025	Adult literacy: Number (000) 1995	Adult literacy: Both sexes increase (%) 1980-95	Adult literacy: Sex ratio of increase female /male 1980-95	GNP per capita: US $ 1994	GNP per capita: PPP[b,c] $ 1994	Speed of integration index[b]	Population below US $ 1 a day (%)[b] 1990-94	Ratio (per 100 000 population) around 1993[b]: Physicians	Nurses and midwives
WHO Member States with values below all three health-for-all targets[d]												
Africa												
Angola	51	61	151	...	...	...	...	...	-0.7	...	...	...
Benin	26	31	75	1 052	199	0.7	370	1 630	-0.8	...	6	33
Burkina Faso	50	57	126	1 090	145	0.4	300	800	-0.2	...	...	...
Burundi	27	31	75	1 215	124	0.6	160	700	-0.5	...	6	17
Cameroon	72	85	210	4 695	122	0.9	680	1 950	-0.7	...	7	...
Central African Republic	19	22	47	1 140	190	1.1	370	1 160	-0.5	...	6	45
Chad	36	42	92	1 732	104	0.8	180	720	-0.3	...	2	6
Comoros	2.9	3.4	9.8	192	135	0.8	510	1 430	...	...	10	33
Congo	13	15	35	1 055	123	1.1	620	1 900	-1.5	...	27	49
Côte d'Ivoire	67	77	195	2 911	172	0.7	610	1 370	-1.1	...	...	...
Equatorial Guinea	2.2	2.4	5.2	178	131	1.0	430	...	...	...	21	34
Eritrea	16	19	45	...	...	...	...	...	...	...	2	...
Ethiopia	244	283	685	10 472	134	0.6	100	430	-0.2	...	4	8
Gabon	10	11	19	508	130	1.0	3 880	...	-1.1	...	19	56
Gambia	6.1	7.2	15.6	253	181	0.6	330	1 100	...	...	2	25
Ghana	89	106	269	6 164	134	0.9	410	2 050	0.6	...	4	...
Guinea	31	36	89	1 272	135	0.5	520	...	-0.2	26.3	15	3
Guinea-Bissau	6.1	6.9	13.5	344	81	0.9	240	820	...	87.0	18	45
Kenya	123	146	442	11 546	140	1.0	250	1 310	0.00	50.2	15	23
Liberia	17	19	48	628	144	0.5	...	...	-1.2	...	...	...
Madagascar	69	83	221	...	...	...	200	640	-0.1	72.3	24	55
Malawi	48	53	114	3 340	129	0.7	170	650	-0.4	...	2	6
Mali	48	56	144	1 758	239	0.7	250	520	-0.2	...	4	9
Mauritania	13	16	35	488	88	0.7	480	1 570	-0.7	...	11	27
Mozambique	79	99	228	3 545	108	0.5	90	860	...	...	...	...
Niger	37	44	112	642	164	0.4	230	770	-0.7	61.5	3	17
Nigeria	576	685	1 658	34 732	151	0.9	280	1 190	-1.9	28.9	21	142
Rwanda	32	37	86	2 598	134	1.0	80	330	-0.1	...	...	...
Senegal	43	51	121	1 524	134	0.7	600	1 580	-0.04	54.0	7	35
Sierra Leone	24	28	59	791	126	0.5	160	700	-1.8	...	...	...
Swaziland	4.2	5.1	14.1	374	105	1.3	1 100	3 010	...	...	...	...
Togo	20	23	59	1 161	140	0.7	320	1 130	-0.4	...	6	31
Uganda	83	94	236	6 735	112	0.9	190	1 410	-0.1	...	4	28
United Republic of Tanzania	134	158	402	10 901	126	1.0	140	620	-0.2	16.4	4	46
Zaire	200	231	591	17 652	104	1.0	...	...	0.1	...	...	...
Zambia	42	48	127	3 889	158	1.0	350	860	-0.6	84.6	...	...
Zimbabwe	56	64	157	5 356	92	1.0	500	2 040	0.03	41.0	14	164
Americas												
Haiti	112	128	285	1 932	88	1.0	230	930	-0.4	...	16	13
Eastern Mediterranean												
Afghanistan	412	559	1 323	3 763	111	0.5	...	...	...	...	...	...
Djibouti	3.9	4.6	9.4	156	214	0.6	...	...	...	...	20	...
Somalia	42	49	123	...	...	...	...	...	-0.8	...	4	3
Sudan	138	162	392	7 282	136	0.8	...	...	-0.6	...	10	70
Yemen	230	291	890	...	...	...	280	...	-0.8	...	26	51
South-East Asia												
Bangladesh	1 285	1 564	4 032	27 790	98	0.6	220	1 330	0.3		18	5
Bhutan	17	19	39	407	97	0.7	400	1 270	...	...	20	6
Myanmar	588	681	1 549	24 205	54	1.1	...	...	-0.4	...	28	43
Nepal	225	263	638	3 476	116	0.4	200	1 230	1.4	...	5	5
Western Pacific												
Cambodia	96	114	283	...	...	...	...	...	...	...	58	136
Lao People's Democratic Republic	81	93	201	1 526	97	0.9	320	...	...	...	...	...
Papua New Guinea	154	181	453	1 877	83	0.9	1 240	2 680	-0.4	...	18	97

Member States[a]	Diabetes mellitus prevalence (000) 1995	2000	2025	Adult literacy: Number (000) 1995	Adult literacy: Both sexes increase (%) 1980-95	Adult literacy: Sex ratio of increase female /male 1980-95	GNP per capita: US $ 1994	GNP per capita: PPP[b,c] $ 1994	Speed of integration index[b]	Population below US $ 1 a day (%)[b] 1990-94	Ratio (per 100 000 population) around 1993[b]: Physicians	Nurses and midwives
Other WHO Member States												
Africa												
Lesotho	11	13	31	846	91	0.9	720	1 730	-0.7	...	5	33
Namibia	8.7	10.2	24.1	...	...	...	1 970	4 320	...	...	23	81
Sao Tome and Principe	0.7	0.7	1.0	...	...	...	250	...	...	...	32	...
Seychelles	4.4	4.8	6.7	...	...	...	6 680	...	...	...	104	417
South Africa	298	346	721	21 274	61	1.1	3 040	5 130	-0.8	23.7	59	175
Americas												
Antigua and Barbuda	3.0	3.5	5.8	...	...	...	6 770	...	...	...	76	233
Bolivia	159	187	449	3 661	71	1.1	770	2 400	0.3	7.1	51	25
Brazil	4 899	5 788	11 603	91 206	67	1.1	2 970	5 400	-0.3	...	134	41
Dominica	3.2	3.7	5.5	...	...	...	2 800	...	...	...	46	263
Grenada	4.1	4.7	7.6	...	...	...	2 630	...	...	...	50	239
Peru	637	761	1 741	13 696	70	1.0	2 110	3 610	-1.0	49.4	73	49
Saint Kitts and Nevis	1.8	2.1	3.2	...	...	...	4 760	9 310	...	...	89	590
Saint Lucia	6.3	7.3	13.4	...	...	...	3 130	...	...	...	35	177
Saint Vincent and the Grenadines	5.0	5.8	9.9	...	...	...	2 140	...	...	...	46	187
Eastern Mediterranean												
Egypt	3 240	3 801	8 802	20 053	91	0.8	720	3 720	-0.2	7.6	202	222
Iraq	561	678	1 739	6 692	136	0.8	...	...	-1.7	...	51	64
Libyan Arab Jamahiriya	126	153	385	2 252	158	0.9	...	...	...	...	137	366
Morocco	608	729	1 747	7 543	137	0.7	1 140	3 470	1.0	1.1	34	94
Pakistan	4 338	5 310	14 523	29 585	130	0.5	430	2 130	0.9	11.6	52	32
Europe												
Monaco	0.5	0.5	0.5	...	...	...	...	...	...	...	300	1 484
San Marino	1.5	1.6	1.5	...	...	...	...	...	...	...	...	...
Turkey	1 841	2 217	4 551	33 705	88	0.9	2 500	4 710	1.9	...	103	151
Turkmenistan	60	70	182	...	...	...	...	...	...	4.9	353	1 195
Yugoslavia	...	...	...	...	...	...	...	...	...	...	...	...
South-East Asia												
India	19 397	22 878	57 243	315 544	83	0.7	320	1 280	0.01	52.5	48	...
Indonesia	4 546	5 396	12 427	110 893	90	1.0	880	3 600	0.8	14.5	12	67
Maldives	2.7	3.2	9.2	127	56	1.1	950	...	...	...	19	13
Western Pacific												
Cook Islands	0.7	0.8	1.4	...	...	...	...	...	...	...	111	537
Kiribati	2.4	2.7	4.5	...	...	...	740	...	...	...	13	193
Marshall Islands	1.2	1.4	2.3	...	...	...	...	...	...	...	...	...
Micronesia, Federated States of	3.3	3.8	6.3	...	...	...	...	...	...	...	46	327
Mongolia	37	45	101	1 239	81	1.0	300	...	...	...	268	452
Nauru	0.6	0.7	1.1	...	...	...	...	...	...	...	...	...
Niue	0.1	0.1	0.2	...	...	...	...	...	...	...	200	1 000
Palau	0.6	0.6	1.1	...	...	...	...	...	...	...	...	...
Samoa	3.3	3.7	18.7	...	...	...	1 000	2 060	...	...	38	186
Tonga	3.4	3.9	6.5	...	...	...	1 590	...	...	...	...	...
Tuvalu	0.2	0.3	0.5	...	...	...	...	...	...	...	89	433

[a] Italics indicate less populous Member States (under 150 000 population in 1990).
[b] For details please refer to the explanatory notes in this annex.
[c] PPP = purchasing power parity ($ denotes current international dollars).
[d] The three targets in WHO's strategy for health for all by the year 2000 relating to health status are: life expectancy at birth above 60 years; under-5 mortality rate below 70 per 1000 live births; infant mortality rate below 50 per 1000 live births.
[e] Value for Belgium includes Luxembourg.
... Data not available or not applicable.

Table B. Analytical tabulations

Indicator	Year	Unit	WHO Member States	Developed world			Developing world		
				Total	Developed market economies	Economies in transition	Total	Developing countries other than LDCs	Least developed countries (LDCs)
Life expectancy at birth	1996	years	65	75	77	69	64	66	52
Increase, male	1980-1995	years	4.4	2.3	3.1	0.4	4.9	4.9	5.6
Increase, female	1980-1995	years	4.9	2.1	2.7	0.9	5.6	5.7	5.8
Under-5 mortality rate	1996	per 1000 live births	81	16	8	30	89	74	153
Decrease, male	1980-1995	average annual rate (%)	2.1	2.3	3.8	1.2	2.2	2.6	1.9
Decrease, female	1980-1995	average annual rate (%)	2.1	1.9	2.7	1.1	2.2	2.6	1.9
Infant mortality rate	1996	per 1000 live births	59	12	6	23	65	55	105
Decrease	1980-1995	per 1000 live births	23	6	5	7	27	28	29
Total population	1996	millions	5789	1219	827	392	4570	3964	605
Average annual growth rate	1980-1995	percentage	1.7	0.6	0.6	0.6	2.0	1.9	2.6
Population aged 65 years and above	1996	millions	379	161	117	44	218	200	18
Average annual growth rate	1980-1995	percentage	2.3	1.5	1.6	1.3	3.0	3.1	2.6
	1995-2000	percentage	2.4	1.3	1.3	1.1	3.1	3.2	3.1
Age and sex standardized death rate	1995-2000	per 100 000 population	880	550	446	800	978	882	1575
Age-specific death rate:									
5-19	1995-2000	per 100 000 population	194	51	36	76	219	161	527
20-64, male	1995-2000	per 100 000 population	558	561	396	936	557	510	941
20-64, female	1995-2000	per 100 000 population	388	262	209	377	428	374	842
65 years and above	1995-2000	per 100 000 population	5971	5413	5104	6235	6375	6280	7419
HIV incidence	1996	millions	3	...	...	...	...	...	...
Leprosy (reported cases)	1996[a]	thousands	937	0.6	0.6	0	936	815	121
Diabetes mellitus prevalence	1995	millions	135	52	34	18	83	78	5
	2000	millions	154	56	37	19	98	92	6
	2025	millions	299	75	50	25	224	210	14
Iodine deficiency disorders-goitre prevalence	1995	millions	760	...	...	...	...	...	...
Vitamin A deficiency prevalence[b]	1995	millions	3	...	...	...	...	...	...
Iron deficiency anaemia prevalence	1995	millions	1789	...	...	...	...	...	...
Adult literacy rate, both sexes	1996	percentage	78	99	...	...	71	74	50
GNP per capita	1994	US dollars	4743	17 317	24 414	2097	1042	1133	210
GNP per capita (PPP[c] estimates)	1994	current international $	5883	15 820	21 091	4113	2846	3007	1056
Speed of integration index[d]			...	...	0.3	...	-0.2	-0.1	-0.4
Physicians	around 1993	ratio per 100 000 population	121	287	252	358	77	84	14
Nurses and midwives	around 1993	ratio per 100 000 population	232	765	742	800	85	96	22
Dentists	around 1993	ratio per 100 000 population	22	50	57	39	12	14	1
Carbon dioxide emissions from industrial processes per capita	1992	metric tons	3.9	11.7	12.2	10.8	1.7	2	0.1
Households: average annual growth rate	1990-2000	percentage	2.1	1.1	1.3	0.8	2.5	2.5	2.7

[a] 1996 or latest available data; includes data for countries with more than 100 registered cases only.

[b] Number of children under age 5 affected.

[c] PPP = purchasing power parity. For details please refer to the explanatory notes in this annex.

[d] Values are the median for all countries in the group. For details please refer to the explanatory notes in this annex.

... Data not available or not applicable.

Index

Main references are in bold type